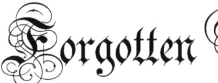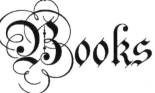

ISBN 978-0-282-17801-7
PIBN 10843974

1 MONTH OF
FREE
READING

at

www.ForgottenBooks.com

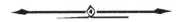

By purchasing this book you are eligible for one month membership to ForgottenBooks.com, giving you unlimited access to our entire collection of over 1,000,000 titles via our web site and mobile apps.

To claim your free month visit:

www.forgottenbooks.com/free843974

English
Français
Deutsche
Italiano
Español
Português

www.forgottenbooks.com

Mythology Photography **Fiction**
Fishing Christianity **Art** Cooking
Essays Buddhism Freemasonry
Medicine **Biology** Music **Ancient
Egypt** Evolution Carpentry Physics
Dance Geology **Mathematics** Fitness
Shakespeare **Folklore** Yoga Marketing
Confidence Immortality Biographies
Poetry **Psychology** Witchcraft
Electronics Chemistry History **Law**
Accounting **Philosophy** Anthropology
Alchemy Drama Quantum Mechanics
Atheism Sexual Health **Ancient History**
Entrepreneurship Languages Sport
Paleontology Needlework Islam
Metaphysics Investment Archaeology
Parenting Statistics Criminology
Motivational

THE TRANSACTIONS

OF THE

MEDICO-CHIRURGICAL SOCIETY OF EDINBURGH.

VOL. XIV.—NEW SERIES.

SESSION 1894-95.

EDINBURGH: OLIVER AND BOYD,

PUBLISHERS TO THE SOCIETY.

1895.

PRINTED BY OLIVER AND BOYD, TWEEDDALE COURT, EDINBURGH.

PREFACE.

The present Volume is the *Fourteenth* of the *New Series*, and contains a record of the work done during the past Session.

That work, as hitherto, embraces the communication of Original Papers; the exhibition of Patients, illustrating rare and interesting forms of disease; and the exhibition of Pathological and other Specimens, so essential to the proper understanding of the morbid changes which take place in the human body.

During the past Session Extra Meetings were held for the purpose of having a Special Discussion on "Cardiac Therapeutics," which occupied three nights. The Discussion was opened by Professor Thomas R. Fraser, followed by Dr George W. Balfour. It is hoped that such Meetings will materially increase the usefulness of the Society.

In an Appendix will be found a paper by Mr F. M. Caird on "Resection and Suture of the Intestine, with Cases."

It is believed that the publication of the Transactions in this permanent form will prove a valuable contribution to medical literature, will encourage the Members to take a more active part in the work of the Society, and will tend in no small degree to increase the influence and usefulness of the Medico-Chirurgical Society of Edinburgh.

WILLIAM CRAIG,
Editor.

October 1895.

235900

Medico-Chirurgical Society of Edinburgh.

INSTITUTED 2ND AUGUST 1821.

OFFICE-BEARERS FOR SESSION 1894-95.

PRESIDENT.

THOMAS SMITH CLOUSTON, M.D., F.R.C.P. Ed.

VICE-PRESIDENTS.

R. J. BLAIR CUNYNGHAME, M.D., F.R.C.S. Ed.
JOHN WYLLIE, M.D., F.R.C.P. Ed.
WILLIAM CRAIG, M.D., F.R.C.S. Ed.

TREASURER.

R. M'KENZIE JOHNSTON, M.D., F.R.C.S. Ed., 44 Charlotte Square.

SECRETARIES.

JAMES W. B. HODSDON, M.D., F.R.C.S. Ed., 52 Melville Street.
GEORGE A. GIBSON, M.D., F.R.C.P. Ed., 17 Alva Street.

EDITOR OF TRANSACTIONS.

WILLIAM CRAIG, M.D., F.R.C.S. Ed.

MEMBERS OF COUNCIL.

HARRY MELVILLE DUNLOP, M.D., F.R.C.P. Ed.
ROBERT WILLIAM PHILIP, M.D., F.R.C.P. Ed.
JOSEPH BELL, M.D., F.R.C.S. Ed.
RUSSELL ELIOTT WOOD, M.B., F.R.C.S. Ed.
WILLIAM BARRIE DOW, M.D., F.R.C.S. Ed., Dunfermline.
WILLIAM RUSSELL, M.D., F.R.C.P. Ed.
ALLEN THOMSON SLOAN, M.D., C.M.
THOMAS M. BURN-MURDOCH, M.B., C.M.

LIST of Presidents, Vice-Presidents, Treasurers, Secretaries, and Editor of Transactions of the Society.

PRESIDENTS.

Note.—The Presidents continue in office two years.

Dr Duncan, Sen.,	1821	Benjamin Bell, Esq.,	1859
James Russell, Esq.,	1823	James Spence, Esq.,	1861
Dr John Thomson,	1825	Sir Douglas Maclagan,	1863
Dr Kellie,	1827	Dr John Moir,	1865
Dr Abercrombie,	1829, 1831	Dr Robert Omond,	1867
Dr Alison,	1833	Dr Bennett,	1869
Sir Robert Christison, Bart.,	1835	Dr Handyside,	1871
William Wood, Esq,	1837, 1839	Dr Haldane,	1873
Dr Maclagan,	1840	Dr Gillespie,	1875
Dr Graham,	1842	Dr Sanders,	1877
Dr Gairdner,	1844	Dr P. H. Watson,	1879
Dr R. Hamilton,	1846	Dr G W. Balfour,	1881
James Syme, Esq.,	1848	Sir Henry D. Littlejohn,	1883
Dr Begbie,	1850	Sir T. Grainger Stewart,	1885
Sir J. Y. Simpson, Bart.,	1852	Dr John Smith,	1887
Dr Seller,	1854	Dr Alexander R. Simpson,	1889
James Miller, Esq.,	1856	Dr Joseph Bell,	1891
John Goodsir, Esq,	1858	Dr T. S. Clouston,	1893

VICE-PRESIDENTS.

Note.—The Vice-Presidents continue in office three years.

Dr James Home,	1821	Sir Joseph Lister, Bart.,	1870
James Russell, Esq.,	1821	Dr R. Paterson,	1871
Dr John Thomson,	1821	Dr P. H. Watson,	1872
Dr John Abercrombie,	1822, 1825	Dr G. W. Balfour,	1873
Dr Andrew Duncan, Jr.,	1823, 1826	Sir Henry D. Littlejohn,	1874
Dr George Kellie,	1824	Dr Keiller,	1875
Dr David Maclagan,	1827	Dr Argyll Robertson,	1876
Sir Robert Christison, Bart.,	1833	Sir T. Grainger Stewart,	1877
William Brown, Esq.,	1839, 1843	Thomas Annandale, Esq.,	1878
Sir Douglas Maclagan,	1850, 1862	Dr Alexander R. Simpson,	1879
Dr Combe,	1851	Joseph Bell, Esq.,	1880
Dr Omond,	1854, 1866	Dr T. R. Fraser,	1881
Benjamin Bell, Esq.,	1856	Dr David Wilson,	1882
James Spence, Esq.,	1857	Dr J. Batty Tuke,	1883
Dr Charles Wilson,	1858	Dr John Duncan,	1884
Dr Inglis,	1859	Dr R. Peel Ritchie,	1885
Dr W. T. Gairdner,	1861	Professor John Chiene,	1886
Dr Andrew Wood,	1862	Dr T. S. Clouston,	1887
Dr P. D. Handyside,	1863	A. G. Miller, Esq.,	1888
Dr Rutherford Haldane,	1864	Dr D. J. Brakenridge,	1889
Dr J. D. Gillespie,	1865	Dr Peter H. M'Laren,	1890
Dr Halliday Douglas,	1867	Dr Claud Muirhead,	1891
Dr W. R. Sanders,	1867	Dr R. J. Blair Cunynghame,	1892
Dr Thomas Keith,	1868	Dr John Wyllie,	1893
Dr Matthews Duncan,	1869	Dr William Craig,	1894

TREASURERS.

James Bryce, Esq.,	1821 to 1826	Joseph Bell, Esq.,	1872 to 1880
Dr Gairdner,	1826 to 1843	A. G. Miller, Esq.,	1880 to 1888
Dr Omond,	1843 to 1854	Dr Francis Troup,	1888 to 1892
Dr John Struthers,	1854 to 1863	Dr R. M'Kenzie Johnston,	1892
Dr George W. Balfour,	1863 to 1872		

Note.—The Treasurer, Secretaries, and Editor of Transactions are elected annually.

SECRETARIES.

Dr Alison,	. . .	1821 to 1823
Dr R. Hamilton,	. .	1821 to 1830
Dr J. C. Gregory,	.	1830 to 1833
William Brown, Esq.,	.	1833 to 1839
Dr W. Thomson,	. .	1833 to 1840
Sir Douglas Maclagan,		1839 to 1864
Dr James Duncan,	.	1840 to 1845
Dr John Taylor,	. .	1846 to 1851
Dr J. H. Bennett,	.	1846 to 1848
Dr Wm. Robertson,	.	1848 to 1851
Dr W. T. Gairdner,	.	1851 to 1857
Dr J. W. Begbie,	.	1852 to 1858
Dr J. D. Gillespie,	.	1857 to 1864
Dr P. H. Watson,	.	1858 to 1867
Dr Dyoer,	. .	1864 to 1867

Sir T. Grainger Stewart,	1867 to 1870
Dr Argyll Robertson,	.	1867 to 1872
Dr Muirhead,	. .	1870 to 1876
John Chiene, Esq.,	.	1872 to 1877
Dr Wyllie,	. .	1876 to 1879
Dr Cadell,	. .	1877 to 1881
Dr Brakenridge,	.	1879 to 1882
Dr MacGillivray,	.	1881 to 1885
Dr James,	. .	1882 to 1886
Dr Cathcart,	.	1885 to 1888
Dr James Ritohie,	.	1886 to 1890
Francis M. Caird, Esq	1888 to 1892
Dr William Russell,	.	1890 to 1894
Dr J. W. B. Hodsdon,	.	1892
Dr George A. Gibson,	.	1894

EDITOR OF TRANSACTIONS.

Dr William Craig, ... 1882

HONORARY MEMBERS.

Professor Rudolph Virchow, M.D., LL.D., F.R.S., Berlin, . .	1869
Sir James Paget, Bart., F.R.C.S. Eng., D.C.L., LL.D., F.R.S., 5 Park Square West, Regent's Park, London, N.W., . .	1871
Professor Kölliker, Würtzburg,	1878
Sir William Jenner, Bart., K.C.B., M.D., D.C.L , LL.D., F.R.C.P. Lond., F.R.S., Greenwood, Bishops Waltham, . .	1884
Charles West, M.D., F.R.C.P. Lond., 4 Evelyn Mansions, Carlisle Place, Victoria Street, London, S.W., . .	1885
Sir Joseph Lister, Bart., M.B., D.C.L., LL.D., F.R.C.S. Eng., F.R.S., 12 Park Crescent, Portland Place, London, N.W., .	1893
Prof. Fr. von Esmarch, M.D., Kiel, ...	1894
Professor Theodor Kocher, M.D., Bern, . . .	1895
John S. Billings, M.D., LL.D., Washington, U.S.A., . .	1895

FOREIGN CORRESPONDING MEMBERS.

M. Louis, Paris, . . .	1857
Prof. Porta, Pavia, . .	1858
Prof. Bouillaud, Paris, . .	1858
Dr Devergie, Paris, . .	1858
Prof. Huss, Stockholm, . .	1861
Prof. du Bois-Reymond, Berlin,	1869
Prof. Kühne, Heidelberg, .	1869
M. Marey, Paris, . . .	1869
Dr C. R. Agnew, New York, .	1877
Dr W. A. Hammond, New York, ...	1877
Dr Edmund Hansen, Copenhagen, ...	1877
Dr D. B. St John Roosa, New York, ...	1877

Dr Henry W. Williams, Boston,	1877
Prof. Stricker, Vienna, . .	1878
Dr Wortabet, Beyrout, . .	1879
Prof. Hegar, Freiburg, . .	1880
Prof. Albert, Vienna, . .	1880
Dr Lewis Sayre, New York, .	1880
Prof. D. W. Yandell, Louisville, Kentucky, ...	1882
Prof. Leon Lefort, Paris, . .	1882
Dr J. Lucas-Championnière, Paris,	1882
Prof. Fran is Franck, Paris, .	1883
Prof. R. Depine, Lyons, . .	1883
Prof. Max von Pettenkofer, Munich,	1884
Prof. L. Ollier, Lyons, . .	1884
Prof. C. J. Ask, Lund, . .	1884

CORRESPONDING MEMBERS IN THE UNITED KINGDOM.

John William Ogle, M.D., F.R.C.P. Lond., 80 Cavendish Square, London, W.,	1869
Frederick William Pavy, M.D., LL.D., F.R.C.P. Lond., F.R.S., 35 Grosvenor Street, London, W.,	1869
David Lloyd Roberts, M.D., F.R.C.P. Lond., F.R.S.E., 11 St John's St., Manchester,	1869
Samuel Wilks, M.D., LL.D., F.R.C.P. Lond., F.R.S., 72 Grosvenor Street, London, W.,	1869
Robert Brudenell Carter, F.R.C.S. Eng., 31 Harley Street, London, W.,	1877
Professor John Burdon Sanderson, M.D., D.C.L., LL.D., F.R.C.P. Lond., F.R.S., 64 Banbury Road, Oxford,	1878
J. Hughlings Jackson, M.D., LL.D., F.R.C.P. Lond., F.R.S., 8 Manchester Square, London, W.,	1878
Sir Thomas Spencer Wells, Bart., M.D., F.R.C.S. Eng., 3 Upper Grosvenor Street, London, W.,	1880
Professor Sir John Banks, K.C.B., M.D., LL.D., D.Sc., F.K.Q.C.P. Irel., M.R.I.A., 45 Merrion Square, Dublin,	1880
Sir Joseph Fayrer, K.C.S.I., M.D., LL.D., F.R.C.P. Lond., F.R.S., 53 Wimpole Street, Cavendish Square, London, W.,	1884
Emeritus-Professor Sir John Eric Erichsen, Bart., F.R C.S. Eng., LL.D., F.R.S., 6 Cavendish Place, London, W.,	1884
Emeritus-Professor John Struthers, M.D., LL.D., P.R.C.S. Ed., 24 Buckingham Terrace, Edinburgh,	1884
Professor William Tennant Gairdner, M.D., LL.D., P.R.C.P. Ed., 225 St Vincent Street, Glasgow,	1884

ORDINARY MEMBERS.

Note.—Those marked with an asterisk have been Members of Council.   Members of Council continue in office two years.

RESIDENT.

		Date of Admission.
**	Professor Sir Douglas Maclagan, M.D., LL.D., F.R.C.P. & S. Ed.,	1834
*	John Moir, M.D., F.R.C P. Ed.,	1836
**	Andrew Halliday Douglas, M.D., F.R.C.P. Ed.,	1842
*	George William Balfour, M.D., LL.D., F.R.C.P. Ed.,	1847
5 *	John Henderson, M.D., F.R.C.S. Ed., *Leith*,	1848
*	William Husband, M.D., F.R.C.S. Ed.,	1849
**	Sir Henry Duncan Littlejohn, M.D., LL.D., F.R.C S. Ed.,	1853
	David Greig, F.R.C.S. Ed.,	1854
*	James Cappie, M.D.,	1855
10 ***	John Smith, M.D., LL.D., F.R.C.S. Ed.,	1856
*	Patrick Heron Watson, M.D., LL.D., F.R.C.S. Ed.,	1856
**	Professor Alexander Russell Simpson, M.D., F.R.C.P. Ed,	1859
*	John Sibbald, M.D., F.R.C.P. Ed.,	1859
*	Sir Arthur Mitchell, K.C.B., M.D., LL.D.,	1859
15 **	Professor Sir Thomas Grainger Stewart, M.D., F.R.C.P. Ed.,	1861
*	Thomas Smith Clouston, M.D., F.R.C.P. Ed., *President*,	1861
*	Douglas Argyll Robertson, M.D., F.R.C.S. Ed.,	1861
*	Robert Peel Ritchie, M.D., F.R.C.P. Ed.,	1862
**	Joseph Bell, M.D., F.R.C.S. Ed.,	1862
20 *	Professor Thomas Annandale, M.D., F.R.C.S. Ed.,	1863
*	John Linton, M.D., F.R.C P. Ed.,	1863
**	John Batty Tuke, M.D., F.R.C.P. Ed.,	1864
	Peter Orphoot, M.D.,	1865
*	Andrew Smart, M.D., F.R.C.P. Ed.,	1865

		Date of Admission.
25	* Professor Thomas Richard Fraser, M.D., LL.D., F.R.C.P. Ed.,	1865
	* Professor William Rutherford, M.D., M.R.C.S. Eng., F.R.C.P. Ed.,	1866
	* Claud Muirhead, M.D., F.R.C.P. Ed.,	1866
	* Alexander Gordon Miller, M.D., F.R.C.S. Ed.,	1867
	* Professor John Chiene, M.D., F.R.C.S. Ed.,	1867
30	* Peter H. M'Laren, M.D., F.R.C.S. Ed.,	1868
	* John M'Gibbon, F.R.C.S. Ed.,	1868
	* John Duncan, M.D., LL.D., F.R.C.S. Ed.,	1868
	* John Wyllie, M.D., F.R.C.P. Ed., Vice-President,	1868
	* Robert J. Blair Cunynghame, M.D., F.R.C.S. Ed., Vice-President,	1868
35	* William Craig, M.D., F.R.C.S. Ed., Vice-President,	1869
	* James Andrew, M.D., F.R.C.P. Ed.,	1869
	* Francis Cadell, M.B., F.R.C.S. Ed.,	1870
	* James Carmichael, M.D., F.R.C.P. Ed.,	1870
	* Peter Alexander Young, M.D., F.R.C.P. Ed.,	1870
40	* John Halliday Croom, M.D., F.R.C.P. Ed.,	1870
	* John J. KirkyDuncanson, M.D., F.R.C.P. Ed.,	1871
	* William Taylor, M.D., F.R.C.P. Ed.,	1871
	* James Ormiston Affleck, M.D., F.R.C.P. Ed.,	1871
	* Archibald Bleloch, M.B., Sc.D.,	1871
45	* James Dunsmure, M.D., F.R.C.S. Ed.,	1872
	* Charles Edward Underhill, M.B., F.R.C.P. Ed.,	1872
	* Ormond Haldane Garland, M.D., F.R.C.P. Ed., Leith,	1873
	* James Ritchie, M.D., F.R.C.P. Ed., F.R.C.S. Ed.,	1873
	* Andrew M. Thomson Rattray, M.D., Portobello,	1874
50	* John Playfair, M.D., F.R.C.P. Ed.,	1874
	* William Alexander Finlay, M.D., F.R.C.S. Ed., Trinity,	1875
	* James Foulis, M.D., F.R.C.P. Ed.,	1875
	* Byrom Bramwell, M.D., F.R.C.S. Ed., F.R.C.P. Ed.,	1876
	* Henry Macdonald Church, M.D., F.R.C.P. Ed.,	1876
55	* Alexander Moir, M.D., L.R.C.P. & S. Ed.,	1876
	* Charles H. Thatcher, F.R.C.S. Ed.,	1876
	* William Allan Jamieson, M.D., F.R.C.P. Ed.,	1876
	** George Hunter, M.D., F.R.C.S. Ed., F.R.C.P. Ed.,	1876
	* James Jamieson, M.D., F.R.C.S. Ed.,	1877
60	* Charles Watson MacGillivray, M.D., F.R.C.S. Ed.,	1877
	* John Brown Buist, M.D., F.R.C.P. Ed.,	1877
	George D. Smith, M.D., M.R.C.P. Ed., Leith,	1877
	** Alexander James, M.D., F.R.C.P. Ed.,	1877
	* Thomas Rutherford Ronaldson, M.B., F.R.C.P. Ed.,	1877
65	Surgeon-Major William T. Black, M.D., F.R.C.S. Ed.,	1877
	William Watson Campbell, M.D., F.R.C.P. Ed., Duns,	1877
	* David Menzies, M.B., F.R.C.S. Ed.,	1878
	* Joseph Montagu Cotterill, M.B., F.R.C.S. Ed.,	1878
	George Mackay, M.B., F.R.C.S. Ed.,	1878
70	* John Graham Brown, M.D., F.R.C.P. Ed.,	1878
	John Fraser, M.B., M.R.C.P. Ed.,	1878
	* Peter M'Bride, M.D., F.R.C.P. Ed.,	1879
	* James Allan Gray, M.D., F.R.C.P. Ed., Leith,	1879
	Andrew Fleming, M.D., Dep. Surgeon-General,	1880
75	* Thomas Duddingston Wilson, M.B., F.R.C.S. Ed.,	1880
	* George Alexander Gibson, M.D., F.R.C.P. Ed.,	1880
	Robert Lawson, M.D., C.M.,	1881
	* Alexander Hugh Freeland Barbour, M.D., F.R.C.P. Ed.,	1881
	John Carlyle Johnstone, M.D., C.M., Melrose,	1882
80	* Francis Mitchell Caird, M.B., F.R.C.S. Ed.,	1883
	* Robert Henry Blaikie, M.D., F.R.C.S. Ed.,	1883
	* R. M'Kenzie Johnston, M.D., F.R.C.S. Ed., Treasurer,	1883
	* Charles Walker Cathcart, M.B., F.R.C.S. Eng. & Ed.,	1883
	* Alexander Bruce, M.D., F.R.C.P. Ed.,	1883
85	* Andrew Semple, M.D., F.R.C.S. Ed., Dep. Surgeon-General,	1883

		Date of Admission.
	John Lyon Wilson, L.R.C.P. Ed.,	1883
	Henry Newcombe, M.D., F.R.C.S. Ed.,	1883
	* Russell Eliott Wood, M.B., F.R.C.S. Ed.,	1883
	John Macdonald Brown, M.B., F.R.C.S. Eng. & Ed., *London*,	1883
90	James William Beeman Hodsdon, M.D., F.R.C.S. Ed., *Secretary*,	1883
	Thomas Francis Spittal Caverhill, M.B., F.R.C.P. Ed.,	1883
	* Robert Alexander Lundie, M.B., B.Sc., F.R.C.S. Ed.,	1883
	Alexander Black, M.B., F.R.C.P. Ed.,	1883
	* Harry Melville Dunlop, M.D., F.R.C.P. Ed.,	1883
95	* George Andreas Berry, M.B., F.R.C.S. Ed.,	1883
	Hamilton Wylie, M.B., C.M.,	1883
	Arthur Douglas Webster, M.D., F.R.C.P. Ed.,	1883
	* Robert William Philip, M.D., F.R.C.P. Ed.,	1883
	* William Russell, M.D., F.R.C.P. Ed.,	1884
100	George Dickson, M.D., F.R.C.S. Ed.,	1884
	Hugh Logan Calder, M.D., C.M., *Leith*,	1884
	Henry Hay, M.B., C.M.,	1884
	R. Milne Murray, M.B., F.R.C.P. Ed.,	1884
	A. S. Cumming, M.D., F.R.C.P. Ed.,	1884
105	John Mowat, M.D.,	1885
	D. Noël Paton, M.D., F.R.C.P. Ed.,	1885
	Michael Dewar, M.D., C.M.,	1885
	Edward M'Callum, F.R.C.S. Ed.,	1885
	John Struthers Stewart, L.R.C.P. & S. Ed.,	1885
110	* Allen Thomson Sloan, M.D., C.M.,	1885
	John William Ballantyne, M.D., F.R.C.P. Ed.,	1885
	George Kerr, M.B., C.M.,	1885
	David Milligan, M.B., C.M.,	1885
	J. Murdoch Brown, M.B., F.R.C.P. Ed.,	1885
115	Robert W. Felkin, M.D.,	1885
	James Haig Ferguson, M.D., F.R.C.P. Ed., M.R.C.S. Eng.,	1885
	Charles Kennedy, M.D., C.M.,	1886
	James Mill, M.B., F.R.C.P. Ed., *Leith*,	1886
	Robert Fraser Calder Leith, M.B., B.Sc., F.R.C.P. Ed.,	1886
120	* Thomas M. Burn-Murdoch, M.B., C.M.,	1886
	Professor William Smith Greenfield, M.D., F.R.C.P. Lond. and Ed.,	1886
	Nathaniel Thomas Brewis, M.B., F.R.C.P. Ed.,	1886
	David Berry Hart, M.D., F.R.C.P. Ed.,	1886
	Robert S. Aitchison, M.B., F.R.C.P. Ed.,	1887
125	John Thomson, M.D., F. .C.P. Ed.,	1887
	T. Brown Darling, M.D., M.,	1887
	Edward Carmichael, M.D., F.R.C.P. Ed.,	1887
	Charles C. Teacher, M.B., C.M.,	1887
	David W. Aitken, M.B., C.M.,	1887
130	John Shaw M'Laren, M.B., F.R.C.S. Ed.,	1887
	George Mackay, M.D., F.R.C.S. Ed., M.R.C.S. Eng.,	1887
	Henry Alexis Thomson, M.D., F.R.C.S. Ed.,	1887
	David Wallace, M.B., F.R.C.S. Ed.,	1887
	James Lockhart Wilson, M.B., C.M., *Duns*,	1888
135	William Booth, F.R.C.S. Ed.,	1888
	George M. Johnston, M.D., C.M., F.R.C.P. Ed., *Leith*,	1888
	George Pirrie Boddie, M.B., C.M.,	1888
	Kenneth Mackinnon Douglas, M.D., F.R.C.S. Ed.,	1888
	George Lovell Gulland, M.D., F.R.C.P. Ed.,	1888
140	William Haldane, M.D., F.F.P. & S. Glasg., *Bridge of Allan*,	1889
	John Hugh Alex. Laing, M.B., C.M.,	1889
	Harold Jalland Stiles, M.B., F.R.C.S. Ed.,	1889
	Allan Cuthbertson Sym, M.D., C.M.,	1889
	Edmund Frederick Tanney Price, M.B., C.M.,	1889
145	William George Sym, M.D., F.R.C.S. Ed.,	1889

		Date of Admission.
	Alexander John Keiller, L.R.C.P. & S. Ed., *North Berwick*, .	1889
	G. Keppie Paterson, M.B., F.R.C.P. Ed., . . .	1889
	William Stewart, M.D., F.F.P. & S. Glasg., *Leith*, . .	1889
	Thomas Proudfoot, M.B., F.R.C.P.Ed., . .	1889
150	Professor William H. Barrett, M.B., C.M., . .	1890
	Dawson Fyers Duckworth Turner, M.D., F.R.C.P. Ed., .	1890
	Edward Farr Armour, M.B., C.M., . . .	1890
	William Guy, F.R.C.S. Ed., . . .	1890
	William Smith, L.R.C.P. & S. Ed., L.F.P. & S. Glasg.,	1890
155	Robert A. Fleming, M.B., F.R.C.P. Ed., . .	1890
	Robert Thin, M.B., F.R.C.P. Ed., . . .	1890
	James Hutcheson, M.D., F.R.C.S. Ed., . .	1890
	A. Cowan Guthrie, M.B., C.M., *Leith*, . . .	1890
	Ralph Stockman, M.D., F.R.C.P. Ed., . .	1891
160	Alexander Lockhart Gillespie, M.D., F.R.C.P. Ed., .	1891
	Stewart Stirling, M.D., F.R.C.S. Ed., . . .	1891
	Francis Darby Boyd, M.D., F.R.C.P. Ed., . .	1891
	J. J. Douglas, M.D., F.R.C.P. Ed., *London*, . .	1891
	Robert Stirling, M.B., C.M., *Perth*, . .	1891
165	J. Y. Simpson Young, M.B., C.M., . . .	1891
	John Macpherson, M.D., F.R.C.P. Ed., *Larbert*, .	1891
	James Smith, M.B., C.M., . .	1891
	Norman Purvis Walker, M.D., F.R.C.P. Ed., . .	1891
	Alexander Miles, M.D., F.R.C.S. Ed., . .	1892
170	Robert Abernethy, M.D., F.R.C.P. Ed., . .	1892
	Arthur Logan Turner, M.D., F.R.C.S. Ed., . .	1892
	T. Herbert Littlejohn, M.B., F.R.C.S. Ed., . .	1892
	G. Matheson Cullen, M.D., C.M., . .	1892
	William George Aitchison Robertson, M.D., F.R.C.P. Ed.,	1892
175	David Middleton Greig, M.B., C.M., F.R.C.S. Ed., *Dundee*, .	1892
	John Stevens, M.D., F.R.C.P. Ed., . .	1892
	James Crawfurd Dunlop, M.D., F.R.C.P. Ed., M.R.C.S. Eng.,	1892
	William Elder, M.B., F.R.C.P. Ed., *Leith*, . .	1892
	Ernest Coleman Moore, M.B., C.M., . .	1892
180	Robert Stewart, M.B., C.M., . .	1892
	William Crawford M'Ewan, M.D., C.M., *Prestonpans*, .	1892
	George R. Wilson, M.B., C.M., . . .	1892
	Richard J. Erskine Young, M.D., C.M., . .	1892
	Richard James Arthur Berry, M.B., C.M., .	1893
185	William Breadon Thompson Gubbin, M.D., C.M., *Portobello*,	1893
	John MacRae, M.D., C.M., *Murrayfield*, . .	1893
	James Harvey, M.B., C.M., . . .	1893
	Henry Anderson Peddie, M.B., C.M., . .	1893
	John Wheeler Dowden, M.B., C.M., . .	1893
190	Alexander Bruce Giles, M.D., C.M., . .	1893
	Thomas Lawson, M.B., C.M., . .	1893
	William Basil Orr, M.D., C.M., . .	1893
	James Aitken Clark, M.B., C.M., . .	1893
	Robert Mackenzie, M.D., C.M., . .	1893
195	William Ford Robertson, M.D., C.M., .	1893
	James Mowat, M.B., C.M., . .	1893
	William Simmers, M.B., C.M., *Crail*, . .	1894
	Charles Arthur Sturrock, M.B., F.R.C.S. Ed., *Dunfermline*, .	1894
	Frederick Maurice Graham, L.R.C.P. & S. Ed.,	1894
200	Claude B. Ker, M.B., C.M., . . .	1894
	Robert Muir, M.D., M.R.C.P. Ed., . .	1894
	John Cumming, L.R.C.P. & S. Ed., . .	1894
	William Fraser Wright, M.B., C.M., *Leith*, .	1894
	Douglas Chalmers Watson, M.B., C.M., . .	1894
205	Archibald Stodart-Walker, M.B., C.M., . .	1894
	James Cameron, M.D., C.M., . .	1895
	James Middlemass, M.B., M.R.C.P. Ed., . .	1895

Date of Admission.

	Lewis Campbell Bruce, M.D., C.M., ...	1895
	Robert Miller Ronaldson, M.D., C.M., M.R.C.S. Eng., .	1895
210	James Scott, M.B., C.M., ...	1895
	John Hardie, M.B., F.R.C.S. Ed., ...	1895
	John Orr, M.B., M.R.C.P. Ed., ...	1895
	James Gibson Cattanach, M.B., C.M., ...	1895
	James Stewart Fowler, M.B., C.M., ...	1895
215	Ernest George Salt, L.R.C.P. & S. Ed., . . .	1895

NON-RESIDENT.

	W. Ord M'Kenzie, M.D., L.R.C.S. Ed., *London*, . .	1845
	W. Judson Van Someren, M.D., L.R.C.S. Ed., *London*, .	1845
	William H. Lowe, M.D., F.R.C.P. Ed., *Wimbledon*, . .	1845
	George Skene Keith, M.D., LL.D., F.R.C.P. Ed., *Currie*, .	1845
220	His Excellency Robert H. Gunning, M.D., LL D., *London*, . .	1846
	Archibald Hall, M.D., *Montreal*, ...	1853
	Sir W. Overend Priestley, M.D., LL.D., F.R.C.P. Ed., *London*,	1854
	Horatio Robinson Storer, M.D., *Newport, Rhode Island, U.S.*,	1855
	James C. Howden, M.D., *Montrose*, ...	1856
225	Thomas Skinner, M.D., L.R.C.S. Ed., *London*, . .	1856
	Professor William Smoult Playfair, M.D., LL.D., F.R.C.P.L., *London*, ...	1857
	J. Ivor Murray, M.D., F.R.C.S. Ed., *Scarboro'*, . .	1857
	Andrew Scott Myrtle, M.D., L.R.C.S. Ed., *Harrogate*, .	1859
	Francis Robertson Macdonald, M.D., *Inveraray*, . .	1860
230	Professor John Young, M.D., *University of Glasgow*, . .	1860
	George Thin, M.D., L.R.C.S. Ed., *London*, . .	1861
	Professor William Stephenson, M.D., F.R.C.S. Ed., *Aberdeen University*, ...	1861
	J. S. Beveridge, M.R.C.P. Lond., F.R.C.S. Ed., *Lochinver*, .	1861
	David Yellowlees, M.D., LL.D., F.F.P. & S. Glasg., *Glasgow*,	1862
235	Prof. Arthur Gamgee, M.D., F.R.C.P. Ed., F.R.S., *Switzerland*, ...	1863
	Professor John Cleland, M.D., LL.D., *The University, Glasgow*,	1864
	Sir R. B. Finlay, M.D., Q.C., M.P., *Middle Temple, London*,	1864
	Stanley Lewis Haynes, M.D., M.R.C.S. Eng., *Malvern*, .	1864
	James Watt Black, M.D., F.R.C.P.L., *London*, . .	1865
240	David Brodie, M.D., *London*, ...	1865
	* John Strachan, M.D., *Dollar*, ...	1867
	Robert Shand Turner, M.D., C.M., *Keith*, . . .	1867
	Peter Maury Deas, M.B., L.R.C.S. Ed., *Exeter*, . .	1868
	Professor J. G. M'Kendrick, M.D., LL.D., F.R.C.P. Ed., *University, Glasgow*, ...	1870
245	Professor Lawson Tait, M.D., F.R.C.S. Ed. & Eng., LL.D., *Birmingham*, ...	1870
	J. G. Sinclair Coghill, M.D., F.R.C.P. Ed., *Ventnor*, .	1870
	* Archibald Dickson, M.D., F.R.C.S. Ed., of *Hartree and Kilbucho*, ...	1871
	James Johnston, M.D., F.R.C.S. Ed., *London*, . .	1871
	J. William Eastwood, M.D., M.R.C.P.L., *Darlington*, .	1871
250	Strethill H. Wright, M.D., M.R.C.P. Ed., *Monmouth*, .	1871
	Charles A. E. Sheaf, F.R.C.S. Ed., *Queensland*, .	1871
	* Alexander Ballantyne, M.D., F.R.C.P. Ed., *Dalkeith*, .	1872
	Professor J. Bell Pettigrew, M.D., LL.D., F.R.C.P. Ed., *University of St Andrews*, ...	1873
	* Andrew Balfour, M.D., C.M., *Portobello*, . . .	1874
255	J. Johnson Bailey, M.D., F.R.C.S. Ed., *London*, . .	1874
	* Robert Lucas, M.D., F.R.C.P. Ed., *Dalkeith*, . .	1875
	John Aymers Macdougall, M.D., F.R.C.S. Ed., *France*, .	1875
	Thomas John Maclagan, M.D., M.R.C.P.L., *London*, .	1875

		Date of Admission.
	Dr Groesbeck, *Cincinnati*,	1875
260	* John Connel, M.D., F.R.C.P. Ed., *Peebles*,	1876
	Professor David James Hamilton, M.B., F.R.C.S. Ed., *Aberdeen University*,	1876
	James Stitt Thomson, F.R.C.P. Ed., F.R.C.S. Ed., *Lincoln*,	1877
	George Herbert Bentley, L.R.C.P. & S. Ed., *Kirkliston*,	1877
	J. Moolman, M.B., C.M., *Cape of Good Hope*,	1877
265	Robert Somerville, M.D., F.R.C.S. Ed., *Galashiels*,	1877
	Graham Steell, M.D., F.R.C.P.L., *Manchester*,	1877
	Frederick William Barry, M.D., D.Sc., *London*,	1878
	John Brown, M.D., F.R.C.S. Eng., *Burnley*,	1878
	James Allan Philip, M.D., *Boulogne-Sur-Mer*,	1878
270	Alex. Robert Coldstream, M.D., F.R.C.S. Ed., *Florence*,	1878
	Professor Johnson Symington, M.D., F.R.C.S.Ed., M.R.C.S.Eng., *Belfast*,	1878
	* William Barrie Dow, M.D., F.R.C.S. Ed., *Dunfermline*,	1879
	Richard Freeland, M.D., C.M., *Broxburn*,	1879
	A. D. Leith Napier, M.D., M.R.C.P.L., *London*,	1879
275	Keith Norman Macdonald, M.D., F.R.C.P. Ed., *Skye*,	1880
	John Home-Hay, M.D., M.R.C.S. Eng., *Alloa*,	1880
	* John Hutton Balfour, M.B., C.M., *Portobello*,	1881
	John Mackay, M.D., L.R.C.S. Ed., *Aberfeldy*,	1881
	William Badger, M.B., C.M., *Penicuik*,	1882
280	* Alexander Matthew, F.R.C.S. Ed., *Corstorphine*,	1882
	John Archibald, M.D., F.R.C.S. Ed., *London*,	1882
	James Rutherford Morison, M.B., F.R.C.S. Ed., *Newcastle*,	1882
	Roderick Maclaren, M.D., *Carlisle*,	1882
	J. Maxwell Ross, M.B., F.R.C.S. Ed., *Dumfries*,	1882
285	* W. Wotherspoon Ireland, M.D., *Polton*,	1883
	F. W. Dyce Fraser, M.D., F.R.C.P. Ed., *Hawthornden*,	1883
	Edwin Baily, M.B., C.M., *Oban*,	1883
	William Hy. Shirreff, M.B., C.M., *Melbourne*,	1883
	John Haddon, M.D., C.M., *Hawick*,	1883
290	A. W. Hare, M.B., F.R.C.S. Ed., M.R.C.S. Eng., *Keyworth*,	1883
	G. Sims Woodhead, M.D., F.R.C.P. Ed., *London*,	1883
	* Alexander Thom, M.D., C.M., *Crieff*,	1884
	T. Goodall Nasmyth, M.D., D.Sc., *Cupar-Fife*,	1884
	Thomas R. Scott, M.D., C.M., *Musselburgh*,	1884
295	F. A. Saunders, F.R.C.S. Ed., *Grahamstown, South Africa*,	1884
	Joseph Carne Ross, M.D., F.R.C.P. Ed., *Withington*,	1884
	G. J. H. Bell, M.B., C.M., *Bengal Army*,	1884
	W. C. Greig, M.B., C.M., *Morocco*,	1884
	J. Craig Balfour, L.R.C.P. & S. Ed., *Belford*,	1884
300	T. Wyld Pairman, L.R.C.P. & S. Ed., *New Zealand*,	1884
	Andrew Brown, M.D., M.R.C.P. Ed., *London*,	1884
	Ernest F. Neve, M.D., F.R.C.S. Ed., M.R.C.S. Eng., *India*,	1884
	James Robertson Crease, F.R.C.S. Ed., *South Shields*,	1885
	T. Edgar Underhill, M.D., F.R.C.S. Ed., *Burnt Green*,	1885
305	S. Hale Puckle, M.B., C.M., *Bishop's Castle*,	1885
	Skene Keith, M.B., F.R.C.S. Ed., *London*,	1885
	G. Hugh Mackay, M.B., C.M., *Elgin*,	1885
	Reginald Ernest Horsley, M.D., F.R.C.S. Ed., *Crail*,	1886
	John Batty Tuke, jr., M.D., F.R.C.P.Ed., *Murrayfield*,	1886
310	Oswald Gillespie Wood, M.D., F.R.C.S. Ed., Surgeon, *A. M. Staff, India*,	1886
	James Hogarth Pringle, M.B., C.M., *Glasgow*,	1886
	Walter Scott Lang, M.D., F.R.C.S. Ed.,	1886
	William Gayton, M.D., M.R.C.S. Eng., *London*,	1886
	A. Bell Whitton, M.B., C.M., *Aberchirder*,	1886
315	J. Walton Hamp, L.F.P. & S. Glasg., L.S.A. Lond., *Wolverhampton*,	1887
	John Keay, M.B., F.R.C.P. Ed., *Inverness*,	1887

		Date of Admission
	John F. Sturrock, M.B., C.M., *Broughty Ferry*,	1887
	Robert Inch, M.B., C.M., *Gorebridge*,	1887
	William Hunter, M.D., M.R.C.S. Eng., M.R.C.P.L., *London*,	1887
320	Sydney Rumboll, L.R.C.P. Ed., F.R.C.S. Ed., *Leeds*,	1887
	George Franklin Shiels, M.D., F.R.C.S. Ed., *San Francisco*,	1887
	D. H. Anderson, M.D., C.M., *Twickenham*,	1887
	J. A. Armitage, M.D., C.M., *Wolverhampton*,	1887
	Thomas Russell, M.B., C.M., *Glasgow*,	1888
325	William Burns Macdonald, M.B., C.M., *Dunbar*,	1888
	Professor John M'Fadyean, M.B., C.M., *London*,	1888
	James W. Martin, M.D., F.R.C.P. Ed.,	1888
	J. R. Home Ross, M.B., F.R.C.P. Ed., *Burmah*,	1888
	John Smith, M.D., M.R.C.S. Eng., *Kirkcaldy*,	1889
330	Benjamin D. C. Bell, L.R.C.P. & S. Ed., *Kirkwall*,	1889
	A. Home Douglas, M.B., F.R.C.P. Ed., *Nice*,	1889
	H. Harvey Littlejohn, M.B., F.R.C.S. Ed., *Sheffield*,	1889
	Surgeon-Captain C. H. Bedford, M.D., M.R.C.S. Eng., *Bengal Army*,	1889
	D. C. Braidwood, M.B., C.M., *Halkirk, Caithness*,	1889
335	Professor J. Berry Haycraft, M.D., D.Sc., *Cardiff*,	1889
	Professor A. W. Hughes, M.B., F.R.C.S. Ed., M.R.C.S. Eng., *Cardiff*,	1889
	Hugh Jamieson, M.B., C.M.,	1889
	Albert E. Morison, M.B., F.R.C.S. Ed., M.R.C.S. Eng., *Hartlepool*,	1889
	James Hunter, M.D., C.M., *Linlithgow*,	1890
340	George M. Robertson, M.B., F.R.C.P. Ed., *Murthly*,	1890
	Charles Templeman, M.D., C.M., *Dundee*,	1891
	Simson C. Fowler, M.B., C.M., *Juniper Green*,	1892
	Robert Dundas Helm, M.D., C.M., *Carlisle*,	1892
	William Gordon Woodrow Sanders, M.B., F.R.C.P. Ed., *Caen*,	1892
345	W. Ramsay Smith, M.B., C.M., *Rhyl*,	1892
	Alexander Peyer, M.D., *Zürich*,	1893
	Alexander Reid Urquhart, M.D., F.R.C.P. Ed., *Perth*,	1893
	F. W. Foxcroft, M.B., C.M., *Wilmslow*,	1893
	William B. Mackay, M.B., M.R.C.S. Eng., *Berwick-on-Tweed*,	1893
350	Alex. Mitchell Stalker, M.D., C.M., *Dundee*,	1893
	D. W. Johnston, F.R.C.S. Ed., *Johannesburg, S. Africa*,	1893
	Frank Ashby Elkins, M.D., C.M., *Sunderland*,	1893
	Philip Grierson Borrowman, M.B., C.M., *Elie*,	1893
	William Craig, M.B., C.M., *Cowdenbeath*,	1894
355	James Mackenzie, M.D., C.M., *Burnley*,	1894
	Charles E. Douglas, M.D., C.M., *Cupar-Fife*,	1894
	Thomas Easton, M.D., C.M., *Stranraer*,	1894
	Gopal Govind Vatve, M.D., *Bombay*,	1895
	John Hosack Fraser, M.B., M.R.C.P. Ed., *Bridge of Allan*,	1895
• 360	John Struthers, M.B., C.M., *South Africa*,	1895

ORDINARY MEMBERS.

ARRANGED ALPHABETICALLY.

RESIDENT.

	Dr R. Abernethy, 12 Alva Street,	1892
	Dr J. O. Affleck, 38 Heriot Row,	1871
	Dr R. S. Aitchison, 74 Great King Street,	1887
	Dr D. Aitken, 17 Hatton Place,	1887
5	Dr James Andrew, 2 Atholl Crescent,	1869

		Date of Admission.
	Professor Annandale, 34 Charlotte Square,	1863
	Dr E. F. Armour, 149 Bruntsfield Place,	1890
	Dr G. W. Balfour, 17 Walker Street,	1874
	Dr J. W. Ballantyne, 24 Melville Street,	1885
10	Dr A. H. Freeland Barbour, 4 Charlotte Square,	1881
	Professor W. H. Barrett, 21 Learmonth Terrace,	1890
	Joseph Bell, Esq., 2 Melville Crescent,	1862
	Dr G. A. Berry, 31 Drumsheugh Gardens,	1883
	Dr R. J. A. Berry, 4 Howard Place,	1893
15	Dr Alexander Black, 13 Howe Street,	1883
	Dr W. T. Black, 2 George Square,	1877
	Dr Robert H. Blaikie, 42 Minto Street,	1883
	Dr Bleloch, 2 Lonsdale Terrace,	1871
	Dr G. P. Boddie, 147 Bruntsfield Place,	1888
20	William Booth, Esq., 2 Minto Street,	1888
	Dr F. D. Boyd, 6 Atholl Place,	1891
	Dr Byrom Bramwell, 23 Drumsheugh Gardens,	1876
	Dr N. T. Brewis, 23 Rutland Street,	1886
	Dr J. Graham Brown, 8 Chester Street,	1878
25	Dr J. Macdonald Brown,	1883
	Dr J. Murdoch Brown, 9 Walker Street,	1885
	Dr Alexander Bruce, 13 Alva Street,	1883
	Dr Lewis C. Bruce, Royal Asylum, Morningside,	1895
	Buist, 1 Clifton Terrace,	1877
30	. M. Burn-Murdoch, 31 Morningside Road,	1886
	Cadell, 22 Ainslie Place,	1870
	Francis M. Caird, 21 Rutland Street,	1883
	L. Calder, 60 Leith Walk,	1884
	James Cameron, 13 Fettes Row,	1895
35	W. Watson Campbell, Duns,	1877
	Cappie, 37 Lauriston Place,	1855
	Edward Carmichael, 21 Abercromby Place,	1887
	Dr J. Carmichael, 22 Northumberland Street,	1870
	Dr H. W. Cathcart, 8 Randolph Crescent,	1883
40	Dr J. G. Cattanach, 3 Alvanley Terrace,	1895
	Dr T. F. S. Caverhill, 8A Abercromby Place,	1884
	Professor John Chiene, 26 Charlotte Square,	1867
	J. A. Clark, 4 Cambridge Street,	1893
	Church, 36 George Square,	1876
45	Clouston, Tipperlinn House, Morningside Place, *President*,	1861
	Cotterill, 24 Manor Place,	1878
	William Craig, 71 Bruntsfield Place, *Vice-President*,	1869
	r Halliday Croom, 25 Charlotte Square,	1870
	G. Matheson Cullen, 48 Lauriston Place,	1892
50	A. S. Cumming, 18 Ainslie Place,	1884
	John Cumming, 94 Gilmore Place,	1894
	R. J. B. Cunynghame, 18 Rothesay Place, *Vice-President*,	1868
	T. B. Darling, 13 Merchiston Place,	1887
	M. Dewar, 24 Lauriston Place,	1885
55	George Dickson, 9 India Street,	1884
	Halliday Douglas, 30 Melville Street,	1842
	J. J. Douglas, 15 Church Road, Upper Norwood, London,	1891
	Kenneth M. Douglas, 26 Rutland Street,	1888
	J. W. Dowden, Lynn House, Gillsland Road,	1893
60	John Duncan, 8 Ainslie Place,	1868
	Kirk Duncanson, 22 Drumsheugh Gardens,	1871
	H. M. Dunlop, 20 Abercromby Place,	1883
	J. C. Dunlop, 24 Stafford Street,	1892
	J. Dunsmure, 53 Queen Street,	1872
65	William Elder, 4 John's Place, Leith,	1892
	Dr R. W. Felkin, 8 Alva Street,	1885
	Dr J. Haig Ferguson, 25 Rutland Street,	1885

		Date of Admission.
	Dr W. A. Finlay, St Helen's, Russell Place, Trinity, . .	1875
	Dr Andrew Fleming, 8 Napier Road, ...	1880
70	Dr R. A. Fleming, 36 Drumsheugh Gardens, . . .	1890
	Dr Foulis, 34 Heriot Row, ...	1875
	Dr J. S. Fowler, 42 Henderson Row, ...	1895
	Dr John Fraser, 19 Strathearn Road, ...	1878
	Professor Thomas R. Fraser, 13 Drumsheugh Gardens,	1865
75	Dr Garland, 53 Charlotte Street, Leith, . . .	1873
	Dr G. A. Gibson, 17 Alva Street, ...	1880
	Dr A. B. Giles, 1 Kew Terrace, ...	1893
	Dr A. Lockhart Gillespie, 23 Walker Street, . .	1891
	Dr F. M. Graham, Cowgate Dispensary, . . .	1894
80	Dr J. Allan Gray, 107 Ferry Road, . . .	1879
	Professor Greenfield, 7 Heriot Row, . . .	1886
	Dr David Greig, 38 Coates Gardens, . . .	1854
	Dr David M. Greig, 25 Tay Street, Dundee, . .	1892
	Dr W. B. T. Gubbin, Selville, Portobello, . .	1893
85	Dr G. L. Gulland, 6 Alva Street, . . .	1888
	Dr A. C. Guthrie, Swanville, Newhaven Road, . .	1890
	Dr William Guy, 11 Wemyss Place, . . .	1890
	Dr William Haldane, Viewforth, Bridge of Allan, .	1889
	Dr John Hardie, 12 Newington Road, . . .	1895
90	Dr D. Berry Hart, 29 Charlotte Square, . .	1886
	Dr James Harvey, 7 Blenheim Place, . . .	1893
	Dr Henry Hay, 7 Brandon Street, . . .	1884
	Dr John Henderson, 7 John's Place, Leith, . .	1848
	Dr J. W. B. Hodsdon, 52 Melville Street, *Secretary*, .	1883
95	Dr George Hunter, 33 Palmerston Place, . .	1876
	Dr Husband, 4 Royal Circus, . . .	1849
	Dr J. Hutcheson, 44 Moray Place, . . .	1890
	Dr James, 10 Melville Crescent, . . .	1877
	Dr Allan Jamieson, 35 Charlotte Square, . .	1876
100	Dr James Jamieson, 43 George Square, . . .	1877
	Dr G. M. Johnston, 9 Morton Street, Leith, . .	1888
	Dr R. M'Kenzie Johnston, 44 Charlotte Square, *Treasurer*, .	1883
	Dr J. Carlyle Johnstone, Melrose Asylum, Melrose, .	1882
	Dr A. J. Keiller, North Berwick, . . .	1889
105	Dr C. Kennedy, 43 Minto Street, . . .	1886
	Dr C. B. Ker, 4 Howard Place, . . .	1894
	Dr George Kerr, 6 St Colme Street, . . .	1885
	Dr J. H. A. Laing, 11 Melville Street, . . .	1889
	Dr Robert Lawson, 24 Mayfield Terrace, . .	1881
110	Dr Thomas Lawson, 16 Dean Terrace, . .	1893
	Dr R. F. C. Leith, 20 Merchiston Terrace, . .	1886
	Dr Linton, 60 George Square, . . .	1863
	Sir Henry D. Littlejohn, 24 Royal Circus, . .	1853
	Dr Herbert Littlejohn, 24 Royal Circus, . .	1892
115	Dr R. A. Lundie, 55A Grange Road, . . .	1883
	Dr P. M'Bride, 16 Chester Street, . . .	1879
	Dr E. M'Callum, 3 Brandon Street, . . .	1885
	Dr William C. M'Ewan, Prestonpans, . .	1892
	John M'Gibbon, Esq., 55 Queen Street, . .	1868
120	Dr MacGillivray, 11 Rutland Street, . .	1877
	Dr G. Mackay, 2A Gilmore Place, . . .	1878
	Dr George Mackay, 2 Randolph Place, . .	1887
	Dr Robert Mackenzie, Napier Villa, Merchiston, .	1893
	Professor Sir Douglas Maclagan, 28 Heriot Row, .	1834
125	Dr J. S. M'Laren, 14 Walker Street, . .	1887
	Dr P. H. Maclaren, 1 Drumsheugh Gardens, .	1868
	Dr John Macpherson, Stirling District Asylum, Larbert, .	1891
	Dr John Macrae, Lynwood, Murrayfield, . .	1893
	Dr D. Menzies, 20 Rutland Square, . . .	1878

130	Dr James Middlemass, Royal Asylum, Morningside,	1895
	Dr A. Miles, 23 George Square,	1892
	Dr J. Mill, 172 Ferry Road,	1886
	A. G. Miller, Esq., 7 Coates Crescent,	1867
	Dr D. Milligan, 11 Palmerston Place,	1885
135	Sir Arthur Mitchell, 34 Drummond Place,	1859
	Dr Moir, 52 Castle Street,	1836
	Dr Alexander Moir, 30 Buccleuch Place,	1876
	Dr E. C. Moore, 2 Coates Place,	1892
	Dr James Mowat, 1 Priestfield Road,	1893
140	Dr John Mowat, 1 Hope Park Terrace,	1885
	Dr Robert Muir, 20 Hartington Place,	1894
	Dr Claud Muirhead, 30 Charlotte Square,	1866
	Dr R. Milne Murray, 11 Chester Street,	1884
	Dr H. Newcombe, 5 Dalrymple Crescent,	1883
145	Dr P. Orphoot, 113 George Street,	1865
	Dr John Orr, 51 George Square,	1895
	Dr W. Basil Orr, 13 Braid Road,	1893
	Dr G. Keppie Paterson, 17 Forth Street,	1889
	Dr D. Noel Paton, 7 Lauriston Lane,	1885
150	Dr H. A. Peddie, 24 Palmerston Place,	1893
	Dr R. W. Philip, 4 Melville Crescent,	1883
	Dr Playfair, 5 Melville Crescent,	1874
	Dr Edmund Price, 1 Middleby Street,	1889
	Dr T. Proudfoot, 13 Lauriston Place,	1889
155	Dr Rattray, Portobello,	1874
	Dr James Ritchie, 22 Charlotte Square,	1873
	Dr R. Peel Ritchie, 1 Melville Crescent,	1862
	Dr Argyll Robertson, 18 Charlotte Square,	1861
	Dr William F. Robertson, Royal Asylum, Morningside,	1893
160	Dr W. G. A. Robertson, 26 Minto Street,	1892
	Dr T. R. Ronaldson, 3 Bruntsfield Terrace,	1877
	Dr R. M. Ronaldson, 17 Morningside Road,	1895
	Dr William Russell, 46 Albany Street, *Secretary*,	1884
	Professor Rutherford, 14 Douglas Crescent,	1866
165	Dr E. G. Salt, 50 George Square,	1895
	Dr James Scott, 32 St Patrick Square,	1895
	Dr Andrew Semple, 10 Forres Street,	1883
	Dr J. Sibbald, 3 St Margaret's Road,	1859
	Dr William Simmers, Denburn, Crail, Fife,	1894
170	Professor Simpson, 52 Queen Street,	1859
	Dr A. T. Sloan, 22 Forth Street,	1885
	Dr Andrew Smart, 35 Lauriston Place,	1865
	Dr G. D. Smith, 148 Ferry Road,	1877
	Dr James Smith, 1 Parson's Green Terrace,	1891
175	Dr John Smith, 11 Wemyss Place,	1856
	Dr William Smith, 14 Hartington Gardens,	1890
	Dr John Stevens, 3 Shandon Crescent,	1892
	Professor Sir T. Grainger Stewart, 19 Charlotte Square,	1861
	Dr J. S. Stewart, 15 Merchiston Place,	1885
180	Dr Robert Stewart, 42 George Square,	1892
	Dr William Stewart, 146 Ferry Road, Leith,	1889
	Dr H. J. Stiles, 5 Castle Terrace,	1889
	Dr Robert Stirling, 4 Atholl Place, Perth,	1891
	Dr S. Stirling, 4 Coates Crescent,	1891
185	Dr R. Stockman, 12 Hope Street,	1891
	Dr A. Stodart-Walker, 30 Walker Street,	1894
	Dr C. A. Sturrock, Dunfermline,	1894
	Dr Allan C. Sym, 144 Morningside Road,	1889
	Dr William G. Sym, 50 Queen Street,	1889
190	Dr W. Taylor, 12 Melville Street,	1871
	Dr C. C. Teacher, 16 Newington Road,	1887

3

		Date of Admission.
	Dr C. H. Thatcher, 8 Melville Crescent, . . .	1876
	Dr R. Thin, 38 Albany Street, ...	1890
	Dr Alexis Thomson, 32 Rutland Square, . . .	1887
195	Dr John Thomson, 14 Coates Crescent, . . .	1887
	Dr Batty Tuke, 20 Charlotte Square, ...	1864
	Dr Dawson Turner, 37 George Square, . . .	1890
	Dr Logan Turner, 2 Coates Crescent, . . .	1892
	Dr Underhill, 8 Coates Crescent, . . .	1872
200	Dr Norman Walker, 7 Manor Place, ...	1891
	Dr D. Wallace, 66 Northumberland Street, . .	1887
	Dr Douglas Watson, 19 Rutland Street, . .	1894
	Dr P. H. Watson, 16 Charlotte Square, . .	1856
	Dr A. D. Webster, Belleville Lodge, S. Blacket Place,	1883
205	Dr George R. Wilson, Royal Asylum, Morningside, .	1892
	Dr J. Lockhart Wilson, Duns, ...	1888
	J. L. Wilson, Esq., 4 Buccleuch Place, . .	1883
	Dr T. D. Wilson, 10 Newington Road, . .	1880
	Dr Russell E. Wood, 9 Darnaway Street, . .	1883
210	Dr W. Fraser Wright, Bonnington Mount, Bonnington Ter.,	1894
	Dr Hamilton Wylie, 1 George Place, . . .	1883
	Dr John Wyllie, 1 Melville Street, *Vice-President*, .	1868
	Dr J. Y. Simpson Young, 14 Ainslie Place, . .	1891
	Dr P. A. Young, 25 Manor Place, . . .	1870
215	Dr R. J. Erskine Young, 14 Ainslie Place, . .	1892

NON-RESIDENT.

	Dr D. H. Anderson, 13 *Montpellier Row, St Margaret's, Twickenham*, ...	1887
	Dr Archibald, 2 *The Avenue, Beckenham, Kent*, .	1882
	Dr J. A. Armitage, 28 *Waterloo Road South, Wolverhampton*, ...	1887
	Dr W. Badger, *Penicuik*, . . .	1882
220	Dr J. J. Bailey, *Piccadilly Club, London, W.*, . .	1874
	Dr Edwin Baily, *Oban*, . . .	1883
	Dr Andrew Balfour, *Portobello*, . . .	1874
	Dr James Craig Balfour, *Belford*, . .	1884
	Dr J. H. Balfour, *Portobello*, . . .	1881
225	Dr Alexander Ballantyne, *Dalkeith*, . .	1872
	Dr F. W. Barry, *Local Government Board, Whitehall, London, W.*, ...	1878
	Surgeon-Captain C. H. Bedford, *Bengal Army, care of W. Watson & Co., 28 Apollo Street, Bombay*, . .	1889
	Dr Benjamin D. C. Bell, *Kirkwall*, . .	1889
	Dr G. J. H. Bell, *Bengal Army*, . . .	1884
230	Dr G. H. Bentley, *Kirkliston*, . . .	1877
	Dr J. S. Beveridge, *Lochinver*, . . .	1861
	Dr J. W. Black, 15 *Clarges Street, Piccadilly, London, W.*,	1865
	Dr P. G. Borrowman, *Elie, Fife*, . . .	1893
	Dr D. C. Braidwood, *Halkirk, Caithness*, . .	1889
235	Dr David Brodie, 12 *Patten Road, Wandsworth Common, London, S.W.*, ...	1865
	Dr Andrew Brown, *London*, . . .	1884
	Dr John Brown, 68 *Bank Parade, Burnley, Lancashire*, .	1878
	Professor Cleland, *The University, Glasgow*, . .	1864
	Dr Coghill, *Ventnor, Isle of Wight*, . . .	1870
240	Dr A. R. Coldstream, 24 *Lung Avno Navvo, Florence, Italy*,	1878
	Dr John Connel, *Peebles*, . . .	1876
	Dr William Craig, *Cowdenbeath, Fife*, . .	1894
	Dr J. R. Crease, 2 *Ogle Terrace, South Shields*, .	1885
	Dr P. M. Deas, *Wonford House, Exeter*, . .	1868
245	Dr Archibald Dickson, *Hartree House, Biggar*, . .	1871

		Date of Admission.
	Dr A. Home Douglas, *Rue Blacas, Nice, France*, . .	1889
	C. E. Douglas, *Cupar-Fife*, . . .	1894
*	W. B. Dow, *Dunfermline*, . . .	1879
	Thomas Easton, *Hanover House, Stranraer*, .	1894
250	J. W. Eastwood, *Dinsdale Park, Darlington*, . .	1871
	F. A. Elkins, *The Asylum, Sunderland*, . .	1893
	R. B. Finlay, Q.C., M.P., *Middle Temple, London*,	1864
	mson C. Fowler, *Juniper Green*, .	1892
	Dr F. W. Foxcroft, *Wilmslow, Cheshire*, . .	1893
255	Dr Glyce Fraser, *Gorton House, Lasswade*, . .	1883
	Dr J. Hosack Fraser, *Bellfield, Bridge of Allan*, .	1895
	Dr R. Freeland, *Broxburn*, . . .	1879
	Professor Gamgee, 8 *Avenue de la Garve, Lausanne, Switzerland*, . . .	1863
	Dr William Gayton, *Bartram Lodge, Fleet Road, Hampstead, London, N.W.*, . . .	1886
260	Dr W. C. Greig, *Tangier, Morocco*, . . .	1884
	Dr Groesbeck, *Cincinnati*, . . .	1875
	His Excellency Dr R. H. Gunning, 12 *Addison Crescent, Kensington Crescent, London, W.*, . .	1846
	Dr John Haddon, *Honeyburn, Hawick*, . .	1883
	Dr Archibald Hall, *Montreal*, . . .	1853
265	Professor D. J. Hamilton, *The University, Aberdeen*,	1876
	Dr J. W. Hamp, *Penn Road, Wolverhampton*, .	1887
	Dr A. W. Hare, *Keyworth, Nottingham*, . .	1883
	Dr J. Home-Hay, *Alloa*, . . .	1880
	Professor J. Berry Haycraft, *Cardiff*, . .	1889
270	Dr Stanley Haynes, *Malvern, Worcestershire*, .	1864
	Dr R. Dundas Helm, 3 *Alfred Street N., Portland Square, Carlisle*, . . .	1892
	Dr R. E. Horsley, *Kirkmay House, Crail, Fife*, .	1886
	Dr J. S. Howden, *Montrose*, . . .	1856
	Professor A. W. Hughes, *Cardiff*, . .	1889
275	Dr James Hunter, *St Catherine's, Linlithgow*, .	1890
	Dr W. Hunter, 54 *Harley Street, Cavendish Square, London, W.*, . . .	1887
	Dr Robert Inch, *Gorebridge*, . . .	1887
	Dr W. Wotherspoon Ireland, *Mævisbush House, Polton, Mid-Lothian*, . . .	1883
	Dr Hugh Jamieson, 13 *Lauriston Place*, . .	1889
280	Dr D. W. Johnston, *P.O. Box 2022, Johannesburg, South Africa*, . . .	1893
	Dr James Johnston, 53 *Princes Square, Bayswater, London, W.*, . . .	1871
	J. Keay, *District Asylum, Inverness*, . .	1887
	Dr George Keith, *Moidart Cottage, Currie*, . .	1845
	Dr Skene Keith, 42 *Charles Street, Berkeley Square, London, W.*, . . .	1885
285	W. Scott Lang, . . .	1886
	Dr Harvey Littlejohn, 13 *Victoria Road, Sheffield*, .	1889
	Dr W. H. Lowe, *Woodcote Lodge, Inner Park, Wimbledon, Surrey*, . . .	1845
	Robert Lucas, *Dalkeith*, . . .	1875
	F. R. Macdonald, *Inveraray*, . . .	1860
290	K. N. Macdonald, *Gesto Hospital, Edinbane, Skye*,	1880
	Dr W. B. Macdonald, *Port Lodge, Dunbar*, . .	1888
	Dr John A. Macdougall, *Cannes, France*, . .	1875
	Professor J. M'Fadyean, 101 *Great Russell Street, London, W.C.*, . . .	1888
	G. H. Mackay, *Elgin*, . . .	1885
295	Dr John Mackay, *Aberfeldy*, . . .	1881
	Dr W. B. Mackay, 18 *Quay Wells, Berwick-on-Tweed*, .	1893

		Date of Admission.
	Professor M'Kendrick, *The University, Glasgow*,	1870
	Dr James Mackenzie, 66 *Bank Parade, Burnley, Lancashire*,	1894
	Dr W. O. M'Kenzie, D.I.G.H., 37 *Belsize Park Gardens, Hampstead, London, N.W.*,	1845
300	Dr T. J. Maclagan, 9 *Cadogan Place, Belgrave Square, London, S.W.*,	1875
	Dr Roderick M'Laren, 28 *Portland Square, Carlisle*,	1882
	Dr J. W. Martin, 16 *Nelson Street*,	1888
	Dr A. Matthew, *Corstorphine*,	1882
	Dr J. Moolman, *Cape of Good Hope*,	1877
305	Dr A. E. Morison, *Brougham Terrace, Hartlepool*,	1889
	Dr J. Rutherford Morison, 14 *Saville Row, Newcastle-on-Tyne*,	1882
	Dr J. Ivor Murray, *Granby House, St Nicholas Cliff, Scarboro'*,	1857
	Dr Andrew Scott Myrtle, *Harrogate*,	1859
	Dr Leith Napier, 67 *Grosvenor Street, Grosvenor Square, London, W.*,	1879
310	Dr T. Goodall Nasmyth, *Cupar-Fife*,	1884
	Dr Ernest F. Neve, *Srinagar, Kashmir, India*,	1884
	Dr T. Wyld Pairman, *H. M. Prison, Lyttelton, New Zealand*,	1884
	Professor Bell Pettigrew, *St Andrews*,	1873
	Dr Alexander Peyer, *Zürich*,	1893
315	Dr J. A. Philip, *Rue Victor Hugo, Boulogne-Sur-Mer, France*,	1878
	Professor W. S. Playfair, 31 *George Street, Hanover Square, London, W.*,	1857
	Sir W. O. Priestley, 17 *Hertford Street, Mayfair, London, W.*,	1854
	Dr J. H. Pringle, 256 *Bath Street, Glasgow*,	1886
	Dr S. Hale Puckle, *Bishop's Castle*,	1885
320	Dr G. M. Robertson, *The Asylum, Murthly, Perthshire*,	1890
	Dr J. Maxwell Ross, *Avenel, Maxwelltown, Dumfries*,	1882
	Dr J. R. Home Ross, *Burmah*,	1888
	Dr Joseph C. Ross, *Withington*,	1884
	Dr S. Rumboll, *Hope Villa, Hillary Place, Leeds*,	1887
325	Dr Thomas Russell, 27A *Westmuir Street, Parkhead, Glasgow*,	1888
	Dr Gordon Sanders, *Cargilfield, Trinity*,	1892
	Dr F. A. Saunders, *Grahamstown, South Africa*,	1884
	Dr Thomas R. Scott, *Musselburgh*,	1884
	Dr C. A. E. Sheaf, *Toowoomba, Queensland, Australia*,	1871
330	Dr G. F. Shiels, 229 *George Street, San Francisco*,	1887
	Dr W. H. Shirreff, *Melbourne, Australia*,	1883
	Dr T. Skinner, 6 *York Place, Portman Square, London, W.*,	1856
	Dr John Smith, *Brycehall, Kirkcaldy*,	1889
	Dr W. Ramsay Smith, *Plas Newydd, Rhyl*,	1892
335	Dr Van Someren, *Goldhurst Terrace, South Hampstead, London, N.W.*,	1845
	Dr Somerville, *Galashiels*,	1877
	Dr A. M. Stalker, 140 *Nethergate, Dundee*,	1893
	Dr Graham Steell, 96 *Moseley Street, Manchester*,	1877
	Professor Stephenson, *University, Aberdeen*,	1861
340	Dr H. R. Storer, *Newport, Rhode Island, U.S.*,	1855
	Dr John Strachan, *Dollar*,	1867
	Dr John Struthers, *Butterworth, Transkei, South Africa*,	1895
	Dr J. F. Sturrock, *Arima, Broughty Ferry*,	1887
	Professor J. Symington, *Queen's College, Belfast*,	1878
345	Professor Lawson Tait, LL.D., 7 *The Crescent, Birmingham*,	1870

		Date of Admission.
	Dr C. Templeman, 8 *Airlie Place, Dundee*, . . .	1891
	Dr Thin, 22 *Queen Anne Street, Cavendish Square, London,* *W.*, ...	1861
	Dr Alexander Thom, *Viewfield, Creiff*, . . .	1884
	Dr J. Stitt Thomson, *The Mount, Lincoln*, . . .	1877
350	Dr J. Batty Tuke, jr., *Balgreen, Murrayfield*, . .	1886
	Dr R. S. Turner, *Keith*, ...	1867
	Dr T. Edgar Underhill, *Dunedin, Burnt Green, Worcestershire*, ...	1885
	Dr A. B. Urquhart, *Murray House, Perth*, . . .	1893
	Dr Gopal Govind Vatve, *care of H.H. the Rajah of Miraj, Bombay, India*, ...	1895
355	Dr A. B. Whitton, *Aberchirder*, ...	1886
	Dr Oswald G. Wood, *Indian Army*, . . .	1886
	Dr G. Sims Woodhead, 1 *Nightingale Lane, Balham, London, S.W.*, ...	1883
	Dr Strethill Wright, *Manor, Monmouth*, . . .	1871
	Dr Yellowlees, *Gartnavel Asylum, Glasgow*, . . .	1862
360	Professor John Young, *The University, Glasgow*, . .	1860

N.B.—*Members are requested to communicate with the Secretaries if they discover any errors or omissions in the List, and also to intimate all changes in their addresses.*

CONTENTS.

I.—ORIGINAL COMMUNICATIONS.

II.—EXHIBITION OF PATIENTS.

III.—EXHIBITION OF PATHOLOGICAL SPECIMENS.

(1.) *Illustrating Parasitical Diseases.*

IV.—EXHIBITION OF MISCELLANEOUS OBJECTS.

(1.) *Mechanical and Surgical Instruments.*

(2.) *Casts, Photographs, Drawings, Microscopic Sections, etc.*

V.—SPECIAL EXHIBITIONS.

TRANSACTIONS

OF

THE MEDICO-CHIRURGICAL SOCIETY

OF EDINBURGH,

FOR SESSION LXXIV., 1894-95.

Meeting I.—November 7, 1894.

Dr CLOUSTON, *President, in the Chair.*

I. ELECTION OF OFFICE-BEARERS.

THE following gentlemen were elected Office-bearers for the ensuing year:—*President*, Dr Clouston ; *Vice-Presidents*, Dr Blair Cunynghame, Dr John Wyllie, and Dr William Craig ; *Coun-cillors*, Dr Melville Dunlop, Dr R. W. Philip, Dr Joseph Bell, Dr Russell Wood, Dr Dow (Dunfermline), Dr William Russell, Dr Sloan, and Dr Murdoch Brown ; *Treasurer*, Dr Mackenzie John-ston ; *Secretaries*, Mr Hodsdon and Dr G. A. Gibson ; *Editor of Transactions*, Dr William Craig.

II. EXHIBITION OF PATIENTS.

1. *Mr Cotterill* showed a young male patient, aged 19, from whose cranium he had removed in May last a large TUMOUR involv-ing the FRONTAL BONE, and necessitating the excision of the greater part of that bone. The tumour was of two years' growth, and presented many of the characters of a sarcoma growing from the diploe. It projected about 1½ inch from the surface of the bone, was soft and elastic in some parts, while in others the thinned outer table of the skull could be felt to crackle under the finger like a broken egg-shell. There was no pain nor tenderness in the growth; no headache, and no optic neuritis. There was nothing in the family or personal history to give any clue. The majority of surgeons who saw the case came to the conclusion that it was

a

sarcomatous, though one or two suggested the possibility of its being tubercular. An incision was made from one external angular process of the frontal over the top of the head to the other; the skin flap was turned down, and the growth, with some three-quarters of an inch of healthy bone all round it, was removed with the saw. The tumour was found to dip down into the left frontal sinus, but was not adherent to it. The growth had also penetrated the inner table at three places, and the dura was visibly affected opposite these points. The affected portions of dura were consequently removed, and the wound stitched up. Healing took place by first intention throughout, and the patient recovered without a bad symptom. As a large part of the brain was exposed by the operation, a celluloid plate has been fitted on under the cap to protect the brain and act as an artificial frontal bone. The growth was found to be tubercular on section and microscopic examination, though to the naked eye it had more of the characters of a fibrous or sarcomatous tumour.

2. *Mr Alexis Thomson* showed two patients after operation for TRAUMATIC MIDDLE MENINGEAL HÆMORRHAGE. The first case was that of a man aged 25, who was admitted to the Infirmary (University Clinical Wards) on the 20th April 1894. On the 12th April, while under the influence of alcohol, he fell off his cart and struck the right side of his head on the ground. When seen by Dr Mathew (of Corstorphine) he was unconscious, and there was a bruise over the right parietal eminence extending down towards the mastoid. He did not fully regain consciousness until the 17th April. On the 20th April Dr Mathew discovered a paralysis of the left arm and of the left side of the face, and sent him into hospital. On admission he was conscious, but for the most part dull and sleepy; from time to time he was restless, and groaned on breathing. There was a very evident bruise over the *right* parietal eminence, and there was discoloration by extravasated blood over the mastoid and between the latter and the auricle. There was motor paralysis of the lower half of the face and of the arm on the *left* side. The tongue, when protruded, pointed to the left or paralysed side. The movements of the left leg were intact, and speech was not affected. The pulse was 66, and the respirations 18. He was ordered to have leeches applied behind the ears, and to have calomel, gr. 8; the head to be shaved and carbolized for operation the following day, the 21st April, when his condition being unchanged, and the lower part of the Rolandic fissure being marked upon the surface, I threw up a large horse-shoe flap of scalp and bone, exposing the areas for the face and arm. In doing so the scalp tissues were seen to be infiltrated with blood. There was no sign of fracture. The dura mater was covered with a thin layer of blood-clot (4 mm. in thickness), which was wiped away with difficulty; there was then some active hæmorrhage at two or

three points from branches of the middle meningeal artery, of which the main trunk or its anterior division ran vertically upwards in a line corresponding to the centre of the area exposed. The artery itself was therefore secured by means of a fine suture at the inferior angle of the wound. As the dura bulged and did not pulsate, a ⊤-shaped incision was made through it and the flaps reflected. The brain bulged, without pulsating, into the gap, and the veins of the soft membranes were enormously congested. One of these veins was pricked with the knife, and the contained blood spurted 1½ ft. into space. Before securing it the veins were allowed to empty themselves, and a quantity of cerebro-spinal fluid drained away; the brain then gradually subsided and began to pulsate. The dura was sutured, the flap replaced and fixed in position with wire sutures through the scalp; at the posterior edge of the flap four threads of silkworm gut were inserted down to the dura to act as drains. Primary healing ensued, and the area of the flap soon became as fixed and rigid as the surrounding skull. The pulse rose from 66 to 110 the night after the operation, and the dressings were changed on the third day, as they had become stained with blood. The mental dulness and fits of restlessness gradually disappeared, and he was up and well on the 21st May, except that *the paralysis of the face, tongue, and arm persisted unchanged until the 1st of June* (forty days after the operation), when he moved the arm for the first time. Thereafter he rapidly and completely recovered. He has resumed his occupation as a carter, for which he regards himself as capable as he was before his accident.

The second case was that of a boy, aged 15, who was admitted to the Infirmary (University Clinical Wards) on the 21st September 1894. Half an hour before admission he was found lying unconscious behind a young horse, which presumably had kicked him. He was bleeding freely from a wound on the left side of the head. On admission he was quite unconscious, throwing himself about and crying out at intervals. He was suffering apparently from concussion and loss of blood. On the left side of the head, about 9 cms. above the auditory meatus, there was a linear bruised wound of the scalp, 4 cms. in length, from which blood was steadily oozing. Around and including this wound there was an area of marked depression of the skull, bounded by the sharp projecting edge of the surrounding bone. There were no signs of compression or of paralysis. He was immediately prepared for operation, and a large horse-shoe flap of the scalp tissues was turned down and secured to the cheek by means of a stitch. The scalp tissues and temporal muscle were infiltrated with blood. An extensive and very considerably depressed " pond-shaped " fracture of the skull was exposed, with strips and shreds of pericranium loosely attached to the depressed fragments, which measured 7·5 cms. in the sagittal and 4 cms. in the coronal plane, and consisted of one piece of bone constituting the floor of the " pond." This was firmly fixed or

wedged by a number of fragments passing almost vertically to the
surrounding bone, these latter fragments constituting the sides of
the " pond." The depressed bone could not be moved at all until
it was divided into two portions by means of the wheel saw
designed by Mr Cotterill; it was then elevated, removed, and preserved. Detached portions of the internal table were then found
beneath the intact external table surrounding the gap in the skull;
these were also removed. When the blood was sponged away, the
brain, covered by dura, gradually rose to its normal level and commenced to pulsate. Blood continued to escape from a small wound
in the dura, implicating the anterior division of the middle meningeal artery; the trunk of the latter was therefore secured by
means of a fine stitch. The exposed dura was then completely
covered with fragments of the portions of bone which had been
removed, and the flap of scalp replaced and secured. The edges
of the original wound in the scalp, caused by the kick of the horse,
were pared and brought together by sutures. Threads of silkworm
gut were inserted at the upper and posterior angle of the flap
wound. The wound healed under the first dressing. He remained
unconscious for a week, and was extremely restless, throwing himself about the bed; the urine had to be drawn off with the
catheter; the bowels were kept freely open with large doses of
calomel. On the 28th inst. (one week after the accident) he spoke
for the first time, and answered questions coherently. At night,
however, he was still very restless, and required to be constantly
watched. On the 6th of October he became more uniformly
sensible, and began to take notice of his surroundings. He suffered from no motor disability whatever. He complained of pain
in the head, and spoke slowly and deliberately with a monotonous
voice, and was on the whole moody, morose, and irritable. On
the 14th October it was noted that he smiled for the first time.
On the 18th he was allowed up, and on the 30th he was sent to
the Convalescent House. The area of the wound, which at the
end of a fortnight after the operation pulsated with the brain
beneath, became gradually hard and rigid like the surrounding
skull, and at present the skin of the flap is freely movable on the
subjacent bone, and one can tap upon it with the knuckles without
causing him discomfort. Mentally he is, so far as one can judge,
as capable as he was before he met with the accident.

Remarks.—Of these two cases, the *second* is chiefly interesting
as an illustration of the success which attends surgical interference
in compound fractures of the skull when one succeeds in
preventing infection of the wound. The absence of paralysis is
explained by the fact that the site of the lesion was anterior to
the cortical motor areas, and the absence of symptoms of compression by the fact that the blood poured out by the ruptured middle
meningeal artery escaped at the external wound in the scalp instead
of accumulating between the skull and the dura mater. The *first*

case is of interest because of the meningeal hæmorrhage taking place without fracture and on that side of the head which had been struck in the fall, and because the symptoms of pressure upon the motor areas did not show themselves until after an interval of eight days.

3. *Mr Hodsdon* showed a man, aged 57, whose LARYNX he had excised. A preliminary tracheotomy was performed on August 27th. On September 26th the tracheal wound was enlarged, a small piece of sponge passed upwards to the cricoid cartilage, and a large tracheotomy tube, surrounded by a thin sponge, introduced. Chloroform was administered through rubber tubing passed into the tracheotomy tube. The soft parts were freely separated through a T-shaped incision, the thyroid cartilage split up, and the interior of the larynx painted with a 10 per cent. solution of cocaine. The entire left half, as well as three-quarters of the right half of the thyroid, and the greater part of the cricoid cartilages, were removed. The wound was stuffed with iodoform gauze, which was renewed every two hours during the first week. The patient's progress was satisfactory. After the first forty-eight hours the temperature did not rise above 99°; solids were swallowed on the fourth day, fluids three weeks after the operation.

The man wears an artificial larynx, made from a pattern obtained from Dr Newman of Glasgow. Articulation is distinct.

Dr Leith has reported the tumour to be " a well-formed epithelioma."

4. *Mr Caird* showed a boy under treatment for UNUNITED FRACTURE by the congestive method.

III. EXHIBITION OF SPECIMENS.

1. *Dr William Russell* showed, for *Dr Gibson*, Photographs from a case of CHYLODROSIS.

2. *Dr Norman Walker* showed DEMODIX FOLLICULORUM *in situ.*

IV. EXHIBITION OF INSTRUMENT.

Dr Bruce showed a new sliding MICROTOME for cutting under spirit.

V. ORIGINAL COMMUNICATIONS.

1. NOTE ON A METHOD OF TREPHINING.

By J. M. COTTERILL, M.B., F.R.C.S. Ed., Assistant Surgeon, Royal Infirmary.

IT has probably happened to some of the surgeons here this evening to meet cases in which patients who have had a considerable portion of the calvarium removed by operation or accident, have either suffered from blows upon such an unprotected part, or have experienced an uncomfortable feeling of vertigo on stooping, due to the normal support of the brain circulation being weakened at this point.

With a view to obviate such discomforts, the plan has been adopted for some years past either of replacing the whole discs of bone removed by the trephine, or better, as has been recommended by M'Ewan, of cutting up the discs into several fragments, and planting these over the exposed surface of dura mater. Both of these plans, however, are open to objection. In the first case, where the whole disc is replaced, it is not uncommon for necrosis to take place; failing this, absorption of the disc, in whole or part, is found to take place. Again, there is the risk that such discs of bone may become depressed below the level of the surrounding skull, may become adherent to the dura mater, and may cause symptoms of irritation of the brain.

I operated some six months ago on such a case. The patient, a soldier who had been wounded at Tel-el-Kebir by a blow on the head with a rammer, had suffered for several years since from Jacksonian epilepsy.

For this condition he was trephined in Glasgow, and the two whole discs of bone were replaced in the wound. The fits left for a time, but subsequently recurred. He was admitted into the Royal Infirmary in a very helpless state. On opening up the wound I found the discs of bone, which I show you, partially absorbed, adherent to the dura, and depressed entirely below the level of the inner table. I removed the discs and the bridge of bone which lay between them; and finding nothing further abnormal after opening the dura, I closed the wound. The fits were at once removed, and had not recurred when I heard of him a few days ago.

Again, the plan of cutting up the disc into small fragments, and planting these, while doubtless better than nothing, does not in any but very exceptional cases give a really firm support; and most certainly does it fail to do so where a large area of bone, of, for example, the size of half the parietal bone, has been removed.

The various heteroplastic methods, either by the introduction of decalcified bone, metal, or celluloid plates, or by transplantation of living bone, have scarcely justified their existence, the results being insufficient, and frequently very unsatisfactory, the old metal plates being probably the best of a bad lot,—they, at least, not being absorbed.

Any plan, then, which will admit of a free access to the brain without the disability of a large actual, or imperfectly closed opening in the skull, would appear to be very desirable.

As long as thirty years ago Ollier suggested an osteoplastic resection of the skull, his idea being to lift up a piece of the skull adherent to a flap of soft parts; but it was not till 1889 that

Wagner first operated on this principle on the living body. Various operations have been practised by different surgeons in the last few years. A large Ω-shaped incision has usually been made, and the bone has been divided round the Ω generally with mallet and chisel. The flap of bone and soft parts has then been turned back, the neck of bone being forcibly smashed across at the base of the flap.

I found by experiment on the cadaver that this method was wanting in accuracy and safety. A great deal of force is required to crack across even a comparatively thin neck of bone, and the result of this violence may be to injure the dura or the vessels with the jagged edge of the broken bone. In one case a long fissure was made, leading down to the base of the skull.

To get over this difficulty I first used a chain saw, passing it below the neck of bone through two trephine openings, and sawing from within outwards. This plan, I find since, has been recommended by Salzer; but I have abandoned it as unnecessary, and rather tiresome in performance.

Various modifications have been proposed by Bruns, Toison, Lauenstein, Chipault, and Müller, but none of them appear to me to be simpler or more effectual than the plan which I had used before studying their methods, and which I now propose to describe shortly.

1. Select as the base of the proposed flap a part of the scalp carrying large vessels, *e.g.*, in front the supra-orbital, at the side the temporal and its branches, posteriorly the occipital.

2. Make two small V-shaped incisions corresponding to the lower ends of the Ω-shaped incision, their angles looking towards each other. Carry these incisions down to the bone, and strip off the pericranium from a small surface of the skull, about the size of a sixpence.

3. Apply a ½-inch trephine at each of these points, and take out the two small discs of bone.

4. Pass a periosteum scraper between these two trephine openings between the pericranium and skull, making a little tunnel.

5. Pass a fine saw (metacarpal) along this tunnel, and saw through the neck of bone lying between the two trephine openings, cutting only down to the level of the inner table. This can be easily enough done, as the difference between sawing the diploe and inner table is quite palpable. (If necessary, a curved director may be passed *under* the bone to protect the brain and dura mater.)

I prefer to do this part of the operation first, as I find one is much less likely in this way to disturb the relation of the flap of soft parts from the bony flap than if one did it at a later stage in the operation.

6. The Ω-shaped incision through the scalp is then completed,

the flap being made of any size or shape that may be thought necessary. The pericranium is then divided all round this line of incision through the scalp, great care being taken not to dislodge the soft parts unnecessarily from the bone.

7. The circular saw is then applied round the circumference of the bony flap to be lifted up, and the saw should be applied obliquely from without inwards, at the expense of the outer table, so that when the window of bone is replaced, it may be prevented by the projection of the inner table from sinking below the level of the rest of the skull.

Though not absolutely necessary, I find it facilitates the use of the saw, in getting round the corners, to take out two small discs of bone with the $\frac{1}{2}$-inch trephine at the upper angles of the flap. It may appear to complicate the operation to have to make four trephine openings; but as a matter of fact, a $\frac{1}{2}$-inch trephine makes a very small hole, and perforates the skull very much more quickly and easily than a larger instrument.

8. The flap of bone is then gently lifted up with four elevators, and the inner table will be found to crack across at the neck with absolute precision along the line at which the outer table and diploe have been already divided with the saw.

The flap of bone being held back, the dura is, if necessary, opened in the same direction as the rest of the incisions, sufficient of an edge being left to enable one to stitch it back into position when the operation is over.

In the cases in which I have done this operation the flap of bone has united satisfactorily; and, as may be seen in the specimen on the table, firm union, partly fibrous, partly osseous, has taken place all round the line of incision, while there is absolutely no roughness on the inner surface, nor at the post-mortem was there found to be any adhesion of the dura to the skull opposite the incision—a most important point.

The case was one sent me by Dr Bramwell of a girl of 16, who had suffered for several months from symptoms of brain pressure and irritation. There was a specific family history, and she had the usual treatment, but continued to grow steadily worse. An exploratory operation was therefore performed. Very advanced degenerative changes were found in the brain, with thickening of the pia mater and other membranes; and the patient, who was a hopeless imbecile at the time of the operation, gradually wasted away, and died in an asylum five months after the operation.

For such satisfactory union to take place in an emaciated and debilitated patient such as this, seems to augur well for the operation in the case of a more robust person.

This form of operation, it need hardly be said, is not applicable in every case of trephining. It is only of use where a large opening must be made in the skull for purposes of diagnosis or for the removal of large cerebral tumours, or diseased portions of the brain. It might also be useful in dealing with intra-cranial hæmorrhage, as likely to afford better access to the wounded vessel than the old operation.

Where it is found that the first flap of bone lifted up does not give sufficient room for the removal of the tumour, etc., there is nothing to prevent a second flap being taken up in a similar manner from the lateral aspect of the original opening.

At first I used the ordinary dental engine, worked by the foot, for the circular saw ; but finding this cumbersome and difficult for any one unaccustomed to the movement to work evenly, I have had made a hand machine which answers the purpose admirably, is more portable, and can be worked smoothly by any assistant.

The operation is neither difficult nor tedious. The first time I performed it the patient was off the table in thirty-five minutes from the commencement of the operation.

Mr Joseph Bell congratulated Mr Cotterill on the success of his method of operating, and approved the plan of incising the outer table of the skull between two small trephine openings instead of the use of the chain saw, which Mr Cotterill had originally advised. Mr Cotterill was original, he believed, in the oblique line of his incision through the skull. His modification of the dental engine was an advantage in being more easily carried about, for a surgeon's armamentarium nowadays was big enough if, as an American surgeon suggests, he should carry about with him a sterilizer and other traps. Mr Bell emphasized the importance of asepsis in justifying such an operation and rendering its results successful. In trephining for injury his experience over a considerable number of cases is that if pericranium is preserved, a great amount of repair takes place from the edges.

Mr Caird expressed his opinion that the dental engine submitted by Mr Cotterill would prove even more serviceable in trephining the mastoid antrum.

Mr Guy suggested the use of an electro-motor.

Dr Byrom Bramwell said that as Mr Cotterill had mentioned his name, perhaps he might be allowed, with the other speakers, to express his admiration of the result of the operation. It seemed to him that the removal of a large area of bone, such as Mr Cotterill's method of operating allowed, would be chiefly useful in dealing with cases of intra-cranial tumour. With regard to the nature of the case itself, he need say little; he had mentioned the particulars in detail at the meeting of the Society at which the subject of intra-cranial tumours was discussed. The case was clearly one of syphilitic brain disease. The patient was paralysed, helpless, and idiotic. The left arm and leg were much more markedly affected than the right; there was, in fact, a condition of left-sided hemiplegia with contracture. The patient complained of great pain in the head; there was optic atrophy, evidently post-neuritic. It seemed certain that there was a widespread syphilitic lesion of the cortex, but the left-sided hemiplegia suggested the possibility of a more localized lesion in the motor area on the right side of the brain. Under these circumstances an experimental operation was abundantly justified. As Mr Cotterill had stated, the patient was neither better nor worse after the operation. The results of the post-mortem seemed to indicate a syphilitic meningo-cerebritis rather than general paralysis of the insane properly so-called; but it was perhaps difficult or impossible in some cases to draw a distinction between the two conditions. The age of the patient, the rapid course of the disease, the marked headache, post-neuritic atrophy, and hemiplegia with contracture, were, he thought, in favour of a coarse meningo-cerebritis rather than of the ordinary form of G.P. He, of course, recognised the important influence which syphilis played in the production of general paralysis of the insane.

Mr Alexis Thomson said that he also had had the advantage of witnessing Mr Cotterill's operations and of using his circular saw. He did not think that the trephine holes at the angles of the flaps were essential, and had omitted them in his own cases, thereby saving time in separating the flap. He had found it easy to overcome the difficulty in completing the sections of the bone at the corners of the flap by means of a small chisel. The argument that the trephine-holes would prove useful in the event of providing an exit for blood did not hold, for the object was satisfactorily carried out by inserting a few threads of silkworm gut at the posterior edge of the flap. From the very free anastomosis of the vessels, he believed the flap would prove as viable when its base was towards the vertex as when it was planned after the manner laid down by Mr Cotterill. In one of his own cases it was found more convenient to turn the flap up instead of down, and the healing left nothing to be desired. It appeared to be simply a question of the presence or absence of septic infection.

Mr David Wallace said that the method of operation devised and carried out by Mr Cotterill with such success would be, he thought, of limited application in recent traumatic cases; but in patients where the procedure was adopted to expose the parts as a diagnostic measure, he believed it would prove most useful. In the latter cases it was undoubtedly advantageous to expose considerable areas of the dura at the outset, and the method under discussion was both speedy and simple. Two difficulties, however, occurred to him,—first, when the surgeon found it necessary to increase the size of the opening; and, second, when the bone varied much in thickness. In the former, if a pathological condition was discovered, but only partly exposed, by the initial removal of bone, it would be necessary to take away more bone, and this latter opening would not only be imperfectly covered, but the support of the bone flap would be interfered with.   In the latter the difficulty of the operation described would be much increased.   To exemplify these difficulties, Mr Wallace quoted a case of intra-cranial tumour upon which he had operated by the usual method.   In this case the symptoms pointed to a small tumour situate in the left arm area, but on exposure of this area the tumour, an endothelioma growing from the dura mater, was found to be very extensive. The bone over it was irregularly and enormously thickened, and it was necessary to increase the opening in every direction, although before the dura was opened the area exposed was two inches by one and a half inch.   The tumour was not removable, and this suggested another point in connexion with Mr Cotterill's method, viz., that in such cases as that referred to it was advantageous to remove the bone, and thus relieve intra-cranial tension, while the risk of hernia cerebri was much lessened by the edge of the large scalp flap being at some distance from the opening.   The greater this distance the less the risk of hernia ; but to operate by Mr Cotterill's method a relatively small flap must be used, and the risk of protrusion was correspondingly increased.   Mr Wallace thought the method would be specially valuable in cases of removal of epileptigenous areas, where it was most desirable that the opening should be closed by bone, but in traumatism or tumours he believed it would be of little practical utility.

Mr Cotterill replied.

2. ON THE TREATMENT OF UNUNITED FRACTURE BY PASSIVE CONGESTION.

By Mr F. M. CAIRD, F.R.C.S. Ed., Assistant Surgeon, Royal Infirmary ; Lecturer on Surgery, Edinburgh School of Medicine.

WHEN Bier of Kiel introduced his excellent method of treating tubercular joint affections by means of passive congestion, he indicated that the method he adopted had been formerly employed by others for the cure of ununited fracture.

This mode of treatment, although apparently well known on the Continent, is somewhat novel here, and the two cases which follow may serve to illustrate the advantage gained by the simple means recommended, namely, the use of a carefully applied flannel roller and an Esmarch's tourniquet.

CASE I.—J. M., æt. 24, a strong healthy miner, was crushed against the wall by a loose hutch, and so got his right thigh broken on March 3rd, 1892.   He was treated at home with the long splint for eight weeks, and at the end of that time was sent in to the Royal Infirmary.   He was then found to have an ununited fracture about the middle of the femur, and was put up in the double long splint with extension, and local splints.

There being no improvement, Prof. Chiene, on 8th June, cut

down on the site of fracture, cleared away a mass of interposed muscle and fibrous tissue, and left the bones in apposition, with a tube leading down to their rawed ends. It was hoped that the tube would promote a local irritation and congestion, leading to union in the manner of the seton.

On August 12th the tube was removed, no improvement having taken place.

On September 2nd,—that is, about six months after the accident, —the lack of union was demonstrated by gently moving the limb. Care was specially taken that no rubbing together of the ends or breaking down of adhesions was practised. A domet roller was then carried from the toes upwards to a point about 3 inches below the fracture, and at a similar distance above it the limb was encircled with a turn of thick elastic tubing. The intervening area then became hard, swollen, and of a bluish-red hue. For a day or two the elastic band was irksome, and then it ceased to prove inconvenient. The long splint was still used. The sinus left by the operation rapidly healed and the congestion abated, but the swelling became firmer. The hair on the congested area showed increase.

Sept. 22.—The bandages were to-day removed; the union was so marked that both fragments moved in unison. From this date rapid improvement followed, and the patient left hospital in November.

CASE II.—J. N., æt. 22, seaman, fell when intoxicated from a window on to the pavement beneath, a distance of 30 feet. He broke his fall by alighting on the heads of two women who happened to be passing at the time. They sustained no serious injury, and, indeed, promptly lodged information with the police that they had been assaulted. The seaman, suffering from a compound comminuted fracture of the right femur, was taken to the Royal Infirmary in an unconscious condition, with a weak, irregular pulse.

On examination the thigh was found to be enormously swollen, and in its outer and upper aspect there was a small semilunar wound, through which the upper fragment had evidently been projected. A corresponding rent was found in the trousers.

The wound was washed out with 1-20 carbolic lotion, its skin edges clipped away, and two portions of bone, about the size of walnuts, felt lying loose between the punctured ends of the femur, were left *in situ*. The wound healed by first intention, and the patient left hospital on November 28th.

He returned again on December 17th, since he was unable to bear his weight on the limb, and now distinct movement was seen at the break. He was accordingly put up in the double long splint for three months, but without avail. On March 24th, 280 days after the receipt of injury, the passive congestion method was tried as in the former case. Unfortunately the elastic was tightened too greatly and a small slough formed, which obliged the discontinuance of the treatment after the fourth day. A dense swollen ring had, however, formed around the site of fracture, and a steady improvement ensued, so that at the end of May no movement could be detected at the seat of injury. The patient was discharged with firm union on June 12th.

I am indebted to Professor Chiene for the opportunity of reporting the above cases, which came under my care when in charge of his wards.

The above method of treating ununited fracture is ascribed by Bier to Dumreicher, and he refers to papers by Nicoladini in the *Wiener med. Wochenschrift* for 1875, and by Helferich in the *Transactions of the German Surgical Congress* for 1887. To the latter paper I have been unable to obtain access. Nicoladini indicates that the object of the treatment is to amass as much blood as possible within a given area, so as to obtain the greatest quantity of nourishment possible for the parts. He holds that something more than œdema results, as is shown by the fact that even two or three days after removal of the tubing there is only a very slight subsidence of the swelling, a firm cartilaginous ring remaining clinging to the bone; and he narrates a case in which he was able to demonstrate that the bone itself, even to its very marrow, responded with a new formation of ossific tissue.

In conclusion, we may note that Nicoladini recommends an interrupted use of the method at intervals of two to six days. He points out that the Esmarch bandage may lead to displacement of fragments in the forearm and leg, while it is more serviceable in regard to the thigh and upper arm. Where two bones are involved, judicious circular padding, the method originally used by Dumreicher, may be substituted. When fully-formed fibrous tissue is the uniting medium we can hardly expect a good result, and this may explain the cause of failure in two cases of ununited fracture of the humerus under our care.

Finally, one has to guard against the evil effects likely to follow in the hands of rash or inexperienced practitioners. Even when the skin subjacent to the elastic band is protected by a layer of lint we have to remember how easily the tender tissues of young people are damaged, and how readily gangrene may be provoked by too great interference with the return circulation. We have, however, certain guides in the sensations of the patient and the frequent inspection of the limb during the first six hours of the application.

The method obviously lends itself to other conditions than those of ordinary ununited fracture. After excision of the knee joint where there is faulty union it may be used with success, and Bier has already indicated its value in various bone and joint lesions.

Mr Cathcart congratulated Mr Caird on the excellent cases which he had brought before the notice of the Society. He thought, however, that the name of the late Mr Owen Thomas should be associated with the method rather than that of Helferich. Under the term "damming," Thomas had advocated a daily temporary venous congestion of the limb in cases of ununited fracture. He had combined it with "hammering" or beating the part to produce mechanical irritation ; but though the details of management might not be identical, the principle of the "damming" process was the same as that used by Mr Caird.

Prof. Chiene said that as the cases described had been in his wards in the Royal Infirmary, he had full opportunities of watching their progress. At first he looked upon the method with some doubt ; to cause venous congestion did not seem to him likely to be a means towards repair. He had now, however, no doubt that the method was a valuable adjunct to the authorized methods of treatment of what were often most troublesome cases. He congratulated Mr Caird on having brought this method of treatment before the profession.

Mr Caird thanked the Society for the reception they had accorded to his communication. In reply to Mr Cathcart, he thought right to state that he had mentioned the names of surgeons who had, prior to Thomas, described and made use of passive congestion in the treatment of ununited fracture. Bier's treatment of tuberculosis of joints had in his hands been always followed by a marked improvement in the condition. He regarded it as a treatment of great value, but had no experience of it in other joint troubles.

Meeting II.—December 5, 1894.

Dr CLOUSTON, *President, in the Chair.*

I. ELECTION OF MEMBERS.

THE following gentlemen were elected Ordinary Members of the Society :—Thomas Easton, M.D., Stranraer ; A. Stodart Walker, M.B., 13 Walker Street.

II. EXHIBITION OF PATIENTS.

1. *Mr Wallace* showed—(*a*) a patient after GASTROSTOMY; (*b*) a case of REMOVAL OF MALIGNANT GOITRE (CARCINOMA).

2. *Dr Sloan* showed a successful case of CARDICENTESIS.

3. *Dr F. D. Boyd* showed a case of DIPHTHERIA TREATED BY TRACHEOTOMY AND ANTITOXIN. The child, aged 3 years, was first

seen on October 1st. There was the history of a cold for two days. There was cough, and the cry and cough had a very laryngeal sound. No obstruction to entrance of air into the chest, and no physical signs in chest. No membrane on fauces, but some enlargement of cervical glands. She was put on the usual treatment, and on the following day seemed a little better. On November 2nd aphonia had developed, and in the afternoon considerable obstructive dyspnœa, the lower part of the chest and epigastrium being drawn in. There was no albumin in urine. There being no improvement by 8.30 P.M., Mr Alexis Thomson performed tracheotomy, and at the same time ♏10 Aronson's antitoxin were injected. No membrane was obtained in opening the trachea. By midnight the temperature had risen to 102°, but the child was sleeping quietly. Some membrane was coming away in small pieces. On November 4th Dr Boyd was sent for at 5 A.M., as the patient had become very restless. A universal erythematous rash had appeared, which was causing considerable irritation. This subsided under treatment in twenty-four hours. As the temperature was still high, on November 5th a second injection (♏5) was given. Some more membrane came away; and on the following day the temperature had fallen, and the patient seemed much better. Recovery after this was uninterrupted. The tube was removed on the tenth day. The child is now quite well. How much of the good result must be ascribed to the antitoxin is difficult to say. Dr Boyd had done a good many tracheotomies, but this was the first in which recovery had taken place. Mr Thomson had had a similar experience. Cultures of the Klebs-Lœffler bacillus inoculated at the Royal College of Physicians' Laboratory from the membrane were shown.

4. *Dr MacGillivray* showed two cases. He remarked,—The first case I wish to bring under the notice of the Society to-night is one of two cases of dentigerous cysts, upon which I have operated during the past six months. They were both of the follicular variety,—namely, growing in connexion with the developmental sac which normally covers the crown of each permanent tooth. The first case was one of a woman æt. 25, who for five years had suffered from a gradually increasing swelling of the upper jaw. When first seen there was a tumour the size of an orange, presenting itself as a translucent swelling, under the upper lip, on the right side. Her teeth were perfect, with the exception of the right central incisor, which was decayed, and obviously a milk tooth. The translucent swelling was opened, and about two table-spoonfuls of glairy fluid evacuated. The interior was lined with mucous membrane, and extended back in the form of an hourglass-shaped sac as far as the last molars, being separated from the antrum by a fibrous membrane; the fang of the decayed incisor projected into the floor; from the roof was seen to be growing a perfectly-formed

permanent incisor, which, together with the milk incisor, was removed. A perfect cure was the result, the cavity gradually contracting. The case I show to-night is a boy aged 6. A similar
tumour began growing five months ago. He had only milk teeth ;
both central incisors were decayed. On opening the tumour under
the upper lip exactly the same conditions were observed ; the root
of the milk incisor projected into the floor of the cavity, and the permanent incisor, perfectly developed as regards its crown, but rudimentary as regards its fang, was growing from the roof. Both were
removed, and a cure is the result. It is interesting to note that
the same irritation which produced the cyst, from the enamel sac,
led to a premature development of the crown, while the fang remained rudimentary.

The points of interest in these cases are—The unusual situation,
the wisdom teeth of the lower jaw being more commonly affected ;
the very complete development of the teeth in the sacs, these being
often rudimentary ; and, lastly, the projection of the fangs of the
milk teeth into the floor of the sacs, which might have led to their
being supposed to be periosteal dentigerous cysts, but for the
presence of the permanent teeth on the roof of the sac.

The next case I wish to show you is one of osseous anchylosis
of the lower jaw, on the left side, in a boy aged 8. It is one of
those cases to which Barker of University College has specially
drawn attention, in which suppurative otitis media, following
scarlet fever, has extended either through the Glaserian fissure or
fibrous membrane, taking the place of the tympanic plate, to the
temporo-maxillary joint, thus leading to suppurative arthritis and
osseous anchylosis. This boy, when 4, had scarlet fever, suppurative otitis, pain and swelling over joint, increase of discharge from
the ear, subsidence of swelling over joint ; in five months absolute
fixation of lower jaw, with interference with development, and continued discharge from ear. When seen six weeks ago, the teeth
on the left side were pressed together, and there was absolutely no
movement ; on the right side they could be forcibly separated to the
extent of admitting a sheet of paper between them. There was no
sign of extra-articular contraction of muscles or fibrous tissue.
The operation, therefore, adopted was that first recommended by
Humphrey of Cambridge for intra-articular fixation,—namely, the
removal of the condyle and neck of the bone by means of an
incision along the lower border of the zygoma, avoiding the temporal artery, and met about the middle by a vertical incision
through skin and fascia only, avoiding the transverse facial artery,
and implicating the facial nerve and parotid as little as possible ;
the masseter is separated from the zygoma, the distorted neck of
the bone cleared and chiselled through. The original site of the
anchylosed joint is then cut through by means of the chisel, being
careful to avoid the internal maxillary artery, some of the soft parts
fixed by suture between the raw surfaces of bone, and the wound

closed, except for a drainage-tube, which was removed the next day. The lower jaw became at once movable, and opened to the extent of more than an inch. Rapid healing resulted, with ability to chew from second day onwards—a result very much superior to Esmarch's operation of removal of a truncated triangle of bone from the body of the jaw anterior to the masseter and internal pterygoid muscles; this operation, however, or some modification, being the only one available in cases of extra-articular, muscular, or cicatricial contraction, leading to permanent closure of the jaws. The slight facial paralysis present after the operation has now almost quite subsided.

5. *Dr Allan Jamieson* showed a case of LUPUS cured after three years' treatment.

III. EXHIBITION OF SPECIMENS.

1. *Mr Stiles* showed microscopic specimen from the case of MALIGNANT GOITRE shown by Mr Wallace, and the naked-eye tumour.

2. *Dr W. Russell* showed a BRAIN with a TUMOUR occupying part of the middle and inferior frontal lobes and part of the ascending frontal on the right side. The dura mater was adherent to it, and the bone over it thickened and softened. The tumour was probably a sarcoma. The man had been for about two years under his care in Queensberry House. There had been no paralysis or paresis or headache, and no eye symptoms. Dr Russell had never seen the patient in a fit, so did not know where the seizure commenced. The patient died a few hours after his last fit, and at the post-mortem examination it was found that the ventricles were inundated with blood, which had coagulated,—this being the immediate cause of death.

3. *Dr G. A. Gibson* showed a card specimen of the microscopic appearances of BLOOD IN CONGENITAL HEART DISEASE.

4. *Dr MacGillivray* showed the OS CALCIS from a case of acute necrosis. The history was one of a kick on the foot in a boy aged 12; slight lameness for a week, then high fever, delirium, great pain and swelling of foot, redness, fluctuation, and abscess opened. Three weeks after original injury admitted to Infirmary; foot swollen, puffy, with stinking discharge; bare bone discovered with probe; incision enlarged, os calcis discovered quite separated, except for slight attachment of tendo Achillis to epiphysis, which was also separated from body and portion of interosseous ligament. Bone removed, as efficient drainage otherwise impossible, and risk of septic inflammation spreading; wound packed with iodoform gauze, to prevent periosteum collapsing. Case going on well.

IV. Exhibition of Instruments.

Dr Lundie showed—(*a.*) Feldbausch's nasal respirator; (*b.*) A feeding-cup designed by Dr F. W. Watt.

V. Original Communications.

1. *Dr Dawson Turner* read the following paper on an electrical theory of the physiology of vision, which was illustrated by experiments:—

According to the late Prof. Clerk Maxwell, light and radiant heat are electro-magnetic waves of the ether, and they only differ from each other as a note of high pitch differs from a note of low pitch. In order that we may be made aware of this wave-motion we must be provided with a proper detector. When the waves are short and of rapid vibration they affect the eye, and we are sensible of light; when they are somewhat longer they affect the cutaneous nerves, and we feel the sensation of heat. But if the waves be still longer, we are not provided with any means of detecting them,—we remain quite unconscious of them. Prof. Hertz and his followers, however, have shown us how to construct detectors of these longer waves, and such detectors I desire to show to the Society to-night.

A tube of iron filings is a bad conductor of electricity, but if an electrical discharge take place in its neighbourhood, then its molecules become so arranged that it becomes a very good conductor. Such a tube can then be used as a detector of electrical discharges; we might call it an electrical eye. At present there is no movement passing through the tube of filings although it is in circuit with a battery. The galvanometer needle, as indicated by the spot of light, is at zero.

If, however, I now cause a few sparks to pass between the terminals of this induction coil,—*i.e.*, if I cause long electro-magnetic waves to be emitted,—then the tube of filings will be stimulated by these waves, and the molecules will become so arranged as to allow a current to pass; this will be rendered evident to us by the movement of the spot of light.

Experiment.—Our electrical eye sees the discharge. If, however, I tap the table the molecules of the filings again become disarranged, and the electrical current no longer passes.

Mr Branly discovered about four years ago this reaction of iron filings to an electrical discharge, and I have worked a good deal at the subject since; and in a paper contributed to the Royal Scottish Society of Arts last winter I showed how such tubes could be used as electrical eyes or detectors, and also the range of their vision (viz., that they respond more readily to long waves than to short ones). It struck me at that time, and also previously, when working with a somewhat similarly sensitive substance (viz., selenium), that the eye might perhaps be constructed on a similar principle. I find that Prof. Oliver Lodge has since, in a paper read before the British Association at Oxford this summer, definitely suggested such an electrical theory of vision. This theory is that in the eye, as he supposes, or in the brain, as I think, there is a source of electrical energy; that a current is, however, prevented from flowing, by reason of certain molecules in the retina being in the condition of the unstimulated iron filings; that when light falls upon these molecules they become so arranged as to be good electrical conductors; and that thus an electrical current is now set up, and that this, either directly or through the intervention of nerve impulses, gives us the sensation of light. In this connexion it is of great interest to learn—and Dr Noël Paton was kind enough to inform me—that there is a complete circuit between the brain and the eye, because efferent nerves have lately been traced to the retina. This circuit would accordingly be made up of the brain, the efferent nerves, the retina with its sensitive molecules, the optic nerve, and the brain.

Darkness may be either due to the simple non-passage of the current in consequence of the rearrangement of the retinal molecules when no light falls upon them, or it may be due to a positive sensation due to the same cause. In some respects the action of selenium affords a better analogy, for, in the first place, it is actually sensitive to vibrations of the same wave length as the eye is sensitive to, viz., to light; and, in the second place, no tapping back or mechanical stimulus is needed to again render it a very bad electrical conductor; an absence of light is all that is required to get the electrical current cut off.

Further, the selenium is most sensitive to exactly the same kind of light that the eye is most sensitive to, viz., to yellow light.

Experiment with coloured lights and selenium.—You observe that the galvanometer needle is most deflected when the selenium is illuminated with yellow light.

Dr Milne Murray said that, according to this theory, the eye was in a state of strain. The waves set up abolished the strain and allowed the current to pass. The defective point in the theory was, that no means were provided by which the state of strain could again be set up. A good shock would be required to re-establish darkness in the eye. The selenium plate was a bad conductor in the dark and a good one in the light. The suggestion that the eye was in a state of electric strain assumed that optic phenomena were due to electric disturbances, a point which, he thought, was a long way from solution. Many experiments had been performed to prove that nervous impulse and electric impulse were the same; but the velocity of the optic impulse was very much less than that of the electric. Until we could explain how electric energy was transformed into nervous energy the theory did not throw much light on the brain. At the same time, it seemed to be a step in the right direction, and showed how the rods and cones could take up the vibrations. It could not be said to be an absolute solution. Dr Turner was to be congratulated on his demonstration, which he (the speaker) could only have undertaken with fear and trembling.

Dr Noël Paton said that they had had a good demonstration of the way in which the optic mechanism *might* act, although it did not prove how it *did* act. It ought to be considered in the light of the lines of the other end-organs.

Dr George Mackay said the temptation was great to compare electrical action and nerve action, but it was merely an analogy. Physiological experiment tended to show that the two were entirely different. Truth, however, was sometimes discovered by following out a theory. Could this theory explain the occurrence of the primary image and the associated after image, perception not merely of white light and its abstraction causing darkness, but of red light and its abstraction producing green; blue followed by complementary sensation of yellow? These and other delicate phenomena must be explained. It would be interesting, however, to experiment with coloured glass between the selenium and the light.

Dr Turner replied, stating that his theory would explain the phenomena of exhaustion.

2. NOTES ON A PECULIAR CASE OF STRICTURE OF THE ŒSOPHAGUS.

By DAVID WALLACE, M.B., F.R.C.S. Ed., M.R.C.S. Eng.

MR PRESIDENT AND GENTLEMEN,—It is not my intention to make remarks on stricture of the œsophagus in general, but rather to draw attention to a peculiar form of the affection illustrated in a patient who has been recently under my care.

It is customary to group strictures of the œsophagus, apart from those due to external pressure, under three headings,—(1), malignant; (2), cicatricial or traumatic; and (3), spasmodic. The case to which I allude differs from all of these. There is no history of traumatism in its accepted meaning,—there is no evidence of malignancy, such as bleeding, tumour mass, or enlarged glands; and the constriction is not, I believe, simply spasmodic. The history of the case is as follows:—Hugh S., an Irishman, æt. 52 years, enjoyed good health until the beginning of June this year. At that time, without any known or discoverable cause, he experienced difficulty in swallowing solids. This difficulty increased rather than diminished under the ordinary treatment used for dyspepsia,—a form of treatment adopted, as the condition was at first looked upon as one of reflex spasm due to gastric irritability brought on by alcoholism. Towards the end of June, no improvement having taken place, an endeavour to pass an œsophageal bougie was made, but the instrument was stopped opposite the cricoid cartilage; eventually a small-sized instrument was passed through this constriction, only, however, to be again stopped, at a distance of 9 inches from the teeth, by a second stricture. The average distance from the teeth to the stomach is 14½ inches, from teeth to cricoid 7½ inches, and therefore from cricoid to stomach 7 inches. The second stricture would therefore be 1½ inch below the cricoid cartilage. It was now found that the patient, who had hitherto said he could swallow liquids but no solids, although able to swallow small quantities of fluid, after a time ejected the greater portion. No "trickling sound" could be heard on auscultation, but some of the liquid food must at this time, and for some weeks later, have passed into the stomach, as he lived for six weeks without any further source of sustenance than that which he took by the mouth. His weight rapidly decreased, and fell from his normal, 13 st. 8 lbs., to 8 st. 13 lbs.

He was admitted into the Royal Infirmary on 15th August 1893. On admission the patient was very emaciated, and from his own statement and the observation of the resident surgeon and nurses, no solid food passed into the stomach, and most of the liquid he swallowed was ejected after a few minutes. Careful examination detected no tumour, and there was no bleeding or sign of ulceration or suppuration. A bougie of small size was passed through the upper stricture, but the lower remained impervious. In the belief that after dilatation of the upper stricture I might be able to pass an instrument through the lower, I passed graduated bougies, and in less than a week the upper was dilated sufficiently to admit a large bulbous bougie. Solid food was now swallowed, but, just as with liquids previously, was ejected in a few minutes. From this I formed the opinion, although no distinct swelling in the neck was felt after the food had been swallowed, that a dilatation of the œsophagus had occurred between the strictures. All efforts to pass an instrument through the lower stricture were still unavailing; and as the patient's strength was visibly failing, I determined to perform gastrostomy. This was done on August 25th by Franks' method. The patient recovered from the operation, and has been fed by the gastric fistula ever since. No evidence of tumour growth was got by examination of the cardiac end of the œsophagus. I hoped, with regard to the gastrostomy, that if the diagnosis of gastric irritation as a source of spasm was correct, that, quite apart from the benefit derived by feeding the patient through the gastric fistula, the stomach would be improved in its tone under treatment, the patient would gain strength, and the œsophagus not being irritated by the lodgement of food, the spasm might pass off, at any rate in part, and treatment by dilatation yet succeed. In that view I was wholly disappointed. During the month that elapsed between the passage of bougies before operation and after operation the upper stricture again contracted, and on its re-dilatation the lower one remained as impervious as ever.

The question, therefore, still remained, What is the nature of the stricture? As I have already said, I exclude traumatic and malignant. I admit that the lower stricture may be due to a scirrhus, much fibrous tissue being present, but no ulceration of the mucous membrane. The situation, however, is against this view, as malignant strictures are usually just at the cricoid or near the cardiac end of the œsophagus. Further, by now some definite evidence of malignancy might be expected to have appeared. I can get no history of syphilis, and certainly no improvement accrued from large doses of iodide of potassium—a drug which was exhibited soon after the gastrostomy was performed. We are thrown back, therefore, to two forms of stricture—the spasmodic or the simple stricture.

In the beginning of this year Dr Morison of Hartlepool published an interesting paper on dysphagia, associated with chronic alcoholism, and from the first occasion when this patient came before me I have had that cause in view. In Dr Morison's cases the patients, three in number, were women; had progressively difficulty in swallowing first solids, second fluids; they had all been addicted to "nipping"—taking the whisky "neat." In all there was an obstruction to the passage of an instrument at a point opposite the cricoid cartilage, but he succeeded in overcoming this by steady pressure, after which the bougie passed easily into the stomach. All the patients died in the course of a few weeks or months after Dr Morison saw them, but in all the history of difficulty in swallowing extended over several years. In one an autopsy was performed, and no organic stricture was present. The patient whose case I have described is a man who has often taken "nips neat," but has been, as far as I can discover, fairly temperate. He has two strictures—not one only at the cricoid. I have been quite unable to overcome the second by steady pressure, although that has been repeatedly tried with bougies of varying size and shape.

In regard to simple stricture, problematically we can think of various causes which might lead to it,—e.g., local ulceration followed by cicatricial contraction. Morell Mackenzie quotes a case of Dr Kendal Franks, in which gradually increasing dysphagia had followed the impaction of a hard piece of bread-crust. He states there was no evidence of hysteria, and that there can be no doubt that the stricture was due to cicatricial thickening at the place of injury, but I can get nothing in this patient's history to point to such an origin. Can it arise in association with spasmodic stricture? Dr Kendal Franks, in the *British Medical Journal* for November of this year, refers to this form as simple stenosis, and relates a case in which he performed œsophagectomy. He refers to nine others, "in all of which it is distinctly affirmed that the tissues at the stenosed portion of the tube were absolutely unaltered." In regard to the etiology, he combats the view of a congenital malformation, points out how the histories quoted show progressive advance of the affection, and remarks that " one of the essentials of a congenital malformation is, that as long as no secondary disease is superadded, the conditions it gives rise to do not vary. The reverse holds good with an acquired malformation ; so long as the originating cause continues to act, so long the malformation increases, and the symptoms it gives rise to become more acute." How, then, he asks, are such strictures acquired ? " The parts involved being found texturely normal, no inflammation or ulcerative process has been at work. The only explanation which can be offered is that it is due to a very localised and very prolonged spasmodic condition of the muscularis mucosæ, or of the circular muscular fibres in the outer coat, which produces shortening of the muscular fibres of a more or less permanent character. Harrison Cripps explains a somewhat similar condition in the rectum in this way." Such a history does not coincide with that of my patient; the dysphagia has been of comparatively short duration—five months; and practically complete obstruction was present in three months.

Can anything further be done to relieve the condition? The patient has now regained much of his former strength, and although three months have elapsed since the operation, no sign of malignancy has appeared. A month ago the patient allowed the tube through which he fed himself to escape into the stomach. An endeavour to ascertain its presence by sounding failed to get any such evidence. Thirty-six hours later I filled the stomach with water, examined the interior with the cystoscope, saw the tube, passed a lithotrite, and with some trouble got the tube end on and withdrew it. As I did so the idea occurred to me that if the difficulty of passing a tube from above the stricture be increased by dilation of the œsophagus or any other cause, could we not pass one from below, and thus having initiated the dilatation, continue it from above, and later close the gastric fistula ? Circumstances have not permitted this endeavour; but at a future time, if no improvement occurs and the patient's health be still maintained, I propose to carry this out. This plan has been tried in at least one other case—Dr Willy Meyer, *Annals of Surgery*, October 1894. I can recall a case of stricture of the urethra where it was impossible to pass an instrument along the urethra into the bladder, even after perineal section. A suprapubic cystotomy was performed, and the stricture successfully treated. This would be more difficult in the case of œsophageal stricture, but it is worthy of trial.

Dr Russell said that, with regard to the pathology of non-malignant stricture, he had looked up his post-mortem records. One case occurred in 1890. There was a constriction behind the aortic arch. When water was poured in, the part of the gullet above that point became distended. The constriction, however, was overcome by putting in water at a high pressure. On slitting it up, no ulceration or thickening was found. The upper part was more congested than the lower. There was no tumour external to œsophagus to account for stricture. In another case there was a very narrow fibroid stricture just behind the thyroid, which gave no evidence of being malignant, yet obstruction was so complete that only a small-sized catheter could have passed. These were the only cases he had examined post-mortem that threw light on the condition.

Mr Caird alluded to a very successful method he had seen in Breslau some years ago. The œsophagus having had sufficient rest after gastrostomy, the patient was encouraged to swallow a long piece of fine silk to which very fine beads or knots were attached. When one end reached the stomach it was pulled out through the wound, and to the other in the mouth a thicker silk thread was attached, and to this a filiform long bougie, and thus eventually the traumatic stricture was dilated.

Dr Bramwell said he had seen two cases of stricture of the œsophagus from enlarged glands at the bifurcation of the trachea. There was no evidence of tumour in the chest, or malignant growth.

Dr Cathcart said it was interesting to have their attention drawn to this form of stricture, with no evidence of injury or malignant disease.

Mr Wallace, in reply, said that the method suggested by Mr Caird was practically the method adopted by Meyer, who attached a piece of thread to a small bullet, which the patient tried to swallow. The stricture was too high up to be accounted for by enlarged bronchial glands. The upper part of the second stricture was about 1 in. above manubrium sterni, 1½ in. below cricoid. There was no evidence of enlarged glands in the neck.

3. CARDICENTESIS—WITH SUCCESSFUL CASE.

(CASE OF ENDOCARDITIS AND PERICARDITIS WITH EFFUSION—ACCIDENTAL TAPPING OF RIGHT VENTRICLE AFTER APPARENT DEATH—RECOVERY.)

By ALLEN THOMSON SLOAN, M.D.

M. B., aged 19 years, a tall, fairly healthy young lady, was seized on 12th May 1894 by a severe attack of erysipelas, which affected chiefly the left side of the face and head, and although it spread over the forehead and part of the right side of the face, was fortunately arrested, under treatment with ichthyol and lanoline externally and iron internally, on the fifth day, and an apparently rapid recovery was about to ensue. The temperature, which at the commencement varied from 103° to 105°, had become normal, all sign of inflammation had disappeared, and a perfect cure seemed established, when suddenly, without any fresh exposure—the patient never having been allowed out of bed—a very severe attack of rheumatic fever developed.

Family History.—To this there was a marked family predisposition, her father having suffered from a prolonged attack of acute rheumatism, which left him a martyr for sixteen years to subacute attacks, and completely deformed him; and her only brother having twice had attacks of rheumatic fever, and suffered frequently from rheumatic sore throat. Her mother and two sisters are alive and well; but her father, who at the time of her attack was suffering from tuberculosis of both lungs—the result of influenza—has since died. Her maternal grandfather and grandmother are octogenarians and in good health, but on the paternal side there is a distinct tendency to phthisis.

Previous Illnesses.—Her previous illnesses all indicate the same susceptibility to rheumatism. When two months old she suffered from bronchitis, which lasted about a fortnight. At five years of age she had rheumatic fever, and two years afterwards suffered from measles, which was followed by a second slight attack of rheumatic fever. Between the ages of nine and ten she had diphtheria, but for the next eight years enjoyed perfect health. In the beginning of February 1893 she was attacked with scarlet fever so severely, that from the onset she was put on a water-bed, and in spite of daily 30-gr. doses of salol and continued lying between blankets, she was seized with a third sharp attack of rheumatic fever, with accompanying endocarditis. This left a well-marked systolic mitral murmur, which, however, in the course of a few months entirely disappeared, and with the exception of slight œdema of the right foot, she enjoyed robust health till within a few weeks of her present attack, when she began to feel her duties as a school teacher rather fatiguing, and doubtless the anxiety regarding her father's health predisposed her to the attack of erysipelas, which was the starting-point of her fourth and most severe attack of rheumatic fever.

Present Attack.—Salicylate of soda, in 10 and then in 15-grain doses every three hours, along with aromatic spirits of ammonia, was substituted for the quinine and antipyrin, which had been given along with the iron during the attack of erysipelas, and had been very badly borne. From the 17th to the 22nd fair progress was made, the temperature varying from 99° to 103°, but with a distinct tendency to an evening rise. No great relief, however, was got from the pains, which were general throughout all the joints, and were most severe in the muscles of the calves. An 8-grain Dover powder was given at bedtime with marked benefit, as a few hours' sleep was induced, and the restlessness, which had been characteristic from the first, somewhat allayed. A daily careful examination of the heart revealed nothing till the morning of the 24th, when slight præcordial pain and a feeling of oppres-

d

sion about the chest was complained of, followed in the evening by
well-marked friction, the " to-and-fro " murmur being audible over
the whole base, but loudest and apparently nearest to the ear over
the pulmonary area.   The dose of salicylate of soda was increased
to 20 grains every four hours, and digitalis added to quieten and
strengthen the pulse, which from the beginning of the attack had
varied from 100 to 116 per minute, but had been of fair strength,
regularity, and volume.   Warm poultices and sinapisms were
applied locally, with the result that in five days the friction had
entirely disappeared, and the patient again seemed in the fair way
of recovery.   Still the temperature kept irregularly rising and
falling in a suspicious manner without sufficient ascertainable
cause, and the muscular pains in the limbs became even worse.
Salicin alone, and combined with antipyrin, was tried, but ineffec-
tually ; and considering the attack to have a possible septic origin,
salol in 12-grain doses every four hours was substituted, with a
slight resulting decrease in fever, but no diminution in pain.   In
fact, the only drug administered with certain benefit was the old-
fashioned but reliable Dover's powder.   During all this time the
services of a skilled nurse had been utilised, and every precaution
as to diet and the general treatment of a patient suffering from
acute rheumatism had been most scrupulously and carefully
observed.   The urine, tested twice a week, presented no abnormality other than scantiness in amount and excess of urates.
From the 28th of May to the 4th of June the condition of the
patient remained much the same, but on the evening of that day
there was a return of the friction, and in addition a well-marked
systolic mitral murmur was audible.   Hourly almost a change
for the worse progressed, hastened by the thought of parting from
a dying father, who was being removed to the country in the vain
hope of prolonging his life, and without an interview.   Every
movement was accompanied by excruciating pain, mostly in the
muscles of the lower limbs ; nourishment was taken with difficulty,
owing to occasional attacks of sickness ; an irritable, hacking cough
developed ; the pulse became rapid—120 to 140 per minute—
feeble, and dicrotic ; and the respirations were greatly increased—
reaching to 30 and 50 per minute.   The livid, anxious countenance,
the pallor of the lips, the working of the alæ nasi, the dilatation of
the veins of the neck, and increased general restlessness, all indicated rapid effusion into the pericardium, which physical examination too truly revealed.   The area of cardiac dulness was greatly
increased, extending fully half an inch to the right of the sternum,
up to the second interspace above, but below and to the left was
indistinguishable from a dulness which extended over the whole
of the left lung, doubtless due to compression from the bulging
pericardium, and probably also to some actual pleuritic effusion, as
all breath-sounds were inaudible over the whole of the left base,
and up to the middle of the scapula.   Friction was still to be

heard, but the actual heart-sounds were distant, feeble, and obscured. From the 8th to the 11th matters got worse, the changing colour of the face indicating the possibility of a fatal faint at any moment, and an ever-present terror of approaching death adding greatly to the patient's discomfort and pain. By this time all anti-rheumatic remedies had been stopped, and stimulants, in the form of champagne and brandy, freely given, while a mixture of strophanthus, strychnine, and iron was added with a view to keep up the heart's action. Two blisters were applied over the præcordium, and sinapisms to the bases of the lungs. Curiously, all the time the patient could only lie in an absolútely recumbent position, any attempt to raise her with a view to ease the breathing having quite the opposite effect. My mind was gradually being made up that tapping the pericardium alone would benefit the patient, so on Tuesday, 12th June, Dr Bramwell was called in consultation. So grave was the patient's condition during the afternoon that the subject of tapping was not even mentioned between us, and the application of another blister was the only remedy suggested. In addition to all the other symptoms, considerable difficulty in swallowing had arisen, showing further increase in the effusion. The blister was applied a little lower down and more to the left than the previous ones, exactly over the apex-beat, which now corresponded to the left nipple.

On the following morning, 13th June, I set up the aspirator and had it ready exhausted in an adjoining room, though the friends of the patient greatly objected to its being used. The pulse, which had been so rapid, had become alarmingly slow—80 per minute— and the nurse was warned if there was further slowing to send at once for assistance.

During the afternoon the patient was seen by Dr Calder of Leith—a personal friend—who was then of opinion that, tapping or otherwise, she had only an hour or two to live.

About 8 P.M., on my way to the house, and whilst about four minutes' walk from it, I was met by a young lady, who told me to hurry, as my patient was just dead. I ran as quickly as possible, and found that Dr James Smith had been summoned, to find her either in a fit or faint. The pulse was uncountable and hardly to be felt, and the livid pallor of the face, profuse, cold perspiration, and changing, startled expression indicated approaching death. First, 30 minims of ether were injected into the arm, and then a sudden dilatation of the pupils and rapid receding of the pulse warned us of further need of stimulation, and 30 minims were injected into the left breast. I proposed tapping; but as the friends were anxious first to see Dr Bramwell, Dr Smith ran to telephone for him. Immediately afterwards the heart and respiration stopped, and in the moment of excitement I jumped up, seized the aspirator, and plunged the needle into the fourth interspace, about half an inch to the left of the sternum and a little below the left nipple. To my astonishment, from 8 to 10 ounces of pure blood flowed rapidly into the bottle of the aspirator and then suddenly stopped, and to my dismay I found I had penetrated a cavity of the heart. As I was slowly withdrawing the cannula, regretfully telling the nurse it was all over, and to close the patient's eyes, to my surprise the heart made first a feeble, irregular movement, then gave a sudden strenuous jump, and finally, like a pendulum regaining its swing or a runner his stride, it started to beat again in the race for life. In moments of intensity, it is difficult to estimate time, but I should say fully half a minute had elapsed between the introduction of the needle and the restarting of the heart-beats. It was an extraordinary sensation to feel the heart beating more and more forcibly against the point of the cannula, which was gradually withdrawn so as not to further injure the heart-wall. I was standing thus, with my thumb on the puncture made by the needle, when Drs Bramwell and Smith made their welcome appearance. My uppermost feeling at first was one of regret that I had converted a patient practically dead into one apparently dying, and sincerely did I lament she had not been left to pass away in peace, for a most pitiful scene was now enacted for an hour. Occasionally there was given a heart-rending shriek, quantities of frothy mucus were half-coughed, half-vomited, and had to be swept out of the mouth with a towel, the blood went ebbing and flowing from the cheeks, which were first ashy-grey, then purplish in hue, the pupils were dilated to their fullest extent, the running, following pulse was quite uncountable, and the patient had every appearance of one dying asphyxiated. Another drachm of ether was injected, with the result that the patient became maniacal, and at Dr Bramwell's suggestion, first $\frac{1}{4}$ and then another $\frac{1}{4}$ of a grain of morphia was administered hypodermically to keep her quiet. This had a slightly soothing effect, and Drs Bramwell and Smith now left, thinking it quite impossible the patient could live through the night. In another hour, however, her aspect had vastly improved, the lividity of the countenance and pallor of the lips had disappeared, the breathing was easier, and the mania was succeeded by the most delightful feeling of intoxication, the patient repeatedly breaking out into ripples of laughter, and saying, "Oh, how nice! What a dear, kind doctor!" "Oh, how funny! Needles and pins, needles and pins running down both legs and arms!" In another half hour she was able to recognise her mother, who had been brought in from the country. The services of two fresh skilled nurses were obtained, and with injunctions that she should be freely stimulated with champagne and brandy, she was left for the night. The blood, which filled one-third of a 30-oz. Winchester jar, had formed a solid clot, and had to be broken up with a stick and dissolved with soda and hot water before the bottle could be cleaned. In it there was no apparent mixture with serum, and clotting had taken place early and was specially firm.   The smallest size of the ordinary aspirating needle was used.

During the night the patient was inclined to wander, and the pulse remained very rapid, changeable, and irregular, while the respirations varied from 22 to 34 per minute, broken at intervals by a prolonged sigh.   Occasionally great anxiety was caused by the deathly pallor of the lips spreading round the angles of the mouth, at which times a little brandy or champagne was administered in teaspoonfuls.   In the morning consciousness completely returned, and the patient was able to take half a cup of tea and a biscuit.   She had no recollection whatever of the dreadful crisis she had passed through, having been quite unconscious during the operation of tapping; and, when puzzled as to the piece of plaster over her left breast, was told it was part of the dressing of her blister, as it was thought wiser to avoid any excitement.   The pulse varied from 118 to 122 per minute, and was still very feeble and irregular, with a long pause at every fourth beat.   The most absolute rest was enjoined; liquid nourishment was given in small quantities frequently, and stimulant only in drachm doses, and with caution, in fear of over-exciting the already too tremulous heart's action.   In the afternoon the temperature rose to 101°·4, but this was accounted for by the exhaustion and the general feeling of soreness, due to continued lying in the same position.   As there was still a tendency to mental excitement, and no further sleep had been obtained, at 12.30 A.M. 15 grs. of bromide of potassium were given, after which she slept till 2 A.M.   At 4.20 there was great restlessness, and other 15 grs. were given, with the result that repeated short sleeps were obtained between the times of administration of nourishment.   Two days after the operation the temperature fell suddenly to normal, and the pulse from 104 to 40, which occasioned great anxiety; and this happened from time to time, till the pericardial effusion cleared away about eight days afterwards, while the slightest movement on the part of the patient caused immediate paling of the lips and face.   It is needless for me to detail the daily progress of the case, which was hourly observed and noted by the two nurses to whose superb after-attention the patient owes her life.   It will suffice for me to point out that after the fifth day there was no rise in the temperature above 99° until July the 2nd, and it was then due to slight gastric disturbance, the consequence of overfeeding, that the pulse first became regular, then gradually slower, till on the 22nd of June it reached the normal rate of 76, and that the respirations, which had varied from 22 to 30, correspondingly declined to 18 per minute.   During the first twenty-four hours no urine was passed, and for seven days after only 12 to 14 ounces daily, thick with urates; but the patient continued at times to perspire so freely that her flannel gowns had to be changed frequently.   The first urine passed contained no sugar nor albumen, but was greatly dis-

coloured, owing to the previous free administration of salol. Solid
food in the form of white fish was first given six days after the
tapping, and the cardiac tonic of arsenic, strophanthus, strychnine,
and iron resumed.   Fruit, in the form of bananas and oranges, was
allowed, and strong soups, flavoured with vegetable juices, given,
with a view to combating the profound anæmia which had ensued.
Stimulants were only given when specially called for, and the
bowels relieved by glycerine enemata.   The only complaint the
patient had was about the soreness of her bones, owing to her great
emaciation ; but an attempt to put her on a water-bed caused such
alarming faintness it had to be abandoned.   It is the most extraordinary fact that here was a case of rheumatic fever, apparently
of septic origin, which no therapeutic agent, with the exception of
the opiate, had done anything to alleviate, which almost nightly
for three weeks had produced a temperature of 104°, and which,
with its complications of endocarditis and pericarditis, had nearly
caused the death of the patient, suddenly and finally arrested by
the heroic process of drawing off 10 ounces of blood direct from
the heart.   At no time afterwards did the patient suffer from the
very slightest rheumatic pain, whilst previously she was practically
never free from such, night nor day.   For the first five days physical observation could only consist of stethoscopic examination over
the heart ; but till Tuesday, the 20th June, the heart sounds were
represented by irregular, muffled thumps, and were quite indistinguishable in any area.   On that day they could be faintly heard
and localized,—the first sound feeble in the aortic, tricuspid, and
pulmonary areas, the second relatively much accentuated ; while
in the mitral area, and especially over the left nipple, a soft blowing systolic murmur was distinctly audible, with a less certain
pre-systolic.   Daily the sounds became clearer, and when the
patient became stronger percussion revealed the gradual disappearance of the pericardial effusion, which was further hastened by
the daily external application of iodine.   A fortnight elapsed
before the lungs could be satisfactorily examined, but at the left
base there was still extensive dulness and absence of breath-
sounds.   Rubbing with turpentine, iodine, and a blister were
successful in removing this, and in three weeks, except for great
debility, the patient was physically perfectly well, the systolic
mitral murmur being the only persistent indication of what she
had passed through.   Dr Bramwell, who daily had looked for some
announcement of the patient's death, kindly re-visited her on
Friday, the 23rd, nine days after the tapping, and found the
young lady whom he had left *in extremis*, apparently without the
faintest hope of recovery, enjoying, through the kindness of a too
indulgent nurse, a plate of strawberries and cream.   In a month
the patient was allowed up on a couch, and in another week to
make personal efforts which had previously been forbidden ; and
it was the utmost gratification to me that within seven weeks from

the time of cardiac aspiration she was able to be driven seven miles into the country to visit her father, the shock of whose death a day or two afterwards she stood remarkably well. A week after this she was sent to the country, and since then has enjoyed perfect health.

December 5th.—The patient continues in excellent health ; she has had no return of the rheumatism, and the cardiac murmur has entirely disappeared.

Cardicentesis.—It is supposed that acupuncture was first employed as a therapeutic agent by the Chinese, who are credited with a special leaning towards tapping internal cavities, the result, however doubtful, being accepted with the philosophy typical of those followers of Confucius. Puncture of the heart by a sharp-pointed body, such as a needle, does not always prove fatal. It was formerly considered that all wounds of this organ were necessarily and instantly mortal ; but cases are on record where, after most extensive injury to the cavities of the heart, life was prolonged for a considerable period ; and even recovery is claimed to have taken place. In Stevenson's edition of Taylor's *Principles and Practice of Medical Jurisprudence* many interesting cases are described, where, after various penetrating wounds of the heart, the patients survived periods extending from four to twenty-eight days ; while out of twenty-nine cases collected by Ollivier and Sanson, only two proved fatal within twenty-eight hours. A case is reported in which a person is stated to have recovered from a punctured wound of the heart (*Medical Gazette,* vol. xvii. p. 82) ; and Tragien met with a case in which a man who had been stabbed in the left ventricle survived *five days* (*Ibid.,* vol. xlvii. p. 42). In the *Transactions of the American Surgical Association* (vol. v. pp. 249-252) many extraordinary cases are referred to, where life was prolonged an incredible time after extensive heart-injury. In the *Surgical History of the War* there is recorded the case of a private who was shot in the chest, the ball entering the right auricle. The patient persisted in sitting up, and walking about his room. He lived for *fourteen* days. A man is stated to have lived twenty days with a skewer through his heart (Ferrus). Mr Durham had a case of bayonet wound of the heart in which the patient survived fifty-six hours. The wound implicated both ventricles, the septum, and the auricle, and the man walked some yards after receiving the injury. In the *Lancet* for January 1879, a case is reported where a man received a shot wound of the left ventricle which did not prove fatal for *fifty-four* days, the patient having in the meantime returned to his work. The Duc de Berri was stabbed in the heart while leaving the theatre in company with his wife. The dagger pierced the heart through, and made a wound several inches in length, yet he lived till six in the morning, and was able to beg that his assassin might be forgiven. In the *New York Medical News* for October 27th, 1894, Dr Church reports a case where the right ventricle of the heart was pierced through by a bullet, the anterior wound being half an inch in diameter, and the wound of exit ⅝ of an inch, and ragged ; and yet the patient lived three hours after the injury. In the same paper the following statistics are given :—In the *Index Catalogue of the Army Medical Museum* there are reported twenty-two cases of direct injury to the heart, all of which lived over three hours ; seventeen lived over three days ; eight lived over ten days; two lived over twenty-five days ; one died on the fifty-fifth day ; and there were three well-authenticated recoveries. Dr S. S. Purple, of New York, gives in the *New York Medical Journal* (vol. xiv. p. 441) an account of a recovery from a wound penetrating both ventricles (confirmation of the diagnosis by post-mortem nine years subsequently), and a tabulated list of forty-two cases which survived injury for from thirty minutes to seventy days. Dr C. E. Lavender, in the *Proceedings of the Medical Association of Alabama* (1851, pp. 104-181), reports a recovery from an incised wound of the heart; and Dr C. L. Ford, in the *New York Medical Record* (1875, p. 173), cites a case of buckshot injury, with recovery. In view of these statistics, Dr Church suggests that it is open to discussion whether a surgeon might not open the pericardium, clean out the clots, close the wound in the heart walls, and give his patient a chance of recovery. Dr Block expressed the belief that death can be averted in many cases of heart-wounds by this procedure, as incision of the pericardium allows escape and extraction of the clots which cause pressure and death. He also stated that he has been able to suture the heart in rabbits, which is quite a simple operation, requiring only three or four minutes ; and that even if cardiac pulsation and respiration stop during this mechanical interference with the heart's movements, death does not necessarily ensue (*American Journal of Medical Science*, January 1883, p. 276). What the surgeons here present might attempt in such cases I do not exactly know ; but, though no harm might actually be done, the prospect of saving the patient's life seems to be unlikely in the extreme, as the majority, from the post-mortem reports, appear to have died from primary hæmorrhage. It is not surprising, when acquainted with such facts, for us to learn that punctures of the heart are apparently not only innocuous, but, in some instances, seem even to be productive of good. In most instances these were performed unintentionally ; but the operation of Cardicentesis—tapping and aspiration of the heart—was originally deliberately proposed and performed by Dr Westbrook, of Brooklyn, in 1882 (*New York Medical Record*, December 23, 1882). His idea apparently was, that it might take the place of venesection, and that the dyspnœa due to a dilated heart, or the pulmonary engorgement of an acute pneumonia, would be more readily relieved by drawing a few drachms of blood direct from the heart, than by taking a similar number of ounces from a vein. He advised that the right auricle should be tapped, and that the proper place to perform the operation was in the third costal interspace, close to the *right* edge of the sternum. Dr J. B. Roberts of Philadelphia, the chief authority on tapping of the pericardium, in his paper on "Heart Puncture and Heart Suture," states he would "prefer to perforate the ventricle of the right heart by introducing the needle through the fourth interspace, about one and a half or two inches to the *left* of the median line of the sternum" (*Transactions of College of Physicians, Philadelphia,* 1883, vol. vi. p. 217). Two cases of cardiac aspiration are reported by Dr C. L. Dana in the *New York Medical Record* for February 1883, but only a veterinary hypodermic syringe was used, and no result followed. He is of opinion that puncture of the right ventricle is neither difficult nor dangerous, and states he has often pricked the heart in cats and dogs, with the result sometimes of stimulating, *never* of checking its action. He would never aspirate the right auricle under any circumstances, as the auricle is chiefly a regulator and reservoir, not a propelling muscle, and the unloading of it could have little effect on the work of the heart. The needle may possibly relieve over-distension, and by its irritation set the heart to work again. Dr Colwin, in the same Journal for March 1883, reports a case where the right ventricle was tapped in the belief that the patient, a victim of kidney disease, was suffering from hydro-pericardium. The post-mortem revealed no such condition, only an enlarged and dilated heart; but though an ounce of blood was withdrawn, he was of opinion that the aspiration had not injured or crippled the heart in any way. He states that he saw and performed cardiac aspiration a number of times where the patient was moribund and the heart ceased to beat, but never saw any benefit resulting from it.

Dr Evans, in the *London Clinical Society Transactions* (vol. viii. p. 169), reports a case of dilated heart, where Mr Hulke inserted a fine trocar and cannula into the fourth interspace, and about a drachm of dark blood was drawn off. Pericardial effusion was thought to exist, but the dulness was found post-mortem to be due to the distension of the heart. Still the patient, who before the operation was almost moribund, rallied after it, expressed herself as being relieved by it, and lived for nearly four weeks, which appears to prove that the right ventricle may be punctured, not only without ill effects, but with the result of relieving the severe distress produced by an over-distended heart.

A most interesting case is detailed by M. Bouchut in the *Gazette des Hôpitaux,* 1873 (vol. xlvi. p. 1130). Here there was a complication of endo-, myo-, and pericarditis, the effusion being hæmorrhagic in character. The pericardium was punctured eight times within a month, with resulting benefit each time, and the heart was twice pierced without any immediate ill-effect, though the patient, a girl aged 11½ years, died from exhaustion three days after the last tapping.

Dr H. Fischer, of Breslau, tried puncture of the heart in a

case of chloroform narcosis, but the patient died, and the post-mortem examination revealed two punctures of the coronary artery, and the pericardium was full of blood. He considers injury to the coronary artery one of the chief dangers of heart-puncture.— *Deutsche Zeitschrift für Chirurgie*, Leipsic, 1879.

Dr Roberts, in the paper already referred to, mentions the following case:—In 1872, Roger, while performing pericardicentesis on a child with pericardial effusion, thrust the needle into the right ventricle and withdrew 6¼ ozs. of pure venous blood. The boy, who was aged five years, became pale, sweated, and had an imperceptible pulse. The withdrawal of the pericardial fluid, accomplished prior to the heart injury, was beneficial; and the cardiac puncture did no permanent mischief, for the patient recovered. Death occurred five months later from long-existing dilatation and valvular disease of the heart.—*Bull. de l'Académie de Médecine*, 1875, p. 1276.

Dr Roberts, in commenting upon this case, says:—"The abstraction of blood seemed to relieve the distended heart much better than phlebotomy would have done, as was evinced by the diminution of threatening symptoms and the decrease of the area of dulness." Of all the cases recorded this most resembles mine, though further research into the literature of the subject only confirms the belief that the young lady whom I had the pleasure of showing you to-night is the only person who has undergone the operation of cardicentesis and continued to live.

If the result, clinically, has been doubtfully encouraging hitherto, that stimulating the heart in such a manner is the proper thing to do under certain circumstances is certainly borne out by experiments on animals. In Landois' *Physiology*, first edition, it is stated that in cases of asphyxia, resuscitation has been induced by compression of the heart. Böhm found that in the case of cats, poisoned with potash salts or chloroform, or asphyxiated so as to arrest respiration and the action of the heart—even for a period of forty minutes, and even when the pressure within the carotid had fallen to zero—he could restore animation by rhythmical compression of the heart, combined with artificial respiration. The compression of the heart causes a slight movement of the blood, while it acts at the same time as a rhythmical cardiac stimulus. After recovery of the respiration the reflex excitability is restored, and gradually also voluntary movements. The animals are blind for several days, the brain acts slowly, and the urine contains sugar. These experiments show how important it is in cases of asphyxia to act at the same time upon the heart. It was by the accidental observation of such an experiment on a bull-dog that Dr B. A. Watson, of Jersey City, was induced to study the possibility of arousing the heart into action, even after the entire cessation of its movements by the introduction of a needle into the organ, and his is by far the most important contribution to this subject. Experiments were made on sixty dogs which were asphyxiated with chloroform, but these are fully detailed in the *Transactions of the American Surgical Association*, vol. v. pp. 275-309. The whole series are most interesting, but it is with the conclusions we have chiefly to deal. These are—(*Firstly*), Puncture of the heart, especially the right ventricle, stimulates muscular contractions, and may be advantageously employed in the treatment of chloroform narcosis. (*Secondly*), The best results are obtained when abstraction of blood from the cavity of the ventricle is combined with the stimulating effects produced by the entrance of the aspirator needle. (*Thirdly*), Puncture of the right ventricle is a safe and more efficient operative procedure than puncture of the right auricle. His reasons for this last conclusion are two. In the first place, the wall of the right auricle is much thinner, and contains less muscular tissue than the wall of the right ventricle. The auricle is in every respect a sort of reservoir for the blood. The propelling power, to a great extent, belongs to the strong muscular walls of the ventricle. There is another reason why we should not puncture the right auricle, for as the wall of the auricle is thin, there is more danger of blood escaping. In no case of puncture of the right ventricle was there any leakage from the interior of the cavity.

By a fortunate accident my case exactly fulfilled all these conditions. Had any blood escaped into the already too full pericardium, instead of freely flowing into the aspirator bottle, death would only have been made more certain. Bleeding from any vein would have been useless, and in such a condition was not to be thought of. The action would have been too slow, valuable time would have been lost, and the very important point of direct stimulation of the heart by the introduction of the needle unavailable.

The practical question to put to ourselves is this: If cardiac tapping can be done successfully by accident, are there any cases where it should be tried as a deliberate remedy? And the answer, I think, must be in the affirmative. In all cases of asphyxia, where the heart's action has stopped, cardicentesis followed by artificial respiration seems the proper treatment. Thus, in cases of suffocation by drowning, accidental hanging, by carbonic acid, carbonic oxide, coal or sulphuretted hydrogen gases, in cases even of still-birth, some good effect might follow the introduction of the needle. It is not always possible to have an aspirator ready for such emergencies; but desperate cases require desperate remedies, and a small trocar and cannula, or the hypodermic syringe, might, if used at the proper moment, have a totally unlooked-for beneficial effect. In cases of chloroform asphyxia it is worth trying, and in some cases of heart affection, of pneumonia, and even of bronchitis, where all other means have failed, and where the patient is evidently dying of engorgement of the right side of the heart, a possible chance of saving life might be lost were cardiac aspiration not attempted. It is not my intention to argue for, or even to suggest its employment in all such cases because a lucky acci-

dent has so marvellously saved one life.   The disappointments
must be many.   I sincerely hope the next successful case will be
recorded by some one else; and that men of greater experience and
knowledge, with larger opportunities, will be encouraged to attempt
what at first may seem hopelessly to fail, but may as unexpectedly
turn out a brilliant success.

My best thanks are due to Drs Bramwell and Smith for their
timely advice and assistance, and to Dr Thin, who not only
repeatedly saw the case for me before and after the operation, but
rendered me invaluable assistance in getting up the literature of
the subject.

_____

Dr Bramwell said he could corroborate Dr Sloan's statement.
The case was a severe one of rheumatic fever with cardiac complications.   When he saw the bottle full of blood, the patient unconscious, with dilated pupils, bringing up frothy mucus, he
certainly thought that she had only a few minutes to live.   No
doubt Dr Sloan had saved her life by tapping the heart.   Whether
the heart ought to be tapped was a difficult question to answer.
He could quite conceive that in desperate cases the expedient
might be employed.   For his own part, he would hesitate to employ it, except in extreme conditions.   He had only once tapped
the heart, and in that case the result was not so fortunate.   The
patient was in Edinburgh Infirmary with ulcerative endocarditis.
The heart was much dilated, but dulness seemed to be too extensive to be accounted for by simple dilatation.   He was under the
belief that there was some pericardial effusion as well.   He determined to tap, and introduced the ordinary diagnostic syringe in
use in the ward.   Instead of entering a dilated pericardium, he
found he had punctured the heart.   He withdrew the syringe full
of blood, and then withdrew the needle.   The patient died in
about half an hour.   Dr Bruce found the pericardium distended
with black blood, and a small wound in the anterior wall of the
right ventricle.   He (Dr Bramwell) supposed that the bleeding
into the pericardium was due to the extremely relaxed and
diseased condition of the cardiac muscle.   There was extensive
ulcerative endocarditis.   That case certainly showed that the
operation was not without danger, and had made him extremely
careful.   He would certainly use the finest needle the blood
would go through.   They were obliged to Dr Sloan for the very
elaborate and exhaustive summary of all that was known of the
operation of tapping the heart in man and animals.

Dr Joseph Bell said the Society was deeply indebted to Dr Sloan
for the exceedingly dramatic and life-like manner in which he had
narrated the case.   He would just record an object-lesson he had
some time ago.   It made him determine that in similar cases he
would open the pericardium thoroughly and drain, as in case of a
surgical wound.   He was sent for to make a post-mortem on a

young man who had been accidentally stabbed with a small
knife by a friend. He opened the body carefully, and found the
pericardium distended with blood, and a small wound in the right
ventricle. The youth had run for some distance before he died.
If the surgeon had simply dilated the wound and cleared out the clot,
he would not have required to suture the wound in the heart; and
he might, by draining under antiseptic precautions, have saved the
man's life. For some time, he thought, it would not be common
to tap the heart intentionally. He had been vainly trying to
remember where Dr John Struthers had published a paper in
which he recommended opening the internal jugular vein for
the purpose of relieving the right auricle in cases of drowning or
chloroform asphyxia.

Dr Taylor said that he would not occupy the time of the Society
by further complimenting Dr Slóan on this classical paper, but he
could not help being struck by the discrepancy in the views expressed by Dr Bell and Dr Bramwell. The lesson Dr Bell had
learned from the case was to open the pericardium freely, so as to
avoid the risk of a clot forming within it by blood oozing from the
puncture in the wall of the heart; whilst Dr Bramwell said that
in dealing with a similar case he would only use a fine needle.
Now this would appear to be the very way to get blood to escape
into the pericardium, and so form a clot within it which would
effectually stop the heart's action. He was of opinion that the
success of Dr Sloan's case was probably due to the aspirator withdrawing 10 oz. of blood from the heart. The patient would be
practically pulseless, and the heart being thus at rest, the internal
wound would have an opportunity of closing, the pressure within
being so much reduced that the contraction of the distended walls
of the heart, when so relieved of pressure, would be sufficient practically to close the opening as soon as the needle of the aspirator
was withdrawn.

Dr Affleck congratulated Dr Sloan on his extremely interesting
paper. The case was eminently worthy of being placed on record.
When he saw the patient in the sideroom he thought of the words
put by Shakespeare into the mouth of Lucentio: " Till I found it
to be true, I never thought it possible or likely; but see." Aspiration was the feature in this case, as also was the considerable
quantity of blood withdrawn. It could not be done except in rare
circumstances,—*e.g.*, immediate presence of the physician, also fluid
state of contents of ventricle. He remembered a case of Mr
Hulke's, of the Middlesex Hospital, in which the patient was much
relieved by the withdrawal of a drachm of blood. A drachm or two
might make all the difference, and save life. Dr Sloan's case
illustrated the difficulty of determining whether we had to do
with a dilated heart or pericardial effusion. Pure blood was withdrawn, so that in this case there was probably no fluid in the pericardium. Heart puncture would not be so suitable for asphyxia,

in which it was the respiration and not the heart that was at fault. He again complimented Dr Sloan on his careful clinical work.

Dr William Russell said he was sure they were all agreed as to the literary and dramatic ability of Dr Sloan's communication. It recalled a discussion that took place in the Society ten years ago on tapping the pericardium, when this difficulty in diagnosis between dilated right heart and pericarditis with effusion was treated of. Dr Sloan's case was apparently mainly a distended heart. In the previous discussion he (Dr Russell) referred to a case in which he made a like mistake, and which he supposed practically every physician had made. He aspirated under the belief that it was a distended pericardium, with the result that he punctured the ventricle. The mark of the needle was distinctly visible on post-mortem examination. Dr Sloan's communication might, to a certain extent, stimulate interference in the direction he had indicated, but even two such cases as Dr Bramwell's and Dr Bell's would make the physician hesitate. There were other considerations. When the heart was in a condition to justify such procedure there was almost always a fibrinous clot extending into the pulmonary artery, in which case tapping the right ventricle would do no good. Dr Sloan's case, however, did hold out encouragement that in certain special cases the physician might adopt this procedure. Yet the instances in which it would be calmly and deliberately recommended must remain rare and exceptional.

Dr Stockman said he agreed very strongly with what Dr Taylor had said as to the aspiration relieving the condition. The right ventricle, when full, normally contained only about 4 oz. In the present case 10 oz. were withdrawn. Puncture disabled the heart rather than stimulated it. Experiments on animals had shown that puncture of the heart produced an arythmic condition which tended to stop the heart. The practice had been the cause of death in cases in America.

Dr Clouston congratulated Dr Sloan. He recalled the case of a lady patient in Morningside Asylum, who transfixed the apex of her heart with a long steel pin, pushing it in almost to its head, with the effect of arresting the rythmical action, and producing apparent death. Dr Joseph Brown discovering the cause, withdrew the pin, and she was none the worse an hour afterwards.

Dr Sloan, in reply, said that whether puncture of the heart would cause bleeding into pericardium would depend on whether or not a cardiac vein were injured in the process. The heart muscle might close the opening. He was still of opinion that his case was one of pericardial effusion, the history being against so rapid and marked a dilatation, and the dulness not disappearing immediately after the operation,—in fact, not till eight days afterwards. He thought the ventricular muscle completely contracted, and on withdrawing the cannula he kept it close against the heart wall. His case was not the only one that lived after the operation. Some other bad cases lived for five weeks, and even longer. That the operation was not in itself fatal had been amply proved.

***

Meeting III.—December 19, 1894.

Dr CLOUSTON, *President, in the Chair.*

I. EXHIBITION OF PATIENTS.

1. *Mr Cathcart* showed two patients illustrating ULCERATIVE FORMS OF SECONDARY SYPHILIS, and remarked that although Jonathan Hutchinson had shown that rupia was not generally a tertiary symptom, the old view was not overthrown, and it might be important medico-legally to ascertain at what periods ulcerative processes might occur. The first case was that of a lad who acquired syphilis in July, and came with a well-developed sore on September 6th, and, although ordered to take mercury, appeared again on November 1st with the most typical rupial eruption Mr Cathcart had ever seen. A cast had been made of it, and was shown. He had been treated in the Lock wards with mercury. The crusts had been poulticed off, and red lotion applied. The sores were healing, although the legs still presented deep ulceration. In this case the hard sore had left no scar. Mr Cathcart was of opinion that in most cases the ordinary hard sore did not leave a scar, although the soft sore did. The second case was that of a young man whose history was not so definite, as he had been exposed to contagion on several occasions. The throat was deeply ulcerated, although the disease seemed only of about three months' standing. In the first case, absence of history of alcoholism or any indication of specially weak constitution confirmed Hutchinson's view that there was predisposition towards syphilis in some cases. Many bad cases, however, were associated with alcoholism.

2. *Dr John Thomson* showed a case of CONGENITAL DEFECT OF THORAX, the left pectorals, major and minor, being absent, and left forearm and hand badly developed.

3. *Dr Allan Jamieson* showed a case of MOLLUSCUM CONTAGIOSUM in a rather anæmic girl, aged 16. No history of communication was obtained. On the left side of the neck were several mollusca the size of a lentil, and a patch behind the ear where the tumours had become aggregated into a patch, somewhat thickened and scaly. At the back of the knee there were two mollusca the size of half a pea, and a nodule twice that size, which she stated had been originally a wart of old standing, but had taken on the molluscous type. The case was interesting from the resemblance to some instances

of Darier's disease. Improvement had already shown itself since the application of boric starch poultices for five days. In reply to Mr Cathcart, he stated that the special features of the diagnosis were—the presence of a conical tumour with a depression on the summit, sometimes pink, oftener of a waxy tint, somewhat like that of a misletoe berry. The period of incubation had been recently ascertained to be from six weeks to two months. Only a few successful inoculations had been accomplished. He believed Dr Paterson of Leith had been the first to inoculate successfully, although the case had not been published. In answer to Dr Littlejohn, he stated that there was no constitutional disturbance.

II. EXHIBITION OF SPECIMENS.

1. *Dr James Ritchie* showed a specimen of CARCINOMA OF THE SPLENIC FLEXURE OF THE COLON.

2. *Dr Bruce* showed a specimen of ANEURISM PERFORATING THE SUPERIOR VENA CAVA.

III. EXHIBITION OF INSTRUMENT.

Mr Cathcart showed a MILK STERILIZER, so constructed as to fit into the size of pot most used by the working-classes, the aperture being plugged with cotton wool. The milk having been boiled, could be drawn off as required through an india-rubber tube below. The advantages claimed were efficiency, ease of working, and small cost.

IV. ORIGINAL COMMUNICATIONS.

1. TWO CASES OF RAYNAUD'S DISEASE OCCURRING IN JAMES MURRAY'S ROYAL ASYLUM, PERTH.

By ALEXANDER REID URQUHART, M.D., F.R.C.P. Ed.

CASE I.—I first saw this patient in consultation with Dr Steele Moon, of Dundee, in November 1893. He was then reported to be childish in manner, usually absolutely taciturn, although cheerful and talkative at times; patellar reflex absent; loss of control of bladder and rectum; walking and standing steadily; occasionally sliding off his chair on to the floor with a thump, and remaining stiff; eyes sometimes open, sometimes closed; no spasm.

I found him in bed, his limbs twitching, and his head thrown back; pulse regular and rather slow; pupils normal. No tender spots on spine. Absolutely taciturn. No ankle clonus. Knee jerk only on *first* trial. Cremasteric reflex normal. Hands clasped on pubes as he lay stretched out. Slightly resistive. Feet very cold, but carefully placed by himself on a hot-water bottle. When got up for further examination, he suddenly and actively popped into bed. No apparent paralysis; no diminution of virile power.

As his wife was a skilled nurse, and able to give him undivided attention, arrangements were made for home treatment; but in a week or two he had become so self-willed, petulant, dirty, and unreasonable, that he was admitted to Murray's Asylum on 24th November 1893.

The following history was then elicited:—Family suffered from rheumatism. Father died from abscess of the brain after an accident. Mother suffered from sciatica. Only sister rheumatic.

The patient had been a medical student, but left the university and enlisted. At that time he was unsettled and intemperate, but having got into the Army Medical Corps, and become an hospital attendant, he was regarded as a reformed character, and was certainly a favourite with the medical officers. His temperament was flighty, always nervous, and easily worried. Seven years before admission he had yellow fever in the West Indies; and in August 1892 suffered from a severe attack of diarrhœa, with hæmatemesis and bloody stools. This severe illness lasted for two months, and left him much enfeebled. In fact, his case appeared hopeless; he became mentally confused, made mistakes with medicines, and complained to his wife that he was unable for work. He often slept in the daytime, and twitched in his sleep. Headaches occurred frequently.

Seven weeks before admission there was a similar, but less urgent, attack of bloody vomit and bloody stools. This was followed by sleeplessness, diarrhœa, want of appetite, and falling off in flesh. His mental habit changed, he became obstinate, resistive, and depressed, and had varying hypochondriacal delusions —that he could not straighten his legs, that he had no feet, that he had no stomach. The delusions were concentrated on his viscera, and after treatment in hospital he was finally discharged from the service.

On admission he was found to be very slightly built and poorly nourished. Height, 5 ft. 9 in.; weight, 9 st. 3 lb. in his clothes age 33. He was anæmic and sallow, with scanty hair and pressure marks over lumbar spine and trochanters. Heart-sounds loud, but not clearly defined at the apex. Breath offensive; bowels constipated. Urine could not be collected owing to his habits. He was either restless or in a stiff attitude. Reflexes normal. Pupils equal, semi-dilated, sluggish.

For the most part he was entirely silent, but was occasionally heard to remark on the number of stones in the building. These symptoms were accompanied by some excitement and evident delusions. At times he was actively resistive, at other times passively resistive. He had a habit of crawling on the floor, squeezing into corners or underneath furniture, and when thus placed lay stark and still. At other times he walked about with a firm step and normal stride. He persistently wet the floor, and required constant attention. He would *not* use closet or chamber.

If not walking or lying as described, he would be found looking out of window, standing on the window seat, or, if possible, on the sill, apparently under the influence of some delusion. In December he picked a sore on the back of his head, which soon healed under appropriate treatment. He also developed hæmatoma auris in both ears.

Jan. 29.—Abstinent, and paler than usual. Evidently much run down. Throwing himself flat on the floor.

Jan. 30.—Bruised side and fractured rib.

Jan. 31.—Bladder enormously distended, urine drawn off by catheter. Right foot swollen, cold, of a dark, earthy colour, especially along the outer side. Left foot desquamated, abraded patch the size of half-a-crown on dorsum. Feet intensely painful. For the first time I heard him speak rationally and emphatically —"For God's sake, don't touch it." Feet soon became hot when wrapped in cotton wool, and the discoloration extended above the ankle. Notwithstanding his prostrate condition he removed the bandages and his night-shirt. No hebetude observed, but rather the reverse.

Feb. 1.—Urine drawn off morning and evening. Right foot warm, and no extension of discoloration. Left foot apparently improved, but dusky purple character of both pronounced. Dressings undisturbed. Temperature normal; pulse 100. Spoke quietly to his sister, saying that he was now comfortable, and wished for nothing except to see his father, who had died many years previously.

Feb. 2.—Features shrunken; skin inelastic. Urine drawn off. Right foot colder; no extension of discoloration, but cessation of pulsation in posterior tibial artery. Left great toe purple. Temperature normal; pulse 80. Respiration became embarrassed in the course of the day. At 4 P.M. a distinct purple line was seen on the front of the tibia, and a dark purple patch over the right patella. No appreciable pulsation at wrists. Death at 6 P.M.

Post-mortem Examination thirty-six hours after death. Body emaciated; subcutaneous fat almost entirely absent. Rigor mortis well marked in lower extremities. Considerable post-mortem discoloration of trunk. Purple colour over the whole of the three outer toes, and external malleolus of right foot. On the dorsal aspect of the third and fifth toes there was a small area, of the size of a threepenny piece, of extremely dark purple colour, within the area of discoloration previously mentioned. On the dorsum of the left foot there was an area about $3\frac{1}{2} \times 1\frac{1}{2}$ inches where the skin was abraded, leaving a dry ecchymosed surface. On the great toe of the same foot there was a purple area of the size of a shilling at the extremity of the plantar aspect. Hæmatoma of both ears; most marked in the right.

Lungs.—Right congested, with several hard masses, and a cavity the size of a bean, containing thick purulent fluid, and several nodules of caseation, varying in size from a pea to a rice grain. *Left* slightly congested, with similar nodules, but fewer in number. A large cavity existed in the upper lobe, containing broken-down caseous material. (No symptoms of this were manifested during life, and adequate physical examination was not possible at any time, owing to the extremely resistive state of the patient.)

Heart contained post-mortem clot, but no lesion of valves. Walls of left ventricle considerably hypertrophied.

Ribs fractured, small and brittle; one where bruised and noted during life, another old with false joint.

Liver (61 oz.) pale and friable. No sign of syphilis.

Spleen (5 oz.) small, soft, flabby; surface wrinkled.

Kidneys.—*Right* (8 oz.) considerably enlarged, but otherwise normal. *Left* (4 oz.) reduced in size; whole interior occupied by a mass of thick, semi-solid, tubercular matter.

Brain small, atrophied; arachnoid cloudy and opaque; convolutions wasted; some congestion of grey matter. Ventricles contained much fluid, and enlarged.

The following parts were sent to Dr Leith, Pathologist to the Edinburgh Royal Infirmary :—1. Medulla, with part of cord. 2. Anterior tibial nerve, with artery and vein (part of). 3. Posterior tibial nerve (part of). 4. Left kidney. 5. Piece of liver. 6. Three toes. 7. Ear.

Dr Leith reports as follows :—

1. *Liver.*—(1.) N.E.: Fairly normal; (2.) M.A.: Normal, no tubercle.

2. *Left Kidney.*—(1.) N.E.: Smaller than normal, about 4 oz. in weight. On section it showed an advanced condition of chronic tuberculosis. There was very little true renal substance.

3. *The Three Outer Toes of Left Foot.*—They were all discoloured, of a purplish colour, and the skin was raised in blebs from the subjacent tissue. On section it was seen that there was blood everywhere between the skin and the bone, most deeply marked just below the skin. This was seen throughout the length of the toe. M.A.: The bloodvessels, especially the veins and capillaries of the subcutaneous tissues, are all seen to be greatly engorged, some of them forming large sinuses. This is most marked in some places just below the skin, in others nearly to the bones. There is not much diapedesis, the appearance of hæmorrhage to the naked eye being brought about by the great engorgement of the vessels everywhere with blood. The structure of the vessels seems everywhere normal, and also of the nerves. There is no sign of any peripheral neuritis or any vascular lesion such as an endarteritis obliterans; and if a general vascular spasm was present during life, it had not persisted, as it must have been followed by great dilatation of both veins and capillaries. The other structures of the digit, skin, fibrous tissues, and bone seem

nearly normal, showing a certain amount of degeneration and necrosis. The bone marrow appears also to show dilated blood-channels and a certain amount of hæmorrhage by diapedesis.

4. *Anterior and Posterior Tibial Nerves.*—N.E. : Only small parts of these were actually sent, as in dissecting them out the vessels had been preserved, but only a small part of the nerves. M.A.: These were examined by Weigert's and other methods, but I have failed to discover any neuritis or degeneration. Both arteries also seem healthy.

5. *Medulla and Pons.*—The condition of preservation of the tissue precluded any examination of the cells, but sections of both medulla and pons were made, to test for degenerations. They were stained by Pal's modification of Weigert's method. So far as I can detect, there is neither sign of degeneration nor neuritis.

6. *Ear.*—Showed a typical hæmatoma auris, viz., a large blood-clot between the cartilage and its perichondrium.

Remarks.—The microscopic appearances do not quite accord with those of an ordinary gangrene. There is practically none of the intertissue hæmorrhage which is seen in such cases. The condition could be accounted for by a vasomotor paralysis; but from the length of time elapsing after its onset we would naturally have expected a considerable amount of diapedesis. If the cause of the lesion were a nervous one, it would be either peripheral or central, but none can be seen. This does not, however, preclude its existence, as a large number of serial sections of the digits have not been made, owing to exceptional difficulties in manipulating the sections. The examination already undertaken precludes the existence of a central (unless it be a cellular) lesion. There was nothing in the sections to preclude a vasomotor spasm of the arteries, or indeed of all the vessels at one time. If this did exist, it was followed, before death, by a paralysis resulting in a dilatation of the veins and capillaries. It is to be remembered that this condition of the vessels is quite consistent with Raynaud's disease, in the later stages of which the spasm may pass away from the veins and capillaries.

CASE II.—I saw this patient in consultation with Dr J. W. Miller, of Dundee. She was then—in February 1892—recovering from an attack of influenza, and labouring under melancholia, excited and delusional, dreading impending ruin, and oppressed by ideas of unworthiness. She was placed in private care with a skilled nurse, but the symptoms increased in severity, rapidly and markedly. Delusions that her life was endangered, that she was to be vivisected, caused her to be so noisy and violent that she was admitted to Murray's Asylum in the same month.

The following is the history of the case:—Father and mother both dead. One sister had puerperal mania; another sister was said to have committed suicide.

The patient was active and clever, a bright and cheerful mother of a large family. Age on admission, 50. She had been particularly healthy, except that she had suffered, when travelling, once from jaundice and once from weakness of the eyes. Mental worry over-taxed her strength in 1891, after an exceptionally happy, useful life. Influenza supervened, and left her enfeebled and depressed.

On admission she appeared prematurely aged and poorly nourished. Heart-sounds normal; pulse 92 per minute under emotional influences. Breath offensive ; bowels constipated. Urine contained abundant lithates. Motor excitability marked. Pupils normal.

From February 1892 till the present time her mental troubles continued marked by the same characteristics,—a noisy, delusional melancholia with suicidal impulses. Change of air and scene was tried in the end of 1892, but without benefit. She has been abstinent and extremely resistive. The delusions are recurrent, if not persistent. There is no apparent dementia. She reads the news-papers furtively, and is aware of all the circumstances of her environment,—so that while her condition remains very un-promising, she cannot be pronounced incurable.

I must not detain the Society with an account of all the variations observed, but will rapidly refer to the symptoms bearing upon the questions immediately at issue.

As in the first-mentioned case, the urine has been retained from time to time, and we have also noticed occasional albuminuria. If the ankles are swollen it sometimes happens that a trace of albumen is discoverable. But we have seen no blood, no casts, and no hæmaturia.

1892, *March* 29.—Left hæmatoma auris, and, within a few days thereafter, œdema of dependent parts of the face and left hand. Heart weaker. Digitaline prescribed.

May 2.—A slight fissure on the right heel.

June 12.—Swelling of left ear and left side of face.

June 19.—Hæmatoma enlarging; face swollen round the right eye.

June 29.—Œdema pedum.

1893, *Jan.* 24.—Re-admitted after six months in private care. Circulation enfeebled. Puffy condition of face. Albumen in urine—a slight trace, which disappeared within a week.

In the summer following there was considerable improvement, mental and physical. Self-control was greater. Œdema pedum was noted once.

1894, *Jan.*—Concurrently with the first described case, similar symptoms were noted in Case No. II. The average temperature was 41·5 maximum and 32·4 minimum during the week before invasion; 40·7 and 30·5 during the week of invasion; and 39·8 and 28·4 during the height of the malady, as recorded on the screen in the Asylum grounds. However, the recurrence of symptoms in the second case in summer-time must be kept in mind. No doubt both patients suffered from " dead fingers ; " and the second case has been observed to be so sensitive to cold after a bath that ablutions have been restricted to tepid sponging.[1]

Jan. 25.—Both feet swollen, and toes blue.

Jan. 29.—Brown patches on toes, as if blisters were threatening.

Feb. 3.—Fresh patches of brown colour appearing.

Feb. 9.—Left foot, faint purple line between first and second toes. Brown patches on dorsum of second toe, large purple patch on plantar aspect of the same toe. Right foot, purple patches on nail and on dorsum of three smaller toes. Roughness of skin of both ankles.

Feb. 15.—Both feet appear "dead."

Feb. 21.—Cutis anserina general and persistent.

Feb. 24.—Spots and areas of discoloration fading.

March 1.—Skin peeling from all the spots, leaving healthy epidermis and no cicatricial marks.

March 8.—No longer confined to bed.

April 22.—Recurrence of œdema pedum, dark purple patches, and unhealthy blisters on heels.

May 11.—Perfect recovery from these symptoms.

May 21.—Purple spots on toes, with œdema pedum.

May 26.—Tendency towards resolution.

June 2.—Toes of a livid colour in the morning, but in the afternoon this had worn off.

Since this date there has been no return of the congestive symptoms, but the appearance of "dead fingers" has been noted.

The treatment adopted was of the routine character—rest, warmth, and gentle friction. The lower limbs were encased in soft lambs'-wool stockings, and special attention was given to proper exercise. Digitaline, lime juice, and stimulants were prescribed, with apparent benefit.

The reported cases of Raynaud's disease are not numerous. These are the only examples which have come under my observation during twenty-one years spent in hospitals for the insane. I have been induced to report them in minute detail, for the study of tropho-neuroses is pregnant with meaning. They testify to the extraordinary ability and acumen which Raynaud brought to bear upon the difficult research he was induced to enter upon.

We have to deal with a malady, to the best of my belief, arising from central lesions. In Case I. we noted a family history of rheumatism, with malarial infection, hæmatemesis, and hæmatoma auris, at no distant date prior to the period of invasion. In Case II. there was an hereditary predisposition to insanity, with great motor excitability, marked trophic changes, and hæmatoma auris. Although these patients presented symptoms of very different

---

[1] It is possible that a morbid dread of water, owing to a delusion of imminent hydrophobia, may have aggravated her condition through emotional influences.

gravity, they suffered in common from symmetrical gangrene, and they may be correlated with cases of general paralysis where intractable bedsores occur in similar symmetrical disposition. Brown-Séquard produced hæmorrhage into the auricle in guinea-pigs by section and irritation of the restiform body in the medulla; and, without laying too much stress on vasomotor influences, or failing to recognise the importance of Dr Goodall's recent researches on othæmatoma (finding staphylococci),[1] it seems to me that the local changes cannot be explained by mechanical obstruction of the vessels or the occurrence of peripheral neuritis. I did not expect that Dr Leith would find arteritis or neuritis in the specimens submitted, believing that the rapid development of the symptoms would negative marked changes in these structures. It is undoubted that neuritis was recorded in the cases reported by Dr Wiglesworth and Dr Affleck, but these were protracted in duration, and the sections were made in the foci of the disease.

I cannot but endorse Raynaud's opinion, that the malady is really "a neurosis characterized by enormous exaggeration of the central grey parts which control the vasomotor innervation." The "dead fingers" of both these cases, and the evident susceptibility to cold in the last recorded, points to a condition of vascular spasm. I regret that it was impossible to obtain ophthalmoscopic information regarding both of these patients, and that electricity as a means of treatment proved unsuitable. We are grievously hampered in diagnosis and treatment by the mental obscuration and other complications in asylum patients. Our reports are necessarily fragmentary, and with those of us who live remote from libraries and specialists these difficulties are still more increased. I feel the need of an apology in describing these cases with omissions that are serious in proportion to the importance of the minute investigation demanded, but at the same time must express my obligations to those who have kept the records and made the observations now digested,—specially to Dr Hay and to Dr Moffat for their untiring attention. The careful noting of the early symptoms in Case II. could only have been possible by a properly trained and observant nurse. Prompt and suitable treatment was thus secured, and resulted, in all probability, in the preservation of a valuable life. We shall continue in the hope that, desperate though the case may be, it will yet prove possible to record a recovery.

Note.—The cases of Raynaud's disease reported as having occurred amongst the insane include several by Dr Southey, one by Dr Wiglesworth, one by Dr Macpherson, and one by Dr Raw. Others have been referred to by Dr Shaw. The late Dr J. E. Morgan collected and analysed ninety-three cases (*vide The Lancet*, 6th July, 1889, *et seq.*), and several have been published since his paper was completed.

[1] *Journal of Mental Science*, October 1894.

Dr Joseph Bell said he had come with the hope of being instructed, and he was satisfied with the clinical account of two excellent cases; but he was no wiser than before as to what, from his point of view, was a most important question, viz., What was to guide the surgeon in considering whether he would take off or leave on a leg or foot in these conditions? He might possibly have been asked to see one of these cases, and he should have felt his own ignorance as to whether to amputate the foot or not. If he had amputated the first foot before the second began, he would have been right. No one could have prophesied that the second foot would have begun so soon. In many cases amputation might be performed with good result; others got better without amputation. He had at present one old lady, a dement, with the toes of both feet affected. She was treated with masterly inactivity. If the affection had been confined to one foot, he would have been strongly tempted to do something for it. He hoped his pathological friends would give some indication as to what was to guide him in considering the question of amputation.

Mr Cathcart did not think it possible to exclude vascular obstruction in the first case, simply because the tibial arteries were not affected. He had often examined legs showing gangrene low down in the foot, and the seat of obstruction at the bifurcation of the popliteal artery. He was not prepared to say that this was a case of arterial obstruction. It was still a moot point; but Dr Bruce had described a case where Raynaud's disease was accompanied with thickening of the coats of the arteries.

Dr Bruce said he had had one case in which toes had to be amputated for necrosis preceded by a cold condition. He supposed that was the case to which Mr Cathcart referred, although it had never been published. In more than one toe there was distinct flattening and closure of the artery. The opposed surfaces of the intima had united, so as to produce a longitudinal cicatrix where the lumen should have been. He quite agreed with Dr Urquhart that the appearance of neuritis in neighbouring nerves might in chronic cases be the result and not the cause of the disease.

Mr Alexis Thomson said he had had an opportunity of examining the posterior tibial nerve in a case in which Mr Duncan had performed Syme's amputation. He did not think the neuritis could be secondary; he did not say it was primary. He had also examined a case of Dr Watson's in which the finger was affected, and which showed very little evidence of neuritis. It was evidently not a constant change, and therefore could not be regarded as the essence of the disease. He quite agreed with Mr Cathcart. In cases of senile gangrene one often found obstruction at the bifurcation, but in most of these cases there was also thrombosis in the vessels below. As to surgical treatment, it was not on a level with senile gangrene. Masterly inactivity was the line of treatment. One was dealing with a condition where there was hope of recovery. If one amputated at all it was after recovery had taken place, and in order to rid the patient of dead tissue.

Dr Sloan said that the case referred to by Mr Alexis Thomson was one of Dr Affleck's. The patient came to consult him (Dr Sloan) complaining of coldness and pallor of the radial side of the fingers, so that the disease was seen at the earliest possible stage. She was sent to Ward 30, and developed the appearance of gangrene of both arms. The treatment simply consisted in wrapping the part in wadding, and she recovered, so that for some months she was able to assist in the work of the ward. She afterwards developed valvular disease of the heart, from which she died. The case had been published by Dr Affleck in the *British Medical Journal.*

Dr Clouston said he had only seen Raynaud's disease in connexion with cases of acute mental affections, and could not speak of its occurrence otherwise. The cases associated with mental disease seemed to divide themselves into two classes,—those of acute mania, an intensely delirious condition, resulting from over-action of the mental part of the cortex to an extreme degree. That could not occur without motor, sensory, and trophic symptoms. The wonder to him was that we had not more trophic symptoms in acute delirious cases. He recalled a case of this character that presented no evidence of neuritis or of such tissue degeneration as usually accompanied hæmatoma auris, but seemed to be a case of intense over-action of the brain cortex, that appeared, from causes that we could not explain, to have specially localized itself in certain twigs of the peripheral nerves. Why it should have done so it was impossible to say. In some cases of insanity there was the greatest possible difficulty in keeping the periphery warm. All kinds of special measures had to be adopted to prevent the lowering of the system which occurred with cold extremities. He had been struck with the procedure of one of the Hospital nurses at Morningside. When she had an excited case to deal with, she took a sheet of cotton wadding, and having made a hole for the head, brought it down over chest and abdomen, and put over all a strong linen dress quilted with flannel and laced behind. Usually in very bad cases she wrapped the limb in wadding, retaining it in position with a surgical bandage. The temperature of the room might be kept up to 60° or 70°, but even then there was an extreme tendency to neurotic coldness, which could, however, be thus counteracted to some extent. He looked on this as being essentially of the same nature as Raynaud's disease. Dr Urquhart's case was more chronic, not an acute delirious mania of a week or two, but with a history of months, and in which we had practically the beginning of the death of the brain cortex as regards its function. He had been much struck with the occurrence of hæmatoma auris in these two cases. In this condition there was actual tissue degeneration of cartilage and of small vessels round it, which he hoped Dr W. F. Robertson would soon be able to demonstrate to the Society. This degeneration evidently occurred from central nervous causes. In fact, we met with all kinds of trophic symptoms from the cortex, and why should we not have localized gangrene as well as hæmatomata and other such lesions? But he had no theory as to why they should be so extremely localized in certain nerve twigs. He did not think Raynaud's disease was allied to ordinary senile gangrene,—the one was central, the other peripheral. In his opinion, masterly inactivity would be the treatment for every case of the former. Amputation would be unjustifiable except in the extreme stage.

Dr Urquhart, in reply, said he was much obliged for the kind way in which his paper had been received. Perhaps Dr Leith, if he had been present, might have suggested that this was not Raynaud's disease. He himself had labelled the cases Raynaud's disease for pigeon-holing purposes. As regards hæmatoma cases and general paralytics with proneness to the symmetrical bedsores that plagued them so much in asylums, he had one case lately where the sores could be counted by the dozen, and were scattered all over the man's body. He would have been disappointed if there had been peripheral neuritis or arteritis in the cases now reported. Dr Weiss seemed to stand alone in claiming it to be a peripheral trouble. In conclusion, Dr Urquhart remarked that he would have expected Mr Bell to inform him whether amputation would be required. He thought the tendency was to recovery, and that they should wait in that expectation.

2. CARCINOMA OF THE SPLENIC FLEXURE OF COLON.

By JAMES RITCHIE, M.D., M.R.C.P. Eng., F.R.C.P. Ed., etc.

THE diagnosis of the exact condition present in chronic obstruction of the bowels is often extremely difficult; it is therefore of advantage that cases exhibiting exceptional symptoms should be recorded. As the following case presented several points of interest, Dr James Ritchie ventured to bring it before the Society.

On the evening of the 18th September he was summoned to see a clergyman who had that day come from London. He stated that he had been travelling in Switzerland, that a week before the date of his return he had been seized with diarrhœa, but that prior to the attack he had been in good health. A dose of castor-oil procured at a chemist's gave temporary relief, but he had quickly relapsed, and now he had not only diarrhœa, but could not retain any food, nor even water.

He was aged 62, short, stout, well nourished, hair iron-grey, face florid, temperature normal. The tongue thickly coated, troublesome flatulence, the abdomen somewhat distended. Pulse 110, rather feeble; the left side of heart dilated and thin walled, the second sound accentuated at apex, but no murmurs. The lungs were normal. The urine high coloured; no albumen. Once overnight there was a small quantity of coffee ground matter in the vomit. A sinapism, hourly drop doses of ipecacuanha wine, bismuth, and small quantities of whey were ordered; the sickness and diarrhœa stopped, the tongue became clean, the appetite returned, and at the end of the week the patient felt so well that he was anxious to return to his ministerial work in Forfarshire, and was with difficulty restrained from indiscretions both in the matter of diet and of going out of doors. At the commencement of the following week he caught a slight cold. On Tuesday he reported that there had been a good motion, but a few days later he had recurrence of gastro-intestinal catarrh with sickness, and now the bowels became constipated. The temperature was normal. Improvement again took place, and on the morning of Saturday the 29th he seemed to be progressing favourably, but on the evening of that day Dr Church, who had seen him in the morning for Dr Ritchie, was hastily summoned because of somewhat copious hæmatemesis; the temperature was for the first time above normal, being 101°, and the pulse 120. The following day Dr Geo. A. Gibson saw the patient in consultation. No cause for the hæmatemesis could be discovered, but as there appeared to be decomposition of the contents of the bowel, and septic absorption, salol was prescribed, and the following morning efforts were made to empty the bowels. These were not effectual. The abdomen was much distended. The condition was now viewed as one of gravity. Careful examination was again made and the whole position reconsidered with care. In the absence of any history of previous illness, the absence of any evidence of organic disease, the having travelled abroad, the recent catarrhal attacks, the temperature now varying from 99° to 101°, the existence of flatulence, the general distension of the abdomen, the urine being high coloured and loaded with urates, on a very spare diet yielding 495 grains urea in twenty-four hours, it was concluded that there was a septic condition of the bowels causing paresis of the intestinal walls, and that this sepsis was probably due to insanitary conditions abroad. A dose of calomel was given, followed by castor-oil, then enema, but no action of the bowels followed. During the succeeding days sulpho-carbolate of soda was given, also morphine and atropine, and on Thursday the 4th October and the following day there were several copious pultaceous motions with small solid portions intermingled. The abdomen became for the time quite flaccid; and as the general condition was improved, with clean tongue and fair appetite, pulse about 80, a more hopeful view was taken. Very soon, however, the epigastrium became prominent because of the distension of some viscus with flatus. The hope that the bowels might now be more regular was disappointed, and after a few days there was sickness at intervals, generally only mucus, but at times all the food which had been taken during many hours came up. Flatulence passed both upwards and downwards, and although not very troublesome it was frequent.

On examination of the abdomen it was found that there was still a considerable amount of fat in the abdominal wall. There was now the suspicion of a small floating movable nodule about the level of and to the left of the umbilicus. Percussion over the prominent epigastrium showed that some viscus was greatly distended with air, and by succussion it was evident that it contained not only air but a considerable quantity of fluid. After consultation with Sir Thomas Grainger Stewart, it was agreed that the physical signs and symptoms warranted the washing out of the stomach. While this was being done, only a little mucus and watery fluid passed out of that organ, and the solution of Condy returned unchanged; it was therefore at once evident that either the stomach was sacculated, or else that it was not the viscus which was dilated. The withdrawal of the stomach-tube produced strong retching, and as only a very small quantity of clear fluid was ejected, it was concluded that there was no sacculation of the stomach, and that the dilatation must be in some part of the intestine. Careful inspection of the abdomen now revealed peristaltic movements of the bowels; these were not very marked, because of the thickness of the abdominal parietes, but they could be faintly seen, and if absent, could be induced by tapping the surface. These symptoms made it tolerably certain that we had to do with obstruction of the bowel, and the suspicious little mass above referred to rendered it probable that the cause was malignant. But where was its seat? Early in the history of the case the rectum had been examined with negative results as far as tumour, hardness, or tenderness were concerned; it was again explored, but the only suspicious condition was a well-marked ballooning of it. Fully three pints of water had on more than one occasion been injected per anum; it seemed probable, therefore, that the obstruction was not in the sigmoid flexure.

The first sound of the heart had been somewhat feeble from the first,—at least there was evidence of a thin-walled heart,—but the pulse had been moderately good; it was easily made faster, but soon returned to its usual rate; now the pulse-rate began to go up a little, it was therefore deemed necessary to give digitalis and nux vomica.

After October 5th there was no satisfactory motion of the bowels; only a small quantity of fæcal matter coloured the water given by enema. Up to the 23rd flatus passed downwards freely, but after that date nothing, unless it were a very small quantity of fæcal matter, just sufficient to stain an enema. Hitherto the general condition had been fairly good; the most troublesome symptom had been eructations of wind; thirst was also sometimes considerable. After that date the tongue became dry and brownish; the pulse gradually, although slowly, increased in frequency. As there was rather less fat in the abdominal parietes, peristalsis was better seen, and the small floating mass to the left of the umbilicus was more evident, but no other tumour could be felt. The question of operation was considered, and on the morning of the 27th, as the examining finger was stained with fæcal matter, Mr Chiene advised that a copious enema be again tried; if this failed, he would operate on the following morning. As the day advanced the patient became suddenly worse from heart failure, and died on the following afternoon.

The post-mortem examination and report was made by Dr Purves Stewart. He found a flattish mass about the size of a dried fig in the great omentum to the left of the middle line. The ascending and transverse colon was much distended. At the splenic flexure there was a hard mass (columnar epithelioma) which completely encircled the gut, and caused great narrowing of its lumen. The descending colon and sigmoid flexure were collapsed and empty. The tumour of the splenic flexure was adherent to the spleen and to the stomach. The stomach was markedly congested at this part, but showed no signs of tumour infiltration.

In this case the hæmorrhage, which occurred twice, once to a large amount, was doubtless due to the rupture of a small vessel in the congested area close to the splenic flexure of the colon. In nearly every case of cancer of the bowels there is peritonitis at the seat of the disease, leading to adhesions to adjacent organs.

Primary cancer of the intestine is most common at orifices and angles; in this case it was an angle—the splenic flexure—but one of the less frequent seats.

Von Ziemssen states that of all deaths from cancer in the Allgemeine Krankenhaus, Vienna, 3·76 were in the intestines; in the rectum and sigmoid flexure, 3 per cent.; and in the intestine, 0·76 per cent.

There is a difference amongst authorities as to the kind of cancer which is most common. Some say scirrhus, but the majority place columnar epithelioma first in the order of frequency. This case seemed to be one of columnar epithelioma with scirrhus change secondarily.

In this, as in other cases of chronic obstruction low down in the intestine, symptoms are usually late in appearing. Dr Ritchie was on one occasion sent for to see a gentleman in a moribund condition with acute peritonitis. He had suffered from constipation for a long period, but had not sought advice for it, and had continued at business up to the time of the fatal seizure. Post-mortem examination revealed ulceration and rupture of the bowel above a cancerous stricture. Such cases are uncommon; usually there is a history of constipation, diarrhœa, or the alternation of these; often paroxysmal pain is present. In the present case it was only at a late date that the friends recalled the fact that occasional abdominal discomfort was complained of in July; no history of constipation or diarrhœa up to the time of the attack in Switzerland could be obtained. There was no cachexia, the face was florid, and the body well nourished, and there was no pain during the illness.

The discovery of a tumour on palpation is in some cases sufficient, along with these symptoms, to establish a diagnosis; but when the splenic flexure is the seat, the tumour being under cover of the ribs, as in this case, is not likely to be discovered, even after the most careful exploration.

Peristalsis visible through the abdominal wall is a very important evidence of obstruction. Hilton Fagge stated that it is rare in obstruction of the large intestine. In the case just recorded the amount of fat in the abdominal wall prevented it from being seen at first, but later it was quite evident, and could be induced by tapping the abdominal wall.

As to the seat of lesion in chronic obstruction, the amount of fluid which can be injected per rectum may give some indication, but it is not an absolute guide; because fluid may pass upward through a strictured portion of bowel and the anatomical arrangements of the elements of stricture may prevent its return. Dr Ritchie did not remember of having seen any case of chronic obstruction having spasm of the bowel below the seat of stricture, but in acute obstruction this is sometimes present and prevents the introduction even of small quantities of fluid. In this case three pints of fluid could be easily injected and returned without trouble; it therefore seemed evident that the obstruction was not in the sigmoid flexure.

As to the ballooning of the rectum, this is sometimes spoken of as evidence of obstruction at the upper part of the rectum or in the sigmoid flexure. May it not be only a late symptom which only occurs after distension of the bowel above the seat of stricture, and that it is produced mechanically by the dragging upwards of the rectum by the distended large intestine? Does this also occur in cases of obstruction of the small intestine?

What is the cause of the dilatation or distension of the bowel above the seat of stricture? Partly the accumulation of the contents of the bowel, and of flatus from their decomposition, but doubtless also partly a paretic condition of the wall of the bowel from septic absorption. Dr James Ritchie had seen a case of malignant stricture at the sigmoid flexure with obstruction, in which, although both flatus and fæcal matter passed in considerable quantity at times, there was nevertheless great abdominal distension. In these chronic cases of obstruction the constitutional symptoms in the later stages are those of septic absorption.

In cases of chronic obstruction, what is the best course to pursue in order to obtain motion of the bowels? In the production of the obstruction there are two factors,—the new growth, and spasm. There are on record cases of complete obstruction in which post-mortem examination showed that the lumen of the bowel at the seat of stricture permitted the passage of the finger, and it is within the experience of most of us that after colotomy for the relief of obstruction apparently complete, motions have after a time passed regularly per anum. The causes of spasm are probably twofold,—viz., local irritation from the new growth, and reflex irritation accompanying an increase of peristalsis. Anything which will increase peristalsis, such as purgatives, should be avoided, and those measures which tend to diminish it should be adopted,—viz., rest, small quantities of those foods which leave little waste material ; and as medicines, antispasmodics, hyoscyamus, morphine, and atropine, also intestinal antiseptics; later, after the spasm has subsided, if no motion takes place naturally, a copious enema may be given.

In the case recorded intestinal antiseptics were given continuously from a very early stage. The copious motions which were obtained followed the adoption of the plan just described. It is a question whether the digitalis and nux vomica which were required for the failing heart, at a later stage of the case, may not have had an unfavourable effect, as far as the muscular wall of the intestine was concerned, increasing the spasm at the seat of stricture, and so preventing evacuation of the bowel. Possibly the increased new growth sufficed to cause complete obstruction.

Dr Joseph Bell said that, as was always the case with Dr Ritchie's papers, it was a model of clinical care, and thoroughly worked up. It had great interest for himself at present, as he had had a case last week in the south of Scotland which to a great extent imitated it. A lady between 60 and 70, who had been very healthy, presented symptoms of chronic obstruction of the bowels. There was no trace of anything per rectum except ballooning. The lower bowel daily admitted three or four pints of water with perfect ease. She had never vomited from beginning to end. She had not complained, but had been taking medicine of her own accord. Three weeks before the end she passed what she told him herself was an excellent large firm stool, about which, however, he had some doubts. The bowel was fairly distended, and he could map out the colon, but could not detect peristalsis owing to the thick parietes. She had been having opium. He recommended strychnia, and gave an injection. There was no difficulty in getting flatus per rectum, and faecal matter also passed, but not in large quantity. The symptoms pointed rather to the ileo-caecal valve than to the lower end. He was sent for a second time, and opened the abdomen. No food had been given. There was very little in the colon. He worked his way down, but could feel no tumour. Then he worked his way upwards, and found a very strong band binding down the caecum firmly. This he separated, tied it in two places, and cut it *secundum artem*. Great relief followed, but the transverse colon did not quite empty itself, and he suggested that it might be safer to make an artificial anus. The relatives, how-ever, were anxious that this should not be done, and against his better judgment he sewed it up. He heard afterwards that flatus was passing freely, but there was no large stool. By the end of the week, before they had time to do anything, there was a fatal issue from heart failure. They made a limited post-mortem, and found a tiny tight cancerous stricture in the sigmoid flexure, very small. The lumen did not quite admit the finger. Dr Boyd reported it to be a slow-growing carcinoma, with colloid degenera-tion. It might have been better if an artificial anus had been made, although death occurred from heart failure.

Mr Hodsdon said he had a case on Friday almost the exact counterpart of Mr Bell's. The patient had suffered from obstruc-tion since the beginning of October. When she came under his care the small intestine showed as distended coils across the abdomen, and the sigmoid appeared to be distended. The difficulty was to locate the site of obstruction, in order to know where to open. He examined per rectum, and found nothing abnormal, and no ballooning. Only a small enema could be retained. He opened on the left side, found a very small malignant stricture, and relieved the obstruction by a colotomy.

He had met with many cases where it was difficult to make up one's mind as to the site of the obstruction. The stricture was, however, so frequently found to be in the sigmoid, that in cases of doubt he opened the abdomen on the left side. If the sigmoid was distended he brought it into the wound and fixed it there; if it was collapsed he closed the wound, made an incision on the right, and stitched the cæcum to the edges of the incision, delaying opening, if possible, until adhesions had formed. His remarks applied to advanced cases of chronic obstruction in old patients.

Dr Ritchie had raised the question of when to operate in cases of chronic obstruction. In his opinion operation was indicated as soon as one was sure that organic obstruction was present. Morphia, while it allayed symptoms, also masked them. Obstruc-tion caused dilatation. Morphia aggravated it to some extent. The more the wall was dilated the greater risk was there, no matter how gently one manipulated, of organisms passing through and setting up peritonitis. We gave the patient a much better chance by operating early. If the cases were seen soon there was a good prospect of successful excision; if that were not possible, the formation of an artificial anus would greatly prolong life. The artificial anus did not cause much inconvenience. He had a patient with one, who now worked as a labourer. In that case the growth had been excised. If the pad were made to fit accurately and lie flat, and did not act as a plug enlarging the opening, patients could follow their occupations without inconvenience.

Dr Ritchie, in reply, said that the remarks of the speakers called for no special reply, except that he thought Mr Bell's case one of great interest.

Meeting IV.—January 16, 1895.

I. ELECTION OF MEMBERS.

The following gentlemen were elected Ordinary Members of the Society :—Gopal Govind Vatve, M.D. Brux., care of H.H. the Raja of Miraj, Bombay ; James Cameron, M.D., 13 Fettes Row ; James Middlemass, M.B., F.R.C.P. Ed., Royal Asylum, Morningside ; Lewis C. Bruce, M.D., Royal Asylum, Morningside ; R. W. Ronaldson, M.B., 2 Bruntsfield Gardens.

II. EXHIBITION OF PATIENTS.

1. *Dr R. A. Lundie* showed the scar on the abdomen of a young woman on whom he had operated for PERFORATING GASTRIC ULCER. Dr Aitken having confirmed his diagnosis, and agreed as to the necessity for operation, he (Dr Lundie) proposed sending the patient to the Infirmary. Dr Aitken, however, pointed out that it would both save time and avoid the increased shock of removal if she were treated at home, and he (Dr Lundie) accordingly undertook the case himself, with Dr Aitken's co-operation. He made a curved incision on the right side, with its concavity towards the middle line. An aperture, small, like the eyelet-hole of a boot, was found well round to the left side on the anterior surface of the stomach. He put in two small stitches through the lips of the opening, and then six Lembert sutures, so that the opening lay at the bottom of a fissure with its sides in contact. The abdominal cavity was washed out with carbolic lotion, about 1 to 120, there being no time to prepare a sterilized lotion. During the process of washing out there was extreme collapse, the patient appearing almost moribund. · But she recovered without any bad symptom. The two points to be emphasized were the desirability of very early operation (in this case the operation was performed ten hours after perforation, and there was already general peritonitis); and, secondly, the use of *antiseptic* fluid for washing out. There were no symptoms of peritonitis after the operation.

Mr Bell congratulated Dr Lundie on having undertaken the case himself.

2. *Mr Caird* showed a man on whom he had operated for REMOVAL OF THE APPENDIX. He found a mass of omentum and some flaky lymph on the organ. Having cleared away the mass of omentum, he removed the appendix, and stitched up. Both before and after operation the patient obtained great comfort from the use of the ice-coil. By stitching the various layers of the abdominal wall separately, the cicatrix was rendered wonderfully firm and resistant.

h

Mr Caird also showed two cases of RESECTION OF GUT, between 6 and 7 inches having been removed. The gut was well pulled down and resected wide of inflamed area, and fairly wide of aperture of exit, and the two ends sutured together. A drainage-tube was inserted, for fear of general peritonitis. Recovery was good. The cases were illustrated with water-colour drawings.

3. *Dr Bramwell* showed two boys who were suffering from PSEUDO-HYPERTROPHIC PARALYSIS. They were brothers of the two girls whom he had shown to the Society during the past session. In the elder boy's case, the symptoms were characteristic of pseudo-hypertrophic paralysis. The buttocks were markedly enlarged, the calves considerably so, the muscles of the upper limb decidedly atrophied; the knee-jerks were absent. The patient often tumbled. He rose from the ground in the characteristic way. His younger brother was affected, but in his case the disease was as yet only in a very early stage. He was unable to run and jump; his knee-jerks were absent; his calves were beginning to be enlarged. These cases were very interesting from the fact that one of the sisters of the patient presented all the characteristic features of the atrophic form of the disease—the form which was sometimes termed "idiopathic muscular atrophy."

Dr Bramwell also showed a patient suffering from the FACIO-SCAPULO-HUMERAL type of the disease. The patient had come under his observation some three years ago. At that time the calves were perhaps relatively large in comparison with the other muscles of the body; but the most striking feature was the muscular atrophy. The deltoids were somewhat enlarged, the upper arms were markedly wasted, the forearms slightly wasted, the calves were atrophied, and the muscles on the front of the thigh were slightly enlarged. The face was markedly affected; the patient was unable to close his lips firmly; he could not whistle; food collected on both sides of the mouth. He was unable to close his eyes firmly. When he laughed the mouth was drawn out transversely. The knee-jerks were absent; the bladder and rectum healthy. There were no sensory disturbances. All the other functions were quite normal. So far as Dr Bramwell knew, this was the first case of the kind which had been met with in Scotland. It was a characteristic example of the Landouzy-Déjerine type of the disease, which seemed to be, comparatively speaking, common in France but very rare in Germany.

4. *Dr MacGillivray* showed a girl, æt. 19, who three years previously began to suffer from severe FACIAL NEURALGIA in the area of distribution of the left infra-orbital nerve. Many remedies were tried without effect, and she was finally admitted into the Royal Infirmary in February 1893, when it was found that she was suffering from abscess of the antrum of Highmore, with discharge from the left side of the nose, and a swollen polypoid

condition in the middle meatus. A decayed tooth was extracted; but as free drainage did not result, an opening was made into the antrum through the canine fossa, and one was enabled to freely syringe through into the nose. As, however, the discharge continued, and the neuralgia was not relieved, the opening was enlarged, the antrum scraped out, the polypi removed, and free drainage established. As she was very anæmic, her general health was attended to, and she finally went home in August 1893, perfectly well, the opening into the antrum having almost closed. She remained well until February 1894, when the neuralgia returned worse than ever, and as nothing seemed to give relief, and the discharge from the nose had recommenced, she returned to the Infirmary in the beginning of November 1894. On November 6th Dr MacGillivray operated, with the intention of excising the nerve far back, along with Meckel's ganglion; this he did by turning up the left cheek, and cutting away the whole front of the antrum. The infra-orbital nerve could not be discovered, the new bone formed after the former operation having pressed upon it and displaced it. The roof and posterior wall of the antrum were cut away, exposing the spheno-maxillary fossa, without being able to definitely make out the nerve. With curved scissors and forceps the tissues in the line of the foramen rotundum were seized and removed, and on examining them he found about an inch of nerve with descending filaments, and, as far as one could make out, some nervous matter, probably Meckel's ganglion. There was smart hæmorrhage, which, however, was easily controlled by pressure. The patient made an uninterruptedly good recovery, has no trace of neuralgia, and is now in every way perfectly well. The facts of interest in the case are:—1st, The cure, for the time at any rate, of the severe neuralgia; 2nd, the fact that any elaborate dissection for the removal of Meckel's ganglion in this operation is quite impossible; 3rd, that no external incision of any kind was required, and thus no deformity resulted.

The second case was one of partial EXCISION OF THE ELBOW JOINT, by subperiosteal removal of the condyles, for unreduced dislocation with fracture of the external condyle. This boy, aged nine, fell while playing football, and his arm doubled under him. A bonesetter attempted to effect reduction, and said he had succeeded. Seven weeks later, as the arm was still slightly flexed, deformed, and stiff, a doctor was consulted. He was sent to the Infirmary nine weeks after the accident. There was no doubt as to the dislocation of both bones backwards, but the external condyle seemed also to be displaced backwards. Even under chloroform reduction was found to be impossible. Dr MacGillivray therefore cut down between the olecranon and the displaced outer condyle, and, as even when one had exposed the parts reduction was still impossible, he proceeded to excise the condyles subperiosteally by the method recommended twenty years ago by Dr Heron Watson for anchylosis of the elbow following fracture of the internal condyle. The external condyle was snipped off by means of bone forceps from above downwards, and removed; then the internal was separated from the shaft from below upwards, the end of the shaft sawn off, and the internal condyle dissected out. The wound was sewed up, extension applied for a week, when the wound was found healed; and now at the end of a month the boy has almost perfect movement, and the removed condyles are largely reproduced by the periosteum.

5. *Dr Norman Walker* showed a woman with typical LICHEN OF FORE-ARM.

6. *Mr Cathcart* showed TWO GELATINE CASTS OF WARTS on female genitals, and one of the condition after removal. The warts, he believed, were due to a special contagious form of poison which might or might not be associated with gonorrhœa. A well-marked COPAIVA RASH was also illustrated with photographs and a water-colour drawing. He also showed a simple form of SPRENGEL PUMP for drainage of bladder, which he had used in several cases, and found to work well. The apparatus was not deranged by the entrance of air into the tube.

7. *Dr Bramwell* showed a patient who presented all the typical physiognomic appearances of CONGENITAL SYPHILIS; also several WATER-COLOUR DRAWINGS of congenital syphilis. The SKULL of one of the patients was also shown.

III. ORIGINAL COMMUNICATIONS.

1. *Mr Caird* read NOTES ON SOME CASES ILLUSTRATING THE SURGERY OF THE INTESTINE, which, with the discussion thereon, will be found in the Appendix.

2. RUPTURE OF AN AORTIC ANEURISM INTO THE SUPERIOR VENA CAVA.

By ALEXANDER BRUCE, M.D., F.R.C.P. Ed., Assistant Physician, Royal Infirmary, Edinburgh; and Lecturer on Pathology, Surgeons' Hall.

CASES of this lesion are of such rare occurrence, that although a very valuable paper by Pepper and Griffith, who have collected and reviewed most of the previously recorded cases, has been published in the *International Journal of the Medical Sciences* for October 1890, it seems worth while to describe a case which came under my observation in the Edinburgh Royal Infirmary, and which presents some special features.

D. W., aged 57, stone-mason, married, was admitted to Ward 26, Royal Infirmary, on Friday, August 3rd, 1894, suffering from great shortness of breath and cyanosis. He gave the following history:—

He has had a cough, more or less constant, for the last five or six years, but never so severe as to keep him off work. During the present summer it has been worse than usual, constant, and accompanied by expectoration. He thinks he caught cold at Musselburgh on Tuesday, July 31st. In the evening the cough became much worse, and he felt very " stuffed up." He states distinctly that on this day there was no history of any extra exertion of any sort. On the following morning, Wednesday, August 1st, he noticed that his face was blue and his breathing rapid and difficult. He went out for about an hour and a half in the morning, but had to return, owing to the difficulty in breathing. This gradually increased, and his face became more cyanotic, and also swollen. On Thursday morning, August 2nd, he sent out for a doctor, and was bled, with slight relief to the dyspnœa. He was admitted to the Infirmary on Friday, August 3rd. His previous history is one of fairly good general health, with the exception of syphilis, contracted eighteen years ago ; cicatrices from old ulcers are still visible on the right side and dorsum of the tongue. He has always had good food, and has been a moderately heavy drinker for many years. His mother suffered from asthma.

When examined, his face was swollen and greatly cyanosed, the colour of his naturally red cheeks being heightened by the lividity present. The ears, especially their lobes, were deeply purple. The neck on both sides was swollen, œdematous, and cyanosed. There was an elastic swelling immediately above each clavicle, rather greater on the right side. The external jugular veins projected like purple cords, with swellings at the valves. They did not pulsate, and they could be emptied of blood by pressure. The thorax and abdomen presented a remarkable contrast. While the skin of the latter presented a perfectly normal colour and appearance, that of the thorax was œdematous, had generally a leaden ground colour, on which there were areas of lividity with distended venules. These formed a broad belt along the line of attachment of the diaphragm to the ribs. Others were over the sternum and to the right of it in the mammary region, in the infra-clavicular area, and above the left clavicle. The left side of the thorax was free from lividity, but it was equally œdematous with the right side. The back of the thorax was also œdematous, and there were irregular areas of distended venules. The œdema and lividity were not circumscribed as in front, but extended down to the loins. The upper extremities were very œdematous, both equally so ; the axillæ were swollen and somewhat tender on pressure, and the veins were felt as distended and apparently solid cords. The lower extremities, like the front of the abdomen, were absolutely free from œdema.

The patient sat propped up in bed, and could not lie down on account of the dyspnœa. The respirations were 32, and the pulse 104 per minute. No palpitation was complained of. There was visible pulsation in the epigastrium. The apex-beat could not be seen or felt. No pulsation or thrill could be felt anywhere on the front of the chest. An area of impaired percussion was made out in front of the upper part of the sternum and adjacent parts of the thorax. It was absolutely dull above the sternum, and became gradually less so in an outward direction on both sides. Owing to the subcutaneous œdema it was difficult to ascertain exactly where the impairment terminated, but several examinations gave an outline corresponding to that represented in Fig. 1. On the right side, at the level of the third rib, it reached about three and three-quarter inches to the right of the mid-sternal line. Above and below this rib the line approached the sternum somewhat. On the left side it just reached the nipple-line at the level of the fourth rib (4 inches from mid-sternum). Above this point it extended towards the junction of the first rib with the sternum. The liver dulness began above at the fifth rib, and extended downwards about 6½ inches. On auscultation *over the base of the heart a peculiar murmur was heard. It was continuous, somewhat resembling a venous bruit, but very loud, having an almost musical, "swishing" character. The sound was most intense during ventricular systole, and gradually died away during the diastole.* Its point of maximum intensity was on the sternum, at the level of the *third* costal cartilage. It was propagated mostly towards the right side of the thorax (see Fig. 2). Its intensity diminished suddenly at the left margin of the sternum, except at a point about opposite the fifth costal cartilage, where it could be fairly well heard for about an inch to the left of the sternum. It was not well heard either at the lower or at the upper end of the sternum. To the right of the sternum it could be fairly well heard over the area indicated in Chart II., which closely corresponds to that of impaired percussion. Beyond this it ceased; but it could be detected faintly in the right interscapular region. The aortic second could be heard free from any diastolic murmur at the apex of the heart, and at the lower end of the sternum. No systolic murmur could be heard in the neck. At the apex both first and second sounds appeared normal, except that the first sound was accompanied by a faint systolic murmur, which was apparently propagated from the base of the heart, and was not continued to the left beyond the apex. There was a slight impairment of the percussion-note in the *right interscapular region* below the spine of the scapula. The breath sounds in front of the chest seemed fairly normal. Posteriorly they were distinctly weaker on the right than on the left side. There were a few fine crepitations at the left base.

The urine was free from albumen or other abnormal constituent.

The following notes of the progress of the case were made by Dr J. V. Paterson, the Resident Physician :—

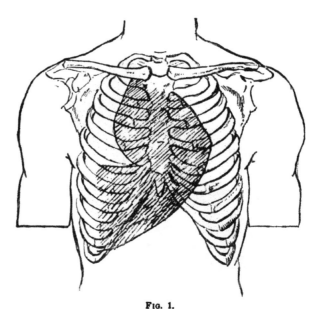

Fig. 1.
To show the area of dulness.

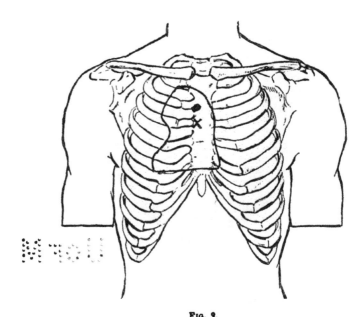

Fig. 2.
The outline bounds the area of distinct audibility of the murmur. The
X shows the first, the ● the second position of maximum loudness
of the murmur.

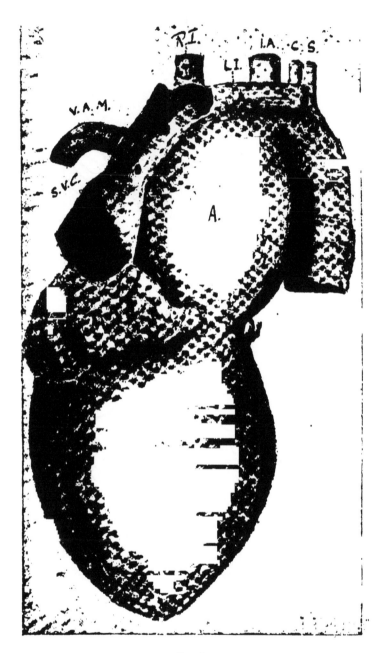

FIG. 3.

A., Aneurism of ascending arch of aorta.
S.V.C., Superior vena cava, stretched over and adherent to the aneurism and showing
    the two positions of rupture, and between them the opening of the (V.A.M.)
    vena azygos major.
R.I., Right innominate vein.
L.I., Left innominate vein, partly adherent to the aneurism.
I.A., Innominate artery.
C., Left carotid; S., Left subclavian artery.
R.A., Right auricle.

hour.

Aug. 11.—Had a pretty good night.
same. General mottling over the fron
tinct. Pulse good. On examination ε
the *point of maximum intensity of the*
of the second right costal cartilage (i.e.,
admission). The murmur still continue
and louder during the systole of the ven
sound is without murmur. On the back
tenth rib, and another, less sharply defin
lower. Whole back œdematous. On p
scapular area perhaps a little duller tha
the level of the base of the spine.

Aug. 12.—Condition unchanged. Ha

Aug. 13, 14.—No marked change.
thorax increasing. Lower extremities
œdema.

Aug. 15.—Says he feels more " stuffe
swollen. Conjunctivæ injected. Slight
discs showed venous congestion. Coa
marked about one inch below left nip
tion, but a slight constant, dull pain ov
at bases of lungs posteriorly. Patient
in his sleep.

Aug. 17.—Very drowsy. Wakes u
drops off to sleep again. Keeps constan
in his sleep. Says he dreams of his
cyanosis and dyspnœa to-day. Marked

of the glottis with the finger. Hooking forward the epiglottis with the finger gave a little relief to the dyspnœa. Did not succeed well in scarifying the glottis. Passed a large catheter into the trachea, but though air came quite freely through it, the breathing grew gradually slower and more gasping in character. Artificial respiration was tried, but natural breathing could not be re-established, and the patient died about three-quarters of an hour after Dr Paterson saw him.

During his stay in hospital the temperature, taken both in the axillæ and in the groins, was sub-normal.

Record of Temperature, Pulse, and Respirations.

Date.	Temperature.		Pulse.		Respirations.	
	Morn.	Even.	Morn.	Even.	Morn.	Even.
Aug. 4.	—	96°·6	—	104	—	32
„ 5.	97°·5	97·5	100	101	30	28
„ 6.	96·8	96·5	102	94	24	28
·„ 7.	96	96·4	86	74	24	28
„ 8.	96	97	104	92	28	22
„ 9.	96·8	96·2	100	100	28	30
„ 10.	96·6	97	100	100	24	40
„ 11.	96·4	97·4	106	108	20	28
„ 12.	97·8	97·7	104	100	26	36
„ 13.	98	98·3	100	—	26	—
„ 14.	96	98·6	88	96	29	28
„ 15.	96	97·8	100	96	20	24
„ 16.	97	97·4	90	80	26	24
„ 17.	97	97	84	70	26	24
„ 18.	97	97·4	79	70	20	24
„ 19.	97	97	60	78	22	26
„ 20.	97	96·8	90	104	24	28

POST-MORTEM REPORT.

Aug. 22.—The cyanosis and œdema had greatly diminished. Œdema of the scrotum still present. Left pleural sac contained about 12 oz. of straw-coloured fluid. The pleura was thickened, especially in the parietal layer, but the two layers were not adherent. On the right side the pleural sac was obliterated by loose connective tissue adhesions, which were very œdematous. The anterior margins of the lungs were only two inches apart, a distance much less than might have been expected from the extent of the impaired percussion-note. The mediastinum was very œdematous, and entirely concealed the great vessels. On dissecting downwards, the tissues in front of the aorta were found to be unusually dense and fibrous. The mediastinal and pulmonary pleuræ were both thickened, of a leathery consistence, and firmly united. The aorta showed an aneurismal dilatation extending from the valves to the origin of the innominate artery. The aneurism projected forwards and to the right, and had pushed the vena cava somewhat backwards. Its size was about half that of an average closed fist. Its walls were thickened, least so the left side. The intima was very irregular, mostly of a greyish colour, with here and there a small, yellow, calcareous-looking area under the epithelium, and here and there a small, shallow, ulcerated, almost circular spot. On the right and posterior aspects were two small perforations into the superior vena cava. They were about three-fourths of an inch apart. The lower of the two was oval, about one-quarter of an inch in diameter, with rounded edges. The upper was three-sixteenths of an inch in diameter, with slightly ragged edges.

The superior vena cava and the left innominate vein, for the first inch of its length, were firmly bound down to the aneurism and flattened against it by very dense fibrous tissue, which could with difficulty be dissected away so as to display the vessels. A very dense fibrous node, in all probability a gumma, lay between the upper end of the superior vena cava, the aneurism, and the trachea, and bound these three structures very firmly together. A considerable amount of fibrous tissue also bound the aneurism to the right bronchus, and apparently to some extent narrowed the latter. The lymph glands near the root of the lungs were greatly enlarged and congested, being of a deep purple colour. The right innominate vein was greatly dilated. The azygos vein appeared as large as an ordinary innominate, and all the veins entering into it, especially the right superior intercostal, were also greatly dilated. The superior vena cava was of normal size for the first inch above the right auricle; then it became suddenly contracted so as barely to admit the tip of the little finger, and this flattening and narrowing continued as far as into the division into the innominate veins. On slitting up the superior vena cava the two perforations were seen on the left aspect of the vessel. The lower perforation was almost opposite the opening of the right azygos vein, and the upper was about three-quarters of an inch below the innominate vein.

The narrowing of the superior vena cava was due to two causes: firstly, it was flattened by the pressure of the aneurism; and, secondly, its closely opposed walls had become organised together over about one-fourth of its circumference. This union was so firm that the walls could not be pulled apart without great force, and it had so affected the opening of the azygos vein as to convert it into a narrow slit.

The heart was almost normal, beyond a very slight thickening of the aortic cusps at their free edges, not sufficient to interfere with the competency of the valves. There was a slight dilatation of the left ventricle.

The lungs showed a few of the fibrous nodules characteristic of silicosis, with some œdema and congestion of the lower lobes. As already mentioned, the right bronchus was slightly pressed upon by the aneurism, and the tissues of the mediastinum were very œdematous.

Remarks.—From the first there was little doubt about the diagnosis. The sudden onset of the symptoms, with the association of dyspnœa with cyanosis, which was localised to the head, upper extremities, and thorax, manifestly suggested a sudden obstruction, or sudden increase of obstruction in the superior vena cava. The nature of this obstruction was rendered evident by the existence of the murmur, with a peculiar continuous character, and the limitation to the sternum and the right side of the thorax.

Like the authors above referred to, I at first considered the possibility of this murmur being due to a mere narrowing of the superior vena cava; but a perusal of the cases they recorded seems to show that this is extremely unlikely, if not altogether impossible. The distribution of the murmur on the right side of the sternum pointed to the vena cava rather than the pulmonary artery as the vessel in which it was produced. In the latter case the murmur would have been loudest on the left side of the sternum; and, moreover, the cyanosis would have affected the lower as well as the upper part of the body, as there would have been no special obstruction in the superior vena cava. A point of great interest with regard to the change in position of the area of the maximum loudness of the murmur deserves mention, although the importance of this did not strike me until after death. On the first examination the maximum intensity was located on the sternum at the level of the third costal cartilage, but on August 11th the murmur was loudest at the sternal end of the second right costal cartilage; that is to say, it had risen by one clear interspace. On the previous day, August 10th, the patient had a sudden attack of dyspnœa with cyanosis, becoming almost black in the face for about a quarter of an hour.

Post-mortem examination showed that there were two perforations into the cava, of which the upper was evidently the more recent, as it had ragged and irregular edges, while those of the lower perforation were rounded off. I think it probable that the sudden attack of dyspnœa and cyanosis on the 10th of August was brought about by the sudden rupture at the upper opening. Such an occurrence would at first greatly increase the backward pressure in the cava, but would gradually tend to be compensated. At the same time a new murmur would be produced, which would be loudest at a somewhat higher level than before.

The state of the superior vena cava produced by its compression and by the adhesion of part of the circumference of its wall must have produced, even before the rupture occurred, a considerable amount of backward pressure; but it is remarkable how much this became increased when the rupture took place. In this connexion it should be borne in mind that the direct line of the blood-stream from the lower opening must have impinged on the button-hole like orifice of the right azygos vein and obstructed it.

With regard to the treatment, the case was so manifestly hopeless from the first, that nothing seemed likely to afford relief so much as bleeding; and in a similar case I should be inclined to bleed much more freely from the arm.

Dr Bramwell considered that they were much indebted to Dr Bruce for bringing this very interesting case before them. Dr Bruce had kindly given him the opportunity of seeing the patient during life, and he had had no difficulty in agreeing that the phenomena could not be accounted for on any other supposition than that which Dr Bruce had advanced, namely, a perforation between the aneurism and the superior vena cava. This was the only case of the kind which Dr Bramwell had seen during life. He had met with several cases in which the superior vena cava had been compressed by large aneurisms and more or less obstructed. He showed the Society a very beautiful drawing of a case of this kind which came under his notice about a year ago. The face was swollen and cyanotic, and the veins of the head and neck markedly engorged. In that case there was no perforation. He had examined several cases post-mortem in which the superior vena cava had been pressed upon. In two, at least, the wall was so thin that it was just on the point of being ruptured, and thrombi had actually formed on the inner surface of the vein at the point of thinning. The absence of pulsation in the distended veins of the neck in Dr Bruce's case struck him (Dr Bramwell) as being a point of special interest and peculiarity.

Dr Gibson desired to concur with Dr Bramwell in his eulogium. He would only make one or two remarks with regard to the symptoms, mainly with regard to those of cyanosis. There were not many cases on record of perforation into the superior vena cava, but it was well known that there was cyanosis in the upper part of the body and a soporose condition of the brain. Dr Bruce had not told them the condition of the aortic cusps—(Dr Bruce, interrupting, said the heart was normal). The mechanism of the murmur, then, was simply this, that the higher presure in the aorta caused the blood to flow into the superior vena cava, and therefore produced a murmur which persisted throughout most of the cardiac cycle. As to the change in the position of the murmur, there could be no reasonable doubt that Dr Bruce's point was proved. He regretted that Dr Bruce had not examined the blood. He would put in a plea for the routine examination of the blood in such cases. He did not know until last year that in severe cases of cyanosis the number of red corpuscles was greatly augmented, sometimes almost doubled. This was just the sort of case to help in the proving or disproving of our theories as to the reason of the doubling of the red corpuscles. Here, again, the aortic cusps dominated the situation. Had they been incompetent there could not have been the same high degree of backward pressure or cyanosis.

Dr Bruce, in reply, said that he did not think the murmur was always continuous in such cases. Cases were described in which there was none, and in which diagnosis must be difficult, if not impossible. The murmur was sometimes systolic in time. He regretted that the blood had not been examined, but the time was unfavourable, being the beginning of the autumn holidays, and he was not then aware of the importance of examining the blood. He omitted to mention the low temperature, which only twice touched the normal. There was absolutely no pulsation, either over the aneurism or in the veins of the neck.

Meeting V.—February 6, 1895.

Dr CLOUSTON, *President, in the Chair.*

DISCUSSION ON CARDIAC THERAPEUTICS.

Prof. Thomas R. Fraser opened the Discussion by reading the following paper on THE REMEDIES EMPLOYED IN CARDIAC AFFECTIONS, AND THEIR INDICATIONS :—

MR PRESIDENT,—When invited by you to take part in a discussion on the subject of Cardiac Therapeutics, I gladly consented, for the subject is one of great importance to all practitioners of medicine, who, also, by the statement of their practical experience, cannot fail to contribute much information useful for guidance in the treatment of heart affections. Cardiac affections, further, are every day before us, and the number of cases seems to be increasing. They nearly always present themselves in circumstances demanding grave consideration; not only because of the disorders produced by a deranged circulation, but also because of the anxiety and distress which are associated with even the less important of their forms.

In the majority of instances, however, they also present themselves as affections in which, notwithstanding associated dangers and anxieties, the physician, by the judicious selection and employment of remedies, can confer more conspicuous benefits than in the case of the greater number of other serious affections.

This gratifying result is most frequently obtained by the administration of substances possessing the fundamental action of digitalis,—the remedy which for the longest period of time has been employed in the treatment of heart diseases, and which, also, has been the substance first used by pharmacologists to define a type of action obviously beneficial in the greatest number of the disorders of the heart. The definition of the action of digitalis, however, was not obtained until many years after it had become widely known as a cardiac remedy, on the recommendations contained in Dr Withering's *Account of the Foxglove and some of its Medical Uses,* published in 1785.

It remained for pharmacological investigators—prominent among whom must be mentioned Claude Bernard—to determine the true action of digitalis; and, indeed, it is only recently that we, as practitioners, have come to understand the action, and thereby to be able to employ this valuable remedy with a precision before unattainable. We now realise that when we administer it we do not, as was formerly supposed, in any true sense produce a sedative action on the heart, but the much more valuable one of strengthening its contractions and thus increasing its capability to overcome causes impeding the circulation of the blood.

This important fact in the action of digitalis having been ascertained, it has since been found that there are many other substances which also are able to produce these effects. While possessing the same chief effects as digitalis, and therefore being properly grouped along with it in action and therapeutic capabilities, it has also been found that differences exist among them in regard to physical properties and pharmacological effects.

Experience has also shown that digitalis does not in all instances succeed in producing the therapeutic benefits that were anticipated, and that its use is not unfrequently attended with inconveniences, and even with unexpected dangers. With the desire, therefore, of obtaining a serviceable substitute, many of the other substances that possess the fundamental action of digitalis have been employed in the treatment of cardiac disease.

The evidence in regard to many of them is, in the meantime, insufficient to decide the great practical question of their relative value, both on positive and negative grounds; but the attention which has been given to their effects, and the endeavours which have been made to define their value in cardiac diseases, has at least had the important result of emphasizing the nature of the fundamental changes of the heart's action which they produce, and which constitute their chief therapeutical value.

n 8.—Fifth day of Strophanthus. Pulse 88, respirations 32,

.—Twentieth day of Strophanthus. Pulse 55, respirations 2

he first six days following the admission
pital, the average daily quantity of urin
following the commencement of treatmei
on the third day, 94 ozs. ; on the fourth d
, 80 ozs. ; and on the sixth day, 70 ozs., be
ial œdema had altogether disappeared.

55, a porter at Bo'ness Docks, was admitte
akness, of being unable to walk without
f breath, sleeplessness, cough, palpitation
. He had been very intemperate in hi
ptoms had followed night-work in v
c weeks before the patient's admission in
ound on examination, that the patien
d bronchitis ; that the liver was consider

and that the heart was dilated, and the mitral orifice incompetent. The urine was scanty in amount, but not albuminous.

On the fifth day after the admission of the patient, he was treated with tincture of strophanthus in doses of 8 minims thrice daily. On the night of the following day, he slept fairly well, and his subjective symptoms had become much lessened, but the cough was still troublesome. The œdema quickly subsided, and the liver dulness gradually diminished; but some enlargement still remained on his leaving the hospital, four weeks after the treatment had been begun. The improvement in the heart's action is shown in the following pulse tracings:—

John B.—Before Strophanthus, five days after admission.   Pulse 84, respirations 24, per min.

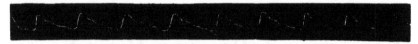

John B.—First day of Strophanthus.   Pulse 88, respirations 24, per min.

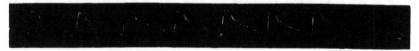

John B.—Fifteenth day of Strophanthus.   Pulse 82, respirations 28, per min.

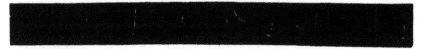

John B.—Twentieth day of Strophanthus.   Pulse 68, respirations 19, per min.

During the four days preceding the first day of the administra-tion of strophanthus, the urine averaged 27 ozs. per diem. On the first day of treatment, the quantity was 46 ozs.; on the following day, 56 ozs.; on the third day, 126 ozs.; on the fourth day, 116 ozs.; on the fifth day, 116 ozs.; and on the eighth day, 70 ozs.; and by this time the dropsy had disappeared.

Combined Mitral and Tricuspid Lesions.

The following case illustrates the therapeutic benefits in the serious condition produced by a combination of mitral and tri-cuspid disease, co-existing with emphysema and bronchitis.

John B., aged 52, a cabman, was admitted into the Royal Infirmary suffering from cough, orthopnœa, general anasarca with great swelling of the legs and scrotum, and extreme weakness. He had not been very alcoholic in his habits, but had necessarily been

.much exposed to cold and wet. Cough had existed for twelve
months, marked difficulty in breathing for six months, and œdema
for eight weeks.

On admission, there were, in addition, cyanosis, an appearance of
great distress, congestion of the superficial veins, with distended
and pulsating jugulars, giving evidence of regurgitation through the
tricuspid orifice; the tricuspid and mitral valves were incompetent;
the heart was dilated and acting feebly ; and there was emphysema
with bronchitis and œdema of the lungs. Six days after admission,
treatment with strophanthus was commenced in doses, during the
first twenty-four hours, of 4 minims of the tincture every two hours,
and, subsequently, every eight hours. An improvement was
manifest in the action of the heart within two hours after the
first dose had been administered, and the improvement steadily
advanced, until on the second day the pulse was 78 per minute
and of good quality, and on the fifth day the left ventricle was
acting with much strength. The quantity of urine became simul-

John B.—Day before Strophanthus, the sixth day after admission.   Pulse 96,
respirations 28, per min.

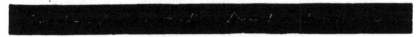

John B.—First day of Strophanthus, two hours after first dose.   Pulse 92,
respirations 25, per min.

John B.—Third day of Strophanthus.   Pulse 78, respirations 21, per min.

John B.—Sixth day of Strophanthus.   Pulse 78, respirations 18, per min.

John B.—Sixth month of Strophanthus.   Pulse 64, respirations 20, per min.

John B.—Seventh month of Strophanthus.

taneously increased, so that on the second day of treatment it amounted to 64 ozs., as contrasted with an average of 15 ozs. daily before treatment, on the third day to 90 ozs., on the fourth day to 60 ozs., on the fifth day to 56 ozs., on the sixth day to 76 ozs., on the seventh day to 79 ozs. At this time, as the supply of tincture with which the patient was being treated had failed, there was substituted for it a tincture dispensed in the Laboratory of the Infirmary. The change was an unfortunate one, for the action of the heart and of the kidneys and the symptoms of the patient soon began to deteriorate. As the addition of acid tartrate of potassium failed to restore the free elimination of urine, and as the œdema and distress of the patient became rapidly aggravated, fluid was drawn from the legs by Southey's tubes, and, soon afterwards, a free discharge of urine occurred, and the patient again steadily improved without any further relapse.

Before passing from the illustration of the valuable therapeutic effects of these agents in auriculo-ventricular lesions, it may be pointed out that the direct and uncomplicated effects of mitral stenosis are not so conspicuously benefited by them as are those of regurgitation. It is obvious that the relatively small muscular structure of the left auricle does not afford much opportunity for the action of a remedy which produces its benefits by increasing the contractile energy of the heart's muscle. Fortunately, however, mitral stenosis is a lesion in which compensation is generally fairly successfully established by spontaneous changes, and if the patient is careful not to over-tax the heart, the asystole of non-compensation and the consequent need for treatment by cardiac tonics of this group may be delayed for many years.

Aortic Lesions.

In this respect, but with a more perfect production of compensation, aortic lesions have a resemblance to the lesion of mitral stenosis. In both stenosis and regurgitation at the aortic orifice the left ventricle usually accommodates itself to the difficulties that are produced, and, especially in stenosis, the compensation thus spontaneously produced may continue for an indefinite time. Injury rather than good is done in these circumstances by the administration of any substance of the group I am now considering. The heart is unduly stimulated and the muscle of the left ventricle becomes hypertrophied beyond the needs of the circulation. The nutritive requirements of the unnecessarily hypertrophied heart become increased, and they may at any moment, and from a diversity of causes, in themselves of trivial importance, become insufficient to maintain the myocardium in a condition of health. Compensation is thus destroyed, and the very evil which should most carefully be guarded against in aortic disease, and which, perhaps, in the course of time inevitably occurs in the majority of cases, is precipitated by improper treatment.

This evil is all the more likely to be produced if the substance administered is not only a tonic of the heart-muscle but also of the bloodvessels; and, even more, if its constricting action on bloodvessels exceeds its power to increase the contractile energy of the heart's muscle,—the characteristics, as I shall afterwards point out, of the action of digitalis.

But even while compensation is being fairly well maintained in aortic disease, the mere mechanical results of the hypertrophy that has produced compensation, the pathological changes that so frequently occur in the hypertrophied muscle long before asystole takes place, and the advance of the arterio-sclerosis so usually associated with aortic disease, originate a group of symptoms widely differing from those encountered in uncomplicated auriculo-ventricular lesions. They constitute the phenomena of that most distressing condition, cardiac angina; but even when present in their most severe type they are not in themselves indications for the administration of cardiac tonics. Their successful treatment, in the absence of independent evidences of non-compensation, is rather to be found in the administration of opium and similarly acting bodies, of nitro-glycerine and nitrites, and of arsenic and iodide of potassium. The most certain of these remedies is opium, but there are circumstances in which the others also are administered with valuable results. As to nitro-glycerine and the nitrites, while recognising their great value in many cases, and especially where the heart symptoms are aggravated by bronchial spasm, I have found that, like probably all other remedies employed to cure a group of symptoms originating from a diversity of causes, they not infrequently fail to give relief. The powerful and rapid action which they possess in dilating bloodvessels is believed to supply the explanation of their therapeutic benefit. In regard to this explanation, and to the spasm of bloodvessels as a cause of the angina, which is implied in the explanation, I have observed angina to occur while the arterial tension remained low, and nitrites to succeed where no obvious effect was produced upon the tension, and I have also observed nitrites to fail where a high tension was greatly reduced by their administration.

As to the administration of iodide of potassium, I am unable to recognise any sufficient modification of the circulation produced by it in therapeutic doses that can afford an explanation of the benefits following its administration. In large doses, it undoubtedly quickens and enfeebles the heart's contractions, but at the same time it renders them irregular; while some experiments which have recently been made in my laboratory by Dr Sillar show that by direct contact, both in large and in small quantities, it produces no marked effect on the condition of the bloodvessels. Its beneficial effects are more probably to be explained by its action on the pathological processes occurring in the aorta and heart, and especially on the fibroid changes that have been there produced. I would, however, leave the further discussion of this subject to Dr George Balfour, from whom we have already learned much regarding the employment of iodide of potassium in aortic diseases.

Still, even on the more characteristic symptoms of aortic lesions, the action of substances acting directly on the cardiac muscle by strengthening its contractions is sometimes found to be a beneficial one, as the following case exemplifies.

Robert L., aged 57, a labourer in an iron foundry, came under my care suffering from precordial pain and intense dyspnœa, both having paroxysmal exacerbations, and from cough, shortness of breath, and anasarca. He had been unusually alcoholic after the death of his wife, which occurred ten weeks before admission; a week afterwards, he strained himself while lifting a heavy weight, when he immediately experienced an aching pain in the chest and sudden general weakness. Five weeks before admission, swelling began in the feet and ankles, and three weeks afterwards a severe cough occurred. All these symptoms having become aggravated notwithstanding treatment, he was sent to the Infirmary by his employers.

On admission, the more striking external morbid phenomena were great œdema of the lower extremities, and marked œdema of the face, which was also cyanosed and jaundiced; enlargement of the abdomen; and an agonizing condition of dyspnœa, preventing sleep, so that, he said, he had slept only six or seven hours in all for the last six days.

He had a characteristic aortic regurgitant pulse, regular and easily compressible, with capillary pulsation, and distended and pulsating veins. The cardiac impact was not visible, but the apex shock could be felt at the sixth rib, nearly two inches to the left of the nipple line. On auscultation, a double aortic murmur was found to be present, and the other valves to be unaffected. Rhonchi and coarse crepitations were heard over a great part of the lungs, and the chest was somewhat barrel-shaped. The breathing was laboured, and it was, by-and-by, observed to have the Cheyne-Stokes characteristics. There was a moderate amount of fluid in the abdomen, but its enlargement was mainly due to an increase in the size of the liver, which measured $9\frac{1}{4}$ inches in the mammillary line.

The case, therefore, presented in an extreme form the symptoms of aortic disease in which compensation had not been established, and in which, therefore, there was occasion to adopt a treatment more generally found beneficial in auriculo-ventricular disease than in the comparatively early stages of aortic lesions. In the first place, however, an attempt was made to relieve the condition by hypnotics, expectorants, and external applications; but as no success was obtained, 5 minims of tincture of strophanthus were administered every four hours on the fourth day after his admission, on the following day every six hours, and on the ninth day every eight hours. Beneficial effects were rapidly produced. On the day before treatment, the pulse-rate was 103. On the day following the commencement of treatment, it had fallen to 70 per minute, and the previous continuous dyspnœa, with frequent intervals of orthopnœa and of Cheyne-Stokes breathing, was rapidly improved, so that on the eighth day of treatment the respiration was quite normal. The anasarca lessened, until on the twelfth day it had altogether disappeared; the enlargement of the liver subsided gradually, so that on the fifth day the length of the line of liver dulness in the mammillary line was 8¼ inches, and on the nineteenth day 5¼ inches, as contrasted with 9¼ on the day before commencing the administration of strophanthus; and the previous weight of 11 stones 4½ lbs. had become reduced on the twelfth day to 9 stones 7¾ lbs.

Although there was no opportunity in the existence of a pulse of aortic regurgitation to produce, by the action of any substance acting on the cardiac contractions in the manner of the strophanthus group, the striking changes often observed in the small, irregular, and weak pulse of auriculo-ventricular diseases, nevertheless an effect, as well marked as in these latter conditions, was produced on the secretion of urine. During the four days preceding the administration of strophanthus, the amounts of urine passed were 26, 24, 18, and 20 ozs., and it contained a little albumen. On the day after administration, the amount was 34 ozs., on the second day 46 ozs., on the third day 100 ozs., on the fourth day 116 ozs., on the fifth day 86 ozs., on the sixth day 62 ozs., on the seventh day 102 ozs., and on the eighth day 102 ozs. Albumen disappeared on the fifth day of treatment. No relapse occurred, but as precordial pain now and then was suffered from, the patient remained in hospital for three months, and during all that time he continued to receive tincture of strophanthus.

But, as I have indicated, almost inevitably, in the course of time, cardiac degeneration occurs in aortic disease. The hypertrophied heart-muscle is no longer able to maintain a sufficient circulation; dilatation with auriculo-ventricular regurgitation frequently occurs; and, whether this complication exist or not, the symptoms of cardiac insufficiency that are produced are indistinguishable from those of auriculo-ventricular regurgitation. It is now that the administration of cardiac tonics is indicated, and in many instances they, for a time at least, produce as remarkable therapeutic results as in the non-compensation of auriculo-ventricular lesions. From many cases in which this complication existed I select the following :—

Combined Aortic and Mitral Lesions.

James M., 65, a tailor, came under my care suffering from general weakness, difficulty in breathing, swelling of the legs and body, and pain over the heart. Many of these symptoms had originated a year previously, but the weakness and cardiac pain had lately much increased.

It was found that the heart was hypertrophied and dilated, that there were systolic and diastolic aortic and systolic mitral murmurs, that the pulse was extremely feeble and its rate between 137 and 146 per minute, and that the arteries were moderately athero-matous. It was considered advisable to treat the cardiac weakness as soon as possible, and, accordingly, on the night of admission tincture of strophanthus was administered in 5 minim doses every four hours. The pulse tracing before treatment was represented by almost a straight line, but it slowly improved, until on the seventh day of treatment a movement of fair amplitude and regu-larity was obtained, but still at the increased rate of 94 per minute.

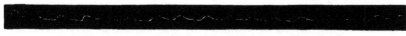

James M.—Before Strophanthus.   Pulse 136, respirations 36, per min.

James M.—Seventh day of Strophanthus.   Pulse 92, respirations 18, per min.

In this case the urine on the day before treatment amounted to only 24 ozs.; in the first twenty-four hours of treatment it had increased to 84 ozs., on the second day to 140 ozs., on the third day to 130 ozs., on the fourth day to 108 ozs., on the fifth day to 120 ozs., on the sixth day to 110 ozs., on the seventh day to 70 ozs., on the eighth day to 80 ozs.; and it afterwards varied from 78 to 40 ozs. That this great diuresis was produced by strophanthus is not, however, so clearly evident as in the former cases, for the preliminary stage of observation without treatment was too brief a one. The patient was dismissed in twenty-eight days free from all urgent symptoms, and able for light work.

Joseph M., 28 years of age, was admitted into the Royal Infirmary with a history of rheumatic fever, which had occurred seven years and also four years previously; and suffering from palpitation, dyspnœa, pain over the heart, cough, weak-ness, and occasional vomiting. The pulse was slow and irregu-lar, but otherwise presented the characters of aortic regurgita-tion combined with stenosis. The heart was much enlarged, with a diffuse apex impact in the 6th interspace, 5½ inches to the left of the mid-sternal line. There was mitral regur-gitation, with both regurgitation and stenosis at the aortic orifice, and a moderate degree of œdema of the base of both lungs, but none elsewhere. On the third day after admission, he was treated with tincture of strophanthus in 5 minim doses thrice daily. The palpitation, dyspnœa, and other symptoms soon subsided, and the pulse became stronger and nearly regular. A distinct effect was also produced upon the urine. During the three days preceding the administration of strophanthus it averaged only 18 ozs. a day; on the day following the administration it had increased to 24 ozs., on the second day to 70 ozs., on the third day to 68 ozs., on the fourth day to 58 ozs., on the fifth day to 62 ozs.; and this satisfactory elimination was maintained so long as strophanthus was being administered. In about a month, however, the condition had so long continued a favourable one that the treatment with strophanthus was stopped. The pulse very soon again deteriorated, and some of the original symptoms returned; but on resuming the treatment the former condition of good health was restored, with a corresponding improvement in the heart's action.

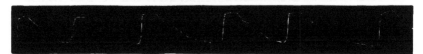

Joseph M.—Before Strophanthus. Pulse, (?); apex shocks about 120 per min. respirations 25 per min.

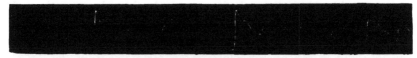

Joseph M.—During Strophanthus, eighth day. Pulse 64, respirations 19, per min.

Joseph M.—Twelve days after Strophanthus stopped. Pulse 91, respirations 22, per min.

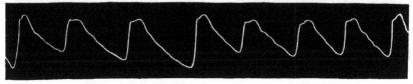

Joseph M.—After resuming Strophanthus. Pulse 64, respirations 20, per min.

Aortic Regurgitation with Cardiac Degeneration.

The final result was not so favourable in the next case of aortic disease.

The patient was a man, George C., 59 years of age, recently a clerk, but formerly a soldier. He was admitted suffering from sleeplessness and intense orthopnœa, with severe attacks of cardiac angina. In early life he had had rheumatic fever. The present acute attack had existed for five days. There was a little œdema of the ankles and of the lungs, the arteries were atheromatous, the heart and aorta were enlarged, and mitral presystolic and systolic and aortic systolic and diastolic murmurs were found. The pulse had the characters of aortic regurgitation, with irregularity; the liver was contracted; and the urine was of moderate quantity, free from albumen, and with a specific gravity of 1020. The condition was not one requiring the administration of a cardiac tonic, but rather of opium. So great was the degree of aortic distress that the patient was unable to remain in bed, and endeavoured to obtain rest and sleep at night sitting propped up in a chair. Accordingly, during the first period of his residence in hospital, morphine was frequently injected subcutaneously, and, although it often caused headaches, its effects were much more satisfactory than those of nitro-glycerine and nitrites. As the heart, however, showed symptoms of increasing insufficiency, and the urine gradually lessened in amount, strophanthus was administered to the patient three weeks after his admission. It improved the heart's strength, and reduced its irregularity. It, at the same time, exerted a diuretic

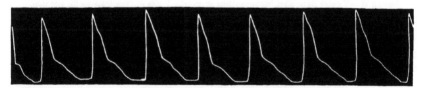

George C.—Immediately before Strophanthus and during Morphine. Pulse 120, respirations 19, per min.

George C.—Second day of Strophanthus. Pulse 96, respirations 24, per min.

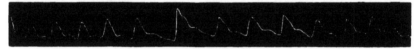

George C.—Third day of Strophanthus. Pulse 88, respirations 18, per min.

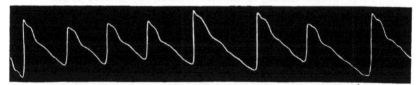

George C.—Eighth day of Strophanthus. Pulse 74, respirations 22, per min.

action; for while during the three days preceding its administration the urine amounted to 35, 30, and 44 ozs., on the day following its administration the urine had increased to 116 ozs., on the second day to 130 ozs., and on the fourth day to 56 ozs. ; and, coincidently, the œdema of the legs had almost disappeared. The improvement, however, was only a temporary one. Orthopnœa persisted, and necessitated the use of opium, iodide of potassium, and nitrites, and although latterly digitalis was also administered, the patient died three and a half months after admission. It was found at the post-mortem examination that the lungs were emphysematous, and in a condition of brown induration, that the aortic and mitral valves were incompetent and atheromatous, that the aorta was much dilated, and that the liver and kidneys were in a state of cirrhotic atrophy.

Grave Cardiac Insufficiency without Valvular Lesions.

Fatty Degeneration of the Heart.—It is not, however, only in the cardiac insufficiency of valvular lesions that the members of this group of substances prove of service. Weakness of the heart's action, producing effects similar to those of the weakness resulting from non-compensated valvular disease, may be caused by degenerative changes in the myocardium itself ; and whether thus caused or not, it may also occur during pyrexia, and there constitute an important danger to life. Fortunately, in both circumstances, efficient remedies are found among the cardiac tonics. My first illustrations are taken from cases in which the weakness of the myocardium was independent of pyrexia.

The patient, Henry B., aged 57, a labourer in a coal-pit, came under treatment suffering from œdema of the legs, scrotum, and abdomen, occasional giddiness, general feebleness, and dyspnœa so great that he could only sleep when well propped up in bed. The dyspnœa and feebleness had prevented him from working for four years, and a fortnight before admission they had so far increased that he was unable to leave his bed. The œdema had been present for about the same time. There was no history of rheumatic fever or of intemperance. Examination of the heart revealed considerable dilation of the right side, the apex shock was not visible, the impact could with difficulty be felt, and the heart sounds were extremely feeble, but without any accompaniments. There was also emphysema and moderate enlargement of the liver, with epigastric pulsation ; but the urine, though rather scanty in amount, did not contain albumen or any other abnormal constituent. The case appeared to be one of cardiac debility, probably due to steatosis of the myocardium. On the third day after admission, treatment was begun with 5 minims of tincture of strophanthus thrice daily. The condition of the patient gradually improved, so that in eight days he could sleep in a normal posture, and walk about the ward without difficulty ; the œdema had disappeared in twelve days, and it was considered unnecessary to continue the treatment longer than three weeks. In six weeks

l

after admission he was sent to the Convalescent Home. The effect in slowing and strengthening the heart's action, and in rendering it more regular, is shown in the following pulse tracings.

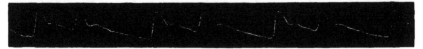

Henry B.—Immediately before Strophanthus. Pulse 96, respirations 34, per min.

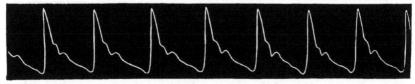

Henry B.—Second day of Strophanthus. Pulse 72, respirations 23, per min.

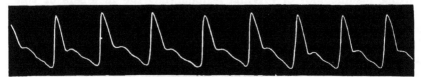

Henry B.—During Strophanthus, twelfth day. Pulse 76, respirations 28, per min.

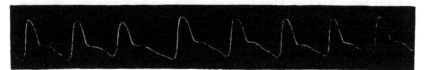

Henry B.—During Strophanthus, third week. Pulse 76, respirations 23, per min.

The diuretic action of strophanthus was also conspicuously produced in this case. During the three days preceding its administration, the urine was of the average daily amount of 33 ozs. On the day following the first administration, the amount was 80 ozs., on the second day 180 ozs., on the third day 260 ozs., on the fourth day 232 ozs., on the fifth day 136 ozs., on the sixth day 220 ozs., on the seventh day 148 ozs., on the eighth day 134 ozs., on the ninth day 80 ozs.; and, indeed, during the remainder of the patient's residence in the hospital the quantity remained above the average, being generally from 52 to 70 ozs.

Some instruction is to be derived from the after-history of this patient. Soon after going to the Convalescent Hospital, on a cold day, he suddenly became sick, and severe pain was felt in the epigastrium. In a few days afterwards, he died of double pneumonia. At the post-mortem examination it was found that the heart was dilated and fatty, especially in the right side, where also there was some interstitial change, and that no valvular disease existed. The kidneys were found to be in a condition of acute inflammation, with slight chronic cirrhosis.

John N., 64, a hawker, formerly a soldier, was admitted suffering from extreme debility, great dyspnœa, cough, and general anasarca. He had all his life, and especially while following the occupation of a hawker, been exposed to fatigue, inclement weather, and insufficient food ; and he admits that he often indulged in large excesses of alcohol.   He had not suffered from rheumatic fever.

Three months before admission, he began to be troubled with a cough, and, soon, his breathing became difficult, and the difficulty increased so that he could not lie in bed, but had to be propped up with pillows.   His symptoms were temporarily relieved by treatment, but by-and-by the cough became more troublesome, and the dyspnœa so distressing, that he often required to get up at night and sleep on a chair, leaning over a table.   During a fatiguing walk, four weeks before admission, his feet and ankles became swollen, and he found himself so feeble that he could complete his journey only at the rate of less than a mile an hour, and he has not since been able to walk.

The œdema having involved the whole body, the patient applied for admission into the Royal Infirmary.

On admission, great dyspnœa was present, and it was soon found that the breathing was, at times, of the Cheyne-Stokes variety. The respirations were rapid, bronchitis with œdema was present, the heart was rapid, weak and irregular in action, and he often suffered from palpitation.   The heart was dilated, but no valvular murmur could be discovered, the only abnormalities being a slight prolongation of the second sound in the aortic area, with reduplication and great weakness of the sounds in all the areas.   The pulse had the characters of that of mitral lesions, in its restricted movements, great feebleness, and irregularity in time and amplitude. The urine was scanty, but no albumen or blood was found in it. The liver was moderately enlarged.   At 2 A.M. on the night of the patient's admission, the resident physician was called to see him because of an alarming attack of cardiac weakness with much increase of dyspnœa.   It was therefore necessary to treat the patient without delay, and alcoholic stimulants were at once administered, with some measure of relief.   During the same day, also, he received 5 minims of tincture of strophanthus every six hours, which was continued for forty-eight hours, and the same dose was then administered every eight hours.   The heart's action was quickly improved, so that on the second day the rate was about 78 per minute, and the ventricular systole was strong, but irregularity remained ; and this irregularity persisted during the two months the patient was under treatment, although other remedies, such as strychnine, were also administered.   On the second day,

John N.—Immediately before Strophanthus. Pulse 144 (?), respirations 41, per min.

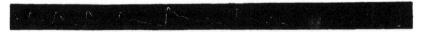

John N.—First day of Strophanthus. Pulse 128, respirations 27, per min.

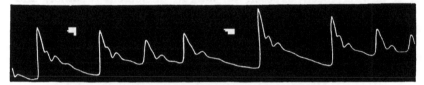

John N.—Second day of Strophanthus. Pulse 78, respirations 33, per min.

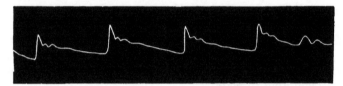

John N.—Fifth day of Strophanthus. Pulse 56, respirations 39, per min.

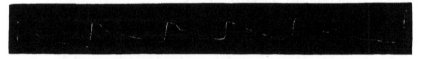

John N.—Eighth day of Strophanthus. Pulse 54, respirations 42, per min.

also, the general condition of the patient was greatly improved, and the breathing was easier.   On the sixth day, the œdema had disappeared everywhere except at the back of the ankles.   It was not until three weeks after admission that the Cheyne-Stokes breathing had so far lessened as to be observable only while the patient was asleep ; and it, as well as irregularity of the heart's action, were the only remaining symptoms when the patient was dismissed from the hospital.

Although the early treatment of the patient rendered necessary by the urgency of the symptoms interferes with the clearness of the evidence, the diuretic return of the remedy was apparently well marked in this case also.   On the day of the first administration of strophanthus, only 16 ozs. of urine were passed.   On the following day the quantity was 40 ozs., on the third day 30 ozs., on the fourth day 44 ozs., on the fifth day 60 ozs., on the sixth day 68 ozs., on the seventh day 80 ozs., on the eighth day 120 ozs., on the ninth day 110 ozs., on the tenth day 112 ozs., and on the eleventh day 80 ozs.

Fibroid Degeneration of the Myocardium.—The patient, Charles S., aged 51, was admitted on 9th February 1895, suffering from great prostration, swelling of the ankles, dyspnœa, sleeplessness, cough with much wheezing respiration.   A complete history could not be obtained because of his condition, but it was ascertained that these symptoms had begun about three weeks ago.

The heart's impact was very feeble, the area of dulness was increased transversely, extending considerably to the right of the sternum, the first sound was extremely feeble, and a faint systolic murmur was heard in the mitral and tricuspid areas; and the pulse was rapid, 130 per minute, and irregular in its rhythm and character. General bronchitis, with considerable pulmonary œdema, and a scanty urine containing much albumen, were also present.

The patient was immediately treated with steam inhalations, poultices, and a cough mixture containing carbonate of ammonium, squill, ipecacuanha and senega; and whisky in small quantities was also administered. Some improvement followed in the breathing and state of general prostration, but as the heart's action did not improve, on the evening of the 12th of February 5 minim doses of tincture of strophanthus were given, and at midnight 10 minims, which latter large dose was repeated every four hours. On the 13th of February, the heart's action was stronger, slower, and less rapid. On the 14th, the improvement was still more marked, the initial rate of 130 per minute having been reduced to 98, while a good pulse expansion with almost perfect regularity had replaced the minute and irregular characters of the pulse of the 12th.

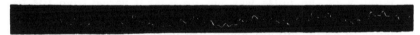

Charles S.—Before Strophanthus.   Pulse 130, respirations 38, per min.

Charles S.—First day of Strophanthus.   Pulse 120, respirations 25, per min.

Charles S.—Second day of Strophanthus.   Pulse 98, respirations 32, per min.

Bronchitis, and especially pulmonary œdema, however, increased, and the patient died suddenly on the 16th of February.

At the post-mortem examination, the diagnosis of enlarged heart, mitral regurgitation, bronchitis, pulmonary œdema, and kidney disease was confirmed. The pulmonary œdema was extreme in both lungs, and had probably been the immediate cause of death.

It was, however, also found that the pericardium was everywhere adherent to the heart, and that extensive chronic myocarditis was present, involving the left ventricle, in patches extending inwards from the pericardium, but nowhere reaching the endocardium, and involving the whole thickness of the wall of the right ventricle from apex to base over a strip from 1 to 1¼ inch wide. The coronary arteries and valves were healthy, and the aorta was very slightly atheromatous, but not dilated.

Notwithstanding this extensive degenerative change in the myocardium of both ventricles, the heart reacted well to the action of strophanthus, and a threatened failure of the cardiac action was promptly prevented, although death afterwards occurred from the asphyxia of increasing pulmonary œdema, which, unfortunately, could not be so favourably modified.

Cardiac Insufficiency during Pyrexia.

In order to illustrate the therapeutic effects in the cardiac weakness of pyrexia, the two following cases are given :—

Pneumonia.—In the first, a double pneumonia existed in a young, non-alcoholic man of 29 years, a labourer (Emmanuel F.).

He came under treatment on the fifth day of the illness, and as the pulse was rapid, feeble, and irregular, on the evening of the seventh day tincture of strophanthus was administered in a dose of 5 minims every four hours, which, on the following day, was increased to 8 minims. On the day on which the treatment was commenced, the heart's action was feeble and irregular, but the rapidity of the pulse was not great, as it varied from 104 to 112 in the minute. On the second day of treatment, the pulse had fallen to 94 per minute, and it had become regular in rhythm ; and on the fourth day of treatment, the pulse was at the rate of 82 per minute, regular and strong, and the heart's apex beat and sounds had become well marked and distinct.

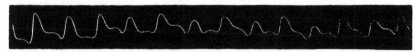

Emmanuel F.—Seventh day of illness. Before Strophanthus. Pulse 104, respirations 56, per min.

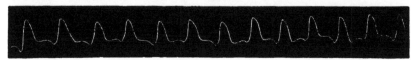

Emmanuel F.—Eighth day of illness. Second day of Strophanthus. Pulse 94, respirations 48, per min.

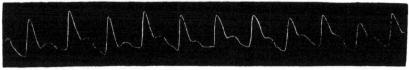

Emmanuel F.—Tenth day of illness. Fourth day of Strophanthus. Pulse 72, respirations 44, per min.

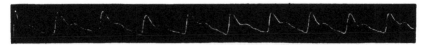

Emmanuel F.—Thirteenth day of illness. Seventh day of Strophanthus. Pulse 78, respirations 30, per min.

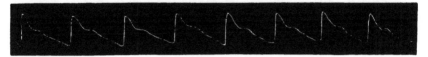

Emmanuel F.—Nineteenth day of illness. Thirteenth day of Strophanthus. Pulse 61, respirations 20, per min.

The progress of the case continued to be uniformly favourable, and the patient left the hospital in less than five weeks after admission.

The improvement in the heart's action in this patient happened to coincide with the first evidences of the termination of the stage of pyrexia, and although during the early portion of the period of apyrexia the heart's strength, contrary to what is usually observed, continued to be maintained without diminution, the former circumstance has to be taken into account in estimating the influence of the treatment.

In the following case, on the other hand, the effects on the heart were obtained during the existence of pyrexia. The patient, John R., 40 years of age, was admitted complaining of severe pain in the chest, with cough and fever, all of which had begun with a severe rigor three days before. He was a strong and muscular man, but there was a definite alcoholic history.

Examination showed that the patient was suffering from pneumonia of both lungs, that his breathing was rapid, that the urine did not contain albumen, that the heart's action was very feeble, and that the pulse was frequent, irregular, and of very low tension. General treatment with expectorants and warm moist applications to the thorax was at once adopted, and on the following day half an ounce of brandy was added, because of the feebleness of the pulse. The pneumonia made slow progress; but as the cardiac action became weaker from day to day, it was determined to administer strophanthus. On the day of the first administration, the seventh day of the illness, the pulse was dicrotic and of the very significant rate of 140 per minute, and the temperature ranged from 100° to 102°. On the second day of administration, the pulse was 112 and the temperature between 99° and 101°; on the third day, the pulse was 84 per minute, with great improvement of strength and entire absence of dicrotism, and the temperature was from 99°·5 to 100°·5; and on the fourth day, the pulse, retaining its improved characters, was 76, and the temperature between 98° and 98°·5. So that, during the existence of pyrexia, an extremely weak pulse of the rate of 140 per minute was in a short time greatly strengthened and its rate reduced to the normal. The after-progress of the patient was favourable, and he left the hospital five weeks after admission.

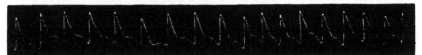

John R.—Seventh day of illness. Before Strophanthus. Pulse 140, respirations 38, per min.

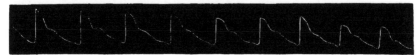

John R.—Ninth day of illness. Second day of Strophanthus. Pulse 84, respirations 32, per min.

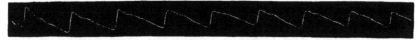

John R.—Eleventh day of illness. Fourth day of Strophanthus. Pulse 76, respirations 30, per min.

John R.—Thirteenth day of illness. Sixth day of Strophanthus. Pulse 78, respirations 28, per min.

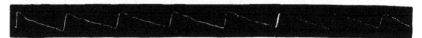

John R.—Sixteenth day of illness. Ninth day of Strophanthus. Pulse 66, respirations 22, per min.

I would add that a distinct diuretic action was produced by strophanthus in this case, although the diuresis did not assume the remarkable proportions often observed in cardiac affections with œdema.

Pleurisy.—I have obtained similar satisfactory results in many other cases of pneumonia, as well as in the pyrexia of phthisis and of pleurisy. In the latter disease, I have been in the habit of using strophanthus for two objects,—in order to restore to normal conditions a weak and dicrotic pulse, and in order to prevent, or at least lessen, the likelihood of recurrence of pleuritic effusions after thoracentesis has been performed, by the stimulation of the kidney action.

The successful attainment of the former object has been frequently demonstrated. It is, however, obviously impossible to demonstrate the successful accomplishment of the latter object, as it cannot be predicted in any case of pleurisy that an effusion will reappear. A scanty elimination of urine has, however, in many instances been changed into a copious one; and thus a condition has been produced unfavourable to a re-accumulation of fluid in the pleural cavity.

I have thus illustrated the therapeutical benefits obtained in the treatment of cardiac affections by the administration of substances whose essential action is to increase the contraction of muscular fibre. It is almost unnecessary to point out that they cannot always succeed in relieving the symptoms of heart disease. Failures are only too frequently encountered; but I believe that the therapeutic efficiency of several of these substances is so great that in only three conditions need failure be anticipated, placing out of consideration opposing conditions outside of the heart, such as great œdema of the lungs, extensive bronchitis, and large pleuritic or pericardial effusions, for whose treatment special measures are required. These conditions are, firstly, degenerations of the myocardium so far advanced that adequate contractions of the heart cannot be originated; secondly, mechanical obstructions of the circulation, caused by valve leakage or stenosis so extreme that no possible increase in the strength of the heart's contractions can produce a sufficient circulation of the blood; and, thirdly, a combination of degeneration and of the mechanical effects of valve lesions, where each separately would be insufficient to cause failure, but where the combination is sufficient to do so.

It may be useful to consider the more important of the other members of this group of remedies, in respect, at any rate, to any special characters which they have been found to possess.

So far as experiment has proceeded, strophanthus occupies the first position in the action which is produced on the contractile power of the cardiac muscle. It increases the contraction of this muscle with a smaller quantity than any other similarly acting substance, and with a rapidity unequalled by any of them. Its energy may be appreciated by the statement, that when a solution containing 1 part of a dry alcoholic extract in 10,000,000 parts of liquid is perfused through the living heart of a frog, the heart is paralysed in extreme systolic contraction in about fifty minutes, and when the solution is one of 1 part of extract in 5,000,000 parts of liquid, such extreme contraction of the cardiac muscle is produced that relaxation occurs only with post-mortem decomposition.

The rapidity of its action finds an explanation in the facts that the active principle is soluble in less than its own weight of water, and that it possesses the diffusibility of a soluble crystalloid.

If, in these respects, it be contrasted with digitalis, it is found that the latter substance has a relatively complex composition, and that several of its active principles are insoluble in water. When the most active of its soluble principles has the energy of its cardiac action tested by passing a solution through the living heart, it is found to have but little effect in a solution of 1 in 50,000, while even a solution of 1 in 5000 is not able to exert on the cardiac muscle so strong an influence as a solution of 1 in 10,000,000 of strophanthus extract.

There is, on the other hand, another aspect of the action of these substances in which the advantage may lie with digitalis. The condition of the circulation is dependent not only upon the contractions of the heart, but also upon the state of the bloodvessels. It has long been known that digitalis possesses the power of causing contraction of bloodvessels, and thus of increasing blood-tension. It is not, perhaps, always appreciated that its action in this respect is probably greater than its action on the heart. Its influence on the bloodvessels is due to a direct effect upon them, and is, therefore, produced even when the bloodvessels are entirely separated from the vascular nerve centres. When contrasted with strophanthus, the most active of the soluble principles of digitalis exerts at least fifty times a greater contractile power upon bloodvessels than extract of strophanthus or than strophanthin. While this difference may constitute an advantage in cases where weakness of the circulation is due more to the state of the bloodvessels than to that of the heart, it is not to be overlooked that it may, in the contrary conditions, constitute a disadvantage, by increasing the difficulties to be overcome by an already enfeebled heart. Although it is not within my experience, still it may undoubtedly occur that the relatively feeble action of strophanthus upon bloodvessels may somewhat restrict its usefulness as a diuretic. On this point practical experience alone can supply evidence. The diuretic action of heart-remedies of this group cannot be satisfactorily determined by pharmacology. None of them has been clearly shown to possess any diuretic action in health, operating in a definite and constant manner. In disease, their diuretic action chiefly depends on the changes they produce in the circulation of the body and of the kidneys. Any of them that, besides, exerts a direct action on the excretory structures of the kidneys will be unable to produce diuresis in conditions of the circulation unfavourable to this action. Even those of them that produce diuresis merely by modifying blood-tension may still fail as diuretics in certain derangements of the circulation locally affecting the blood supply of the kidneys. Unfortunately, it is impossible to determine in patients the condition of the kidney blood supply, and, therefore, there must always occur a certain proportion of failures in the diuretic use of each of these remedies, and, therefore, also circumstances, which may be regarded as accidental, are likely to produce erroneous impressions regarding their relative value as diuretic remedies.

But while in some cases a diuretic action may possibly be more successfully obtained by an agent which increases the contractility of the muscles of bloodvessels more than of the muscle of the heart, the contrary is not unusually observed. For instance, in a patient, William W., 64 years of age, suffering from mitral incompetence, with dropsy and dyspnœa, the administration of tincture of strophanthus during seven days failed to increase the quantity of urine above a daily average of 40 ozs.; sodium nitrate, in doses of half a grain four times daily, was then given along with the previous doses of tincture of strophanthus, and on the first day after this addition the quantity of urine was 40 ozs., on the second day 55 ozs., on the third day 104 ozs., on the fourth day 85 ozs., on the fifth day 114 ozs., on the sixth day 115 ozs., on the seventh day 110 ozs., and so on, for several more days.

For similar reasons, it may happen that better results will be obtained by combining together two or more of these substances than by giving one alone, as has been illustrated by Dr Brakenridge in the diuretic effects produced by the combination of digitalis and caffein.

At the same time, disappointments will be produced if it be not apprehended that usually no remarkable diuresis is caused by remedies of this class in the absence of cardiac insufficiency, and that the great flow of urine, such as might occur after the removal of an obstruction or the opening of a sluice, exemplified in several of the cases I have narrated, only occurs when, in patients suffering from cardiac insufficiency, general œdema shows that much liquid has accumulated in the body.

It is unnecessary to make more than a brief reference to the more commonly used of the other substances which possess this fundamental action of increasing the contraction of the heart muscle.

The more important of them are caffein, convallamarin, helleborein, scillitoxin, and adonidin. It may be interesting to remark that when the energy of their action on the heart is determined by perfusion experiments, strophanthus extract is found to be 8 times more powerful than adonidin, scillitoxin and erythophlein, 20 times more powerful than helleborein, 30 times more powerful than convallamarin, 300 times more powerful than some specimens of digitalin, 3000 times more powerful than others, and 30,000 times more powerful than caffein. .

None of them, however, acts so powerfully upon bloodvessels as digitalin.

As to spartein, it slows the heart rather by weakening its systole and thus delaying the cardiac contractions, than by increasing the strength of the contractions. Its action is not, therefore, of the same kind as that of strophanthus and the other substances that act as it does. It has no direct action on the myocardium, but only on its regulating nerves; and even this can be produced only by large doses. By this regulating action, however, it may prove useful in certain forms of cardiac insufficiency, and may also increase the flow of urine.

I have thus made some reference to the more important members of the most important group of cardiac remedies. Notwithstanding the infinite variety of conditions presented by heart diseases, the simple indication for their use is the existence of *cardiac insufficiency*. The selection of any one of them to overcome this insufficiency may be based on considerations such as those which I have stated. It is also to be recollected that the practitioner can generally best use for any definite purpose the remedy in whose use he has most fully trained himself by practical experience. I have, for instance, in my own experience with strophanthus, extending over a large number of cases, never been disappointed in any reasonable expectation; but, because of that gratifying experience, I should be unwilling to assert that successful results are not obtained by other practitioners with some other of these cardiac remedies.

I have not discussed many therapeutic measures which are every day usefully adopted in the treatment of heart diseases, such as special measures for increasing the removal of accumulated liquid, both pharmacological and mechanical, venesection, and, in the absence of marked phenomena of non-compensation, the employment of arsenic, strychnine, and graduated physical exercise. In association with these latter measures, and exceeding them all in importance, I would, in conclusion, enforce the importance of *rest*. It is not only a requisite in the more severe, but also in the mildest forms of non-compensated cardiac disease; and it has over and over again come under my observation that, with the simple aid of a regulated dietary, it has been sufficient to remove, not only the cardiac symptoms of mild non-compensation, but also those of more aggravated cardiac insufficiency, including even œdema of a limited part of the body. And by *rest* I also mean the avoidance of the unnecessary exertion of the heart, only too frequently produced by the administration of digitalis, or some other similar substance, whenever a cardiac bruit is detected, and without due regard to the actual requirements of the circulation.

―――――

Dr G. W. Balfour remarked that it was rather a wide subject to enter upon, the Therapeutics of Cardiac Disease. With regard to the last few sentences, he was entirely at one with Prof. Fraser. He entirely agreed that rest and diet were well fitted to cure a large number of cardiac affections, and that digitalis was not necessary for all. He had been educated first of all in veterinary medicine, and having thus had the inestimable advantage of having dumb patients, he early learned the advantage of exact observation for therapeutics as well as for diagnosis, and from the peculiar idiosyncrasies of these animals he also learned to distrust all experiments upon the lower animals. The discrepancies between the action of drugs on various of the lower animals and man were so very great that all pharmacological experiments on lower animals were to be received with a certain amount of distrust. That might account for some discrepancies that arose between himself and Dr Fraser. Of course, Dr Fraser had given them a great pæan on the use of strophanthus, which he need not say that he did not intend to follow. Strophanthus had rather disappointed him, and especially in one respect, probably from its want of action on the bloodvessels, and the blood-supply of the heart being thus at a lower pressure than when digitalis is given. He had found it very uncertain in its action. That might be due partly to the tinctures not being so carefully prepared as those prepared and used by Dr Fraser himself. He had another objection, which was, perhaps, more worthy of consideration, and that was that he was very early taught by Dr Fraser's predecessor that of two drugs with similar actions, one indigenous and the other foreign, it was much better, for many reasons, to use the indigenous. He rather agreed with Sir Robert Christison, and thought that because strophanthus came from abroad they did not always get it so pure as it might be. He had had no difficulty in getting the heart to do anything he chose with digitalis. They were far too much afraid of digitalis nowadays compared with what they used to be long ago. In former days the doses were very much larger, and given very much oftener. The infusion then contained 3 grs. in every half-ounce, double the strength of the ordinary Pharmacopœia preparation, and was given in double the dose up to as much as 12 grs. every four hours. He did not counsel use of such excessive doses, because they must always employ it in every case with great caution and an accurate idea of what they desired. Like many other drugs, it was cumulative, and might produce disagreeable, he did not say dangerous, symptoms, because they had always sufficient warning to avoid that. When they wished tonic action alone they must employ it in sufficiently small doses to allow a sufficient period to elapse between the first dose and the next following one to allow the drug to be entirely eliminated and leave only its effect behind; then they had no cumulative action. Such doses could be continued for many months or years. According to his experience, one grain every twelve hours was quite enough to ensure tonic action on the heart, given as powder, or in any of the other forms, infusion or tincture. This might be administered, certainly for many months, even for many years. When they wished to use it for other purposes,—to contract the heart or to produce diuretic action,—then they must give it in much larger doses, so as to have a certain amount of cumulative action. Where there was considerable general œdema from weakness of the heart, it was better to give large doses freely and at short intervals, so as to have a rapid action; then diuresis set in at once, and they were more quickly warned as to the commencement of cumulative action. For this purpose it was better to give digitalis in doses of from 3 to 5 or 7 grs., or even more, every four hours, and it should be continued until diuresis set in, or until symptoms occurred which indicated saturation. There were seldom any indications of saturation until 30 or 40 grs. had been employed. If after giving that amount diuresis went on comfortably, the drug should be stopped; and if sickness and nausea occurred after administration of 30 or 40 grs. in any shape, either as infusion or tincture, the drug should be stopped as a rule, and in the course of the next few hours a copious diuresis set in. Digitalis might be stopped for a day or two; then, when diuresis began to fail, commenced again in more moderate doses, so as to keep up the action of the drug. By careful watching they avoided all difficulty in regard to dangerous saturation of the system. When, however, smaller doses (ordinary British Pharmacopœia doses of ½ oz. of infusion every three, four, six, or eight hours) were employed, the action of digitalis set in gradually and slowly,—not the copious diuresis of large doses. The slight diminution of urine and slowing of the pulse that happened when saturation commenced were scarcely noticed,—they were suddenly brought face to face with the rapid and more or less irregular cardiac action of digitalis poisoning. This poisonous action of digitalis was more likely to follow the giving of small doses for more or less prolonged intervals than the large full doses formerly recommended. There was no difficulty in avoiding the danger of saturation, for as soon as sickness or nausea set in, or even rapid, irregular action of the heart,—he did not consider slowing of the pulse a thing of any great consequence: that generally occurred early in treatment,—all they required to do was to keep the patient recumbent, and in the course of twelve hours he was all right again. Slowness of the pulse might continue for a very much longer period. He had seen a patient who swallowed a whole ounce of the tincture, and the only result was a pulse of 40 for a week. Digitalis in pretty full doses not only caused contraction, but kept the heart contracted, if given in sufficient quantity, and this was important in those cases of aortic regurgitation where compensation failed. In all cases of cardiac disease, they must remember that compensation was for ever failing,—there was no such thing as perfect compensation. From the very commencement of regurgitation or obstruction, heart failure commenced; and it was well in all these cases to take time by the forelock, to be forewarned by results, and use cardiac tonics of proper character to feed the heart and tone it up, and thus postpone the occurrence of serious symptoms, and sometimes prevent them altogether. In all classes of cases this held,—even in mitral stenosis. In mitral stenosis very often the heart presented no symptoms of any consequence. Sooner or later, after over-exertion or a bad cold, they had a slight amount of cardiac failure. Then it was desirable to commence, and continue more or less ever afterwards, the use of cardiac tonics of some kind or other. Digitalis was not always requisite, but strychnia or arsenic were more usually the kind of tonics that were of greatest use in such circumstances. When they had free regurgitation either from mitral or aortic valve, it was of great importance not only to use tonic doses to tone and strengthen the heart, but to use contractile doses to contract the cavity and prevent dilatation. This was specially true in aortic regurgitation, where, from the hydraulic laws which governed the circulation, they had a column of blood by its weight more or less rapidly dilating the ventricle, it was important, for the patient's comfort, to contract the heart at once, and thus relieve more urgent symptoms. Get the patient laid down, and some of the hydraulic pressure was at once removed and the patient made more comfortable. No doubt by the use of morphia they could quiet the heart and enable the patient to lie down; but this was done at a certain amount of risk. Morphia had no effect in strengthening the heart, and none in contracting it. By teaspoonful doses of the tincture, or ounce doses of the strong infusion, or 10 grs. of the powder, they got the heart, after a few doses, contracted, firmed, toned, and strengthened, so that it resisted the evil effects of the hydraulic pressure; after a time they were enabled to diminish these doses, and to continue the tonic action by giving the drug more moderately. Of course, in all those cases where they had obstruction in front in the shape of diseased arteries that had lost tone and acted as an obstruction, they must be careful to secure that the blood-flow into the veins was as perfect as possible. Otherwise they put an already weakened and partly dilated heart in the position of being between the devil and the deep sea. It might become irritable and irregular in consequence of being thrown into a state of strain or exertion for which it was unfit. They could always manage this by employing some of the vascular stimulants which had been referred to. He preferred iodide of potassium, because he found it efficacious. He found it answered the purpose, and he concluded that it acted as he believed, given along with infusion of digitalis in those cases in which digitalis alone throws the heart into an irritable and often irregular condition, and made the patient uncomfortable. In doses of 2 or 3 grs., iodide quieted the action of the heart and soothed it, and the reasonable deduction was that it prevented the action of digitalis on the arterioles, and allowed the blood to pass more readily into the veins. It was therefore extremely advantageous in all such cases. Nitrites and some other drugs had a similar effect. But the action of iodide was more permanent, and answered the purpose better. A dose of the iodide allowed the free passage of the blood for about eight or twelve hours. Other drugs acted more rapidly, but not for so long,— e.g., nitro-glycerine, which did not act, in full doses, longer than from four to five hours, and the nitrites had even a less permanent action. Iodide given in moderate doses dilated the arterioles and reduced blood-pressure, and this was its apparent mode of action in the treatment of aneurism. They saw the pulsation diminishing and the sac to a certain extent slowly contracting. Up to a certain dose the heart slowed, and remained steady. But if the dose of the iodide was increased beyond this, they had blood-pressure apparently falling too low, and thereupon the heart's rate rose, and all the benefit from the use of the iodide was lost.   At first, when he employed iodide for aneurism he did not know this action on the arterioles, and he was tempted to give it in large doses, thinking it had an action on the sac and its coverings ; but he found that the patients took a very long time to get better.   He had known patients remain in bed for more than a year.   Afterwards, when he adopted the idea that the iodide lowered blood-pressure by unlocking arterioles, he put the patient to bed, took the recumbent pulse-rate, and by gradually increasing the dose of the iodide until the pulse began to rise, he got the exact dose necessary to dilate the arterioles and enable the sac to contract. In two months' time he had seen large aneurisms quite contracted and the patients comfortable.   They did not get all the benefit they would ultimately obtain in two months' time, but sufficient to enable them to move about out of bed.   He had had one patient with an aneurism in the posterior mediastinum on the left side. She had been treated for many a long day by many drugs of no consequence,—at least with no result.   The consequence was that the aneurism ate into the spinal column, pressed on the cord, and produced violent nerve storms down the left side of the body from crown to sole.   By long-continued perseverance with iodide in moderate doses, she had now got rid of her nervous symptoms, could move about, and for the last four or five years had been comparatively well, although the aneurism still pulsated.   Before sitting down he might say that, with regard to the treatment of cardiac disease of all kinds, it was of extreme importance, first of all, to make an accurate diagnosis.   He supposed there was no one in that room who could not diagnose an ordinary valvular murmur. These constituted the great bulk of cases they saw in the wards of a hospital, but did not constitute the bulk of the cases seen outside. There they had every variety of cardiac disease and symptom, and it was of the utmost importance, if they were to do any good to the patient at all, to make a very accurate diagnosis of what the affection was of which the patient complained, and then to discover, as far as possible, the cause upon which that affection depended, and, finally, to select their remedy for the removal of that cause or the prevention of its action, in whatever way might seem to be best. Neither digitalis nor strophanthus was always necessary for the treatment of cardiac disease ; and there were many other remedies which they scarcely regarded as cardiac remedies at all which came to be of very great service.   Take one symptom,—palpitation. What did patients mean by it ?   Why, palpitation meant half a dozen different things.   Each required different treatment and different drugs.

Prof. Sir Thomas Grainger Stewart said he counted it a great privilege that he had had an opportunity of hearing these admirable addresses on the treatment of cardiac diseases from the distinguished masters of our school, who had each in his own way contributed so much towards our knowledge of that subject. Every member must have been gratified with the opportunity of hearing a deliberate statement with regard to the general principles and lines of practice. It was also agreeable to find that, to a large extent, their experience corresponded with his own. He thought he could verify a large proportion of the statements that each of the speakers had made. As to their differing, he did not think they were fundamentally different in general line of treatment, although one of them was so convinced of the worth of that invaluable friend digitalis, and another thought strophanthus in his hands so powerful. He had very little to add to what had been said on the department of cardiac therapeutics that had been selected for discussion, except this. He was, like Dr Balfour, more successful with digitalis than with strophanthus. He believed that, probably, to a large extent that was to be explained by the fact that most of us probably worked with an inferior article to that which Prof. Fraser prepared and used; otherwise they should probably have results as good as his. He should accept that as the whole explanation, were it not for another thing. According to his experience, there was one particular in which strophanthus surpassed digitalis —that was, for meeting an emergency. He found that in an extreme case of cardiac failure strophanthus helped more than digitalis, although for ordinary work-a-day heart troubles digitalis was his best friend. In addition to those considerations mentioned by Prof. Fraser forbidding the use of the cardiac tonic group, they had no doubt he held the same view as to the great importance of not using cardiac tonics if there were very active changes going on in the valves. He never liked, even in cases where the heart muscle was growing very feeble, to increase the force of the contraction if the patient had crumbling valves. If he had anything like ulcerative endocarditis, malignant or simple, if he had had a tear of the valve, or if that seemed likely to take place, he avoided cardiac tonics, and rather turned to the other favourite remedy of Dr Balfour, and used iodide of potassium in order to quiet the heart's action and prevent damage to the valve. He believed that in practice that was in certain cases of vital importance. It was important to avoid cardiac tonics if there was anything like acute inflammatory action going on, however feeble the heart might be. One other remark he should like to make was, that indications for cardiac tonics, according to his experience, were precisely those which Prof. Fraser had stated. They should be given wherever the heart muscle is feeble. They could be used then with safety and advantage. He could not understand what anybody could mean by saying that in aortic disease they must not use cardiac tonics. Having referred to Dr Brakenridge's paper on Caffein, and the value of that preparation as a cardiac tonic, he spoke of the great advantage of combining the use of arsenic, strychnine, and, above all, iron with the cardiac stimulants. There was a type of cardiac disease he often saw in hospital, and not unfrequently in private practice too, where anæmia of the brain was the most distressing element,—insomnia, headaches, and all sorts of discomfort attending upon it. Note the value of iron in such cases to combat the anæmic element, not only the actual anæmia, but helping to fill up the arteries better, to nourish the brain better. The last point he wished to make was this. He thought in his practice he attached a great deal more importance than most physicians here did to mechanical relief, aiding the patient by tapping the pleura especially. It was not, of course, to be relied on as the main treatment, but it acted by removing a certain amount of obstruction, and thereby helping the feeble heart. Wherever one found in a case even a limited area of dulness at the base of the lung behind—even 1 in. of dulness—he thought it was a wise plan, if there was much dyspnœa, to put in a needle and see whether there was fluid to be got off. If fluid was got off, very often it happened that by aspiration we could draw off, say 10, 12, 20, or 40 oz., and give most marked relief to respiration at the time, marked relief to the heart always. Many patients had been sent out of the Infirmary during the last twenty years who, so far as he could judge, undoubtedly owed their lives to repeated tappings, along with the use of cardiac tonics. They all knew how disappointments came, sudden failures of the heart occurred. That might happen to their patient at any time; but he must speak in the strongest terms of the value of constantly repeated tapping. The removal of even 6 oz. from the pleura sometimes produced distinct benefit, and if they took more, they got a corresponding improvement. He did not intend to enter upon subjects not dealt with by the previous speakers, and thanked the gentlemen who had spoken for their instructive remarks.

Dr J. O. Affleck said he had very little to add to what Dr Fraser, Dr Balfour, and Sir Thomas Grainger Stewart had said. He had only to express his general concurrence with the statements made. He would have been glad if the discussion had taken a little wider area than the mere comparison of the relative value of two drugs,—if it had included the means of treating symptoms of cardiac disease, such as dyspnœa, insomnia, and many other distressing symptoms. He hoped others would allude to them that night. The value of a discussion of this sort consisted in bringing forward the results of our observations of cardiac disease in practice. Every cardiac case required to be considered by itself. When treatment became indicated by evidence of failing compensation, they very often found that other organs had taken on a diseased action as well as the heart. They had to address themselves to the consideration of this state of matters, and that very condition of the organs so affected might to a large extent interfere with the application of cardiac remedies. The importance of trying to make out, not merely the existence of a valvular lesion, but the actual state of the cardiac wall, lung, kidneys, and liver, was obvious, if they were to deal effectively with the case. With regard to the relative usefulness of digitalis and strophanthus, his own experience had been rather in favour, on the whole, of digitalis; and he thought the profession generally had more confidence in that drug as a cardiac tonic. At the same time, he believed that was, very likely, due to the fact that they had not an opportunity of working with a certain strength of strophanthus. He had been very much impressed with Prof. Fraser's results. He found strophanthus useful in emergencies, as Prof. Grainger Stewart had said. Often, also, it was valuable in cases where digitalis had produced gastric disturbance and other symptoms. In the forefront of all remedies he would place rest, the value of which could not be over-estimated. There were conditions of cardiac disease, however, where exercise was very valuable. Rest in aortic regurgitation, where the heart was acting too rapidly, he had seen produce extraordinary effects where there was risk of dilatation. Diet was also very important. The points alluded to in Dr Balfour's recent book on diet in heart disease were well worth the attention of the profession. It was all very well to administer drugs, but they should attend to hygiene and the patient's general condition. As to dyspnœa, they should note the value of dry cupping over chest and back. He had found marked relief from application of dry cups to the back when there was great pulmonary engorgement. The use of *moderate* bleeding was advocated by one who was the master of many of us—Professor Hughes Bennett. It was one of the few things he would allow bleeding in. Moderate bleeding, then, often gave marked relief. He had used it over and over again,—either leeching the præcordia, or wet-cupping or venesection. They must guard against the production of anæmia, however. He referred to the insomnia of cardiac disease, which was very distressing, and very hurtful to the heart itself. He had used a great many sedatives. He always trusted to a very favourite one, which often gave relief. Equal parts of Liquor morphinæ and Chloric ether, āā ʒss., gave wonderful relief, whether the lesion be mitral or aortic. Paraldehyde also gave very good results; but morphia and chloric ether, or spirit of ether, or some of the diffusible stimulants, produced marked effects. One other point he alluded to: the condition of the heart in acute diseases, as in fever, pneumonia, or any other acute case where danger threatened from the heart. Cardiac danger belonged to some of these diseases—*e.g.*, pneumonia, some of the fevers, to diphtheria, and some other acute diseases. Sometimes it was predisposed to by interference with the temperature at the outset of the case. It was risky to interfere with the temperature at the outset by use of strong antipyretics. He had reason to believe that in not a few instances where antipyretics had been given too liberally at the outset of acute disease, we sent the heart on the down grade. We should watch threatened cardiac failure, also, towards the crisis. It was important to note the cardiac failure that sometimes occurred in delirium tremens. He was in charge of Ward 6 in the Infirmary for several years, and he had seen strong men suddenly collapse in an hour or two, nothing being found to account for death but a dilated heart and congested lungs. Dr Bramwell, who was pathologist at the time, examined not a few cases, where they found absolutely nothing to account for death but this condition of the heart. In cases of that kind we should carefully watch the heart, and, if necessary, administer cardiac tonics from the beginning. It was well known that digitalis had been used as a remedy for delirium tremens in large doses. Without going the length of these doses, it was well to remember the toxic action of alcohol on the cardiac branches of the vagus, and to direct our treatment, if need be, to this condition.

Dr C. E. Underhill said those who had practised much among children saw the beginning of many heart cases, and had therefore an opportunity of checking the advance of the disease, and possibly preventing serious results. He had seen principally two forms of heart trouble in the young; one which was common in connexion with rheumatism, and possibly also with influenza, a disease which was connected with rhematism, which was organic and lasting. He had seen in children approaching adult life another form of heart trouble, not connected, he believed, with anæmia to a marked extent, which was curable. As regarded the rheumatic form, he believed almost all the cases of heart disease arising in later life were rheumatic in origin. The onset of rheumatism in a young child is very insidious, the pain slight, the fever trifling. Mothers and nurses called them growing pains very frequently. He was very pleased to hear Dr Balfour and Prof. Fraser express an opinion on the value of rest, because he was quite certain that the best treatment of these cases in the young was prolonged rest in bed and the greatest care. He meant rest not for a few days or a few weeks, but for months or years. He was quite certain that if they carried out this, they did more to save the child from subsequent troubles than by any use of drugs whatever, and if they did not carefully watch this they might fail, with the best of therapeutic treatment, in saving the patient. He had a lamentable instance of this which occurred some years ago. The child had the slightest amount of fever, with growing pains, and just a suspicion of impurity in the first sound. He saw the child two or three times, and told the mother there was a suspicion of impending rheumatism. She was evidently of opinion that the pains were of no importance. He was told not to call until sent for. About six weeks later he was sent for. The child had gone about in the meantime, had fallen down in a fit of dyspnœa when running upstairs, got blue in the face, and very nearly died. The heart was dilated, there was a loud mitral murmur, and in six months the child was dead. Not only must the patient rest until the symptoms had disappeared and compensation was established, but great care must be exercised against any violent exertion. The young heart was a delicate organ, and had to develop and grow. It was easily distended and easily dilated, and they must put as little strain as possible on it, by reducing strain of circulation to a minimum. They might allow the patient to walk, but not to run upstairs or play violent games. In addition to rest they required to see that ordinary nutrition was carefully carried out. He believed in such drugs as iron and arsenic in the treatment of the young, and hitherto he had almost always employed digitalis as a heart tonic. He had not had much opportunity of using strophanthus. It was best to use the drugs they were accustomed to if they answered the purpose. There was another form of heart trouble, namely, weakening of the heart in growing boys and girls about the age of puberty. He believed it was due very largely to overstrain of mental or physical work during the time of rapid growth. A boy was brought to them, and they found a soft blowing mitral murmur. No history of rheumatism, and no disease about him. Perhaps he was anæmic and rather feeble. That case also required a modified form of rest, and the patient must avoid the strain of competitive athletics. He was quite sure that compulsory games and races now and then seriously damaged the hearts of growing boys. Allow them, however, to walk about, and in course of time they got quite well, but it might take months or years. These were cases which required a great deal of attention. One point in Prof. Fraser's address he should like to notice,—i.e., the value put on opium in cases of angina. One risk in the use of opium for angina in elderly people was that the case might be of a gouty character, and complicated with gouty disease of the kidneys. An old lady sent for the speaker in a hurry. She had had some anginous attacks. She had run upstairs, and on coming down had a violent attack of pain. She was ordered opium pills, with the result that she became, not comatose, but slightly delirious, and died in a few hours. Only after she had taken the pills was it discovered that she had had a great deal of albumen in her urine. Another case seen last year was that of a young man—generally speaking, in excellent health—who had a severe attack of angina. He had had one or two before. He said morphia had done him good. Morphia was injected and he got well. This case puzzled him much; nothing was found wrong with the heart or lungs, but it was discovered that he smoked a great deal of very strong tobacco. When the tobacco was cut short he had no more attacks. Dr Underhill had been much impressed by the excellent addresses they had had from their seniors.

Dr T. R. Ronaldson remarked that he found his views with regard to the treatment of cardiac disease had altered much from the experience of the past years. Though in suitable cases the direct cardiac tonics were needful, there was a large field for helping the heart by shielding it from direct and reflex nervous disturbances, and by making its work in various ways easier. As an example, he narrated the case of a lady with cirrhotic Bright and secondary heart affection, who with absolute certainty brought on an attack of cardiac asthma if she indulged in late supper. The same patient afforded an example of how the heart could be helped by its work being made easier. At one time she required a cardiac tonic; digitalis was prescribed, and she improved. When seen again, however, after some weeks, the pulse had become of very high tension, and the heart thumping, and there was great general discomfort. On stopping the digitalis and substituting nitro-glycerine, marked improvement set in. The keeping of her arteries dilated, and thereby lightening the work of the heart, made all the difference between an uncomfortable and a comfortable existence, with the prospect of some prolongation of life. A second case was narrated where diminution in obesity, the result of thyroid extract administered for psoriasis, produced the greatest benefit in a case of cardiac dilatation. Other examples of the importance of keeping in mind the principle of relieving cardiac disease by diminishing the work of the heart were given. The speaker advised great care of all pulmonary catarrhs, strict attention to diet with regard to the kind of food, the frequency of meals, the hour of the last daily meal, and the amount of fluid drunk, the quantity of alcohol and tobacco allowed, and the condition of the liver and bowels, all being important either in the way of removing disturbing influences or of easing the heart's work. With regard to the direct cardiac tonics, he preferred digitalis, though strophanthus had frequently proved useful. He thought if we could get good strophanthus it would take the place of digitalis to a great extent, as it did not tighten up the arterioles, but had a powerful tonic effect on the heart itself.

Dr John Moir remarked that much had been properly said by former speakers as to the necessity of lightening the work of the heart and removing all obstruction to its free working. No notice, however, had been taken of œdema of the lower extremities,—a very serious complication in many cases. Very many years ago he had begun to suffer from slight irregularity of the heart's action. About ten years ago these became aggravated, accompanied by slight œdema of feet and ankles. He then began to bandage his legs up to the knees with Dummette or thin flannel bandages every morning before getting out of bed—taking them off on retiring to rest. This he had continued regularly all these years up to the present day, and felt satisfied that it had been a great relief to him —chiefly by facilitating the heart's action. He believed that practitioners would find it a great relief to their patients, if resorted to early, and faithfully and carefully carried out.

On the motion of *Dr Young* the discussion was adjourned.

Meeting VI.—February 20, 1895.

Dr CLOUSTON, *President, in the Chair.*

DISCUSSION ON CARDIAC THERAPEUTICS—*Continued.*

Dr Byrom Bramwell continued the Discussion by reading the following paper on TREATMENT OF THE DISEASES OF THE HEART :—

MR PRESIDENT AND GENTLEMEN,—The subject selected for this discussion—the treatment of the diseases of the heart—is so extensive that it is impossible for any individual speaker to attempt to consider it fully and adequately in all its details.

In his introductory address, to which I need not say I listened with the greatest pleasure and profit, Prof. Fraser chiefly limited himself to the consideration of the digitalis group of remedies, and to the treatment of cases of cardiac valvular disease after the breakdown of compensation. That, no doubt, is the period during which active drug treatment is most required, and digitalis and strophanthus are without doubt the remedies which, under such circumstances, are best fitted to tone up the enfeebled and failing heart. But, after all, that is only one, though a very important, part of the subject. I wish that the time at his disposal had permitted Prof. Fraser to have considered in the same able, thorough, and truly scientific manner the many other and no less important parts of the subject. I am sure that every member of the Society will agree with me when I say that we would have liked to have heard his opinion as to the value of the many other drug remedies and means of treatment which we are in the habit of employing in the treatment of cases of heart disease.

In the remarks which I am about to make, I propose, in the first place, to consider some of the general principles which I am in the habit of taking as my guide in the treatment of cases of heart disease ; and, in the second place, to refer, so far as the time at my disposal will allow, to the remedies and means of treatment which I find most serviceable in practice.

I will premise what I have to say by endorsing Dr Balfour's statement, that the first essential for the successful treatment of every case of heart disease is a correct diagnosis. And by a correct diagnosis I mean as exact an opinion as the circumstances of each individual case will allow of—(1.) The nature, severity, and extent of the lesion, and whether it is progressive or stationary ; (2), the condition of the cardiac muscle ; (3), the condition of the arteries ; (4), the condition of the tissues and organs as a whole ; and (5), the special peculiarities and surroundings of each individual patient.

The condition of the cardiac muscle is the key to cardiac therapeutics. And this statement applies not only to those diseases in which the myocardium is the primary seat of the lesion, but to almost every form and kind of *heart* disease. Every one will, I suppose, allow that in most cases of cardiac disease (I do not, of course, include aneurisms of the aorta or large bloodvessels) the condition of the heart muscle is of far greater importance than the condition of the valves. It is unnecessary to say that murmurs are very deceptive guides, and the man who prescribes digitalis or strophanthus in a routine way simply because a loud cardiac murmur or a cardiac valvular lesion is present, is anything but a judicious and reliable practitioner.

The determination of the exact condition of the cardiac muscle is in many cases one of the most difficult problems in the whole range of diagnosis. In trying to arrive at a correct conclusion on this most difficult but most important point, two sets of facts have to be taken into account.

In the *first* place, we must endeavour to form an opinion as to the exact condition of the heart muscle by observing—(*a*), the size of the heart; (*b*), whether hypertrophy or dilatation is predominant; (*c*), the way in which the heart is acting and contracting, whether forcibly, irregularly, and the like; (*d*), the condition of the peripheral, arterial, venous, and capillary circulations; (*e*), the way in which the circulation is carried on, as indicated by the presence or absence of symptoms indicative of cardiac embarrassment or distress (dyspnœa, palpitation, cardiac pain, etc.), not only during rest, but also under strain, and under conditions which put the heart muscle, as it were, on its mettle; and (*f*), the way in which the heart muscle responds to tonic remedies.

I lay special stress upon the two latter points, for the amount of reserve force which the heart muscle possesses—an all-important point for the purposes of successful treatment—can in many cases only be determined by observing the way in which the heart acts under strain and difficulty, and by noting the way in which it responds to such remedies as digitalis and strophanthus.

In the *second* place, we have to observe the state of the organism as a whole, and in particular whether the conditions for the nutrition of the cardiac muscle are satisfactory or not. And in this connexion it is particularly important to note the condition of— (1), the blood; (2), the aorta and the peripheral arteries (for the condition of the aorta and peripheral vessels in many cases gives us a clue—and it is often the only certain clue—to the condition of the coronary arteries,—the nutrient arteries of the heart); (3), the stomach, liver, and digestive organs; (4), the intestine; (5), the kidneys; and (6), the nervous system.

I need not add that the condition of the lungs is also of importance, since emphysematous and other pulmonary lesions which impede the blood-flow through the lungs throw a strain on the right heart, the activity of which is, in the case of mitral lesions, of so much importance for satisfactory compensation.

Further, the natural disposition and temperament of the patient
—whether he is hopeful or gloomy, whether he is a good or
bad patient, together with his social circumstances and surroundings, his ability and willingness to do what he is told, and
to protect himself from injurious conditions—must be taken into
account.

Every one who has had much experience in the treatment of
cardiac diseases will admit that each and every one of these points
may be of great importance in the treatment of individual cases,
and that in many cases of heart disease the success of the treatment depends quite as much upon the careful regulation of the
whole mode of life of the individual, and upon attention to the
minute, but none the less important, details of every-day life (diet,
rest, exercise, and the like), as upon the administration of drug
remedies—necessary and all-important as drug remedies in many
cases are.

The paramount importance of the condition of the heart muscle
and of the many different factors which go to form the personal
equation of each individual patient, as it may be termed, is clearly
demonstrated by the different results which the same diseased conditions produce in different individuals.

Every now and again, for example, we see patients with marked
valvular lesions, and in some cases with large hearts (the enlargement, of course, showing that the valvular lesion is a severe one),
living for many years in comparative comfort, able not only to
enjoy life, but to lead useful, busy, and it may even be active lives.
In cases of this kind the disease may go on for twenty, thirty, or
even forty years,—until, in fact, senile and degenerative changes
begin to interfere with the compensatory changes, or until the
progress of the disease is interrupted by the development of some
acute complication or intercurrent affection. If time had permitted, I would have liked to have given you the details of some
striking cases of this kind which have come under my own
notice.

On the other hand, we more frequently see cases in which, with the
same or even less severe valvular lesions, all the well-known symptoms of grave cardiac disease are rapidly developed, and in which,
notwithstanding our best efforts, death takes place at a comparatively early stage of the case.

Now, the explanation of the very different course which the
disease pursues in these two classes of cases is usually to be found
in the condition of the cardiac muscle, or in some one or other of
the factors which go to form what I have already termed the
personal equation. In the cases which survive and do well it will
usually be found either that the lesion, though perhaps considerable, is stationary and inactive; that the heart muscle is sound;
that the tissues and organs are healthy, and the conditions for the
nutrition of the heart muscle are satisfactory; that the circumstances

and surroundings of the patients are good; that the patients are of an equable, placid mental temperament; or that they inherit longevity, or, to put it in another way, that they do not inherit a tendency to premature arterial degeneration and decay. And *vice versâ*, in the cases which do badly, that the reverse conditions or some of them are present.

It is needless to say that tissue degeneration of any kind, and especially arterial degeneration, exerts a very deleterious influence on the course of cases of heart disease, and heavily handicaps the efforts of the physician. In this connexion I attach special importance to excessive and long-continued muscular strain, syphilis, alcohol, and gout,—the chief causes (leaving hereditary predisposition out of account) of premature arterial degeneration and decay. The age of an individual should, as Sir James Paget has well remarked, be measured not by the number of the years he has lived, but by the condition of his arteries.

Again, as more than one of the speakers has already pointed out, the all-important influence of the cardiac muscle is strikingly demonstrated by observing the effects of acute disease, such as pneumonia or influenza, in different individuals.

In old people, even a limited croupous pneumonia, which in young persons whose hearts are healthy would almost certainly be recovered from, is often fatal. In the observation of cases of pneumonia in old people, nothing has impressed me more than the fact, that in many cases in which the disease pursues a perfectly satisfactory course for several days without any urgent or alarming symptom, rapid failure of the heart and collapse—I do not, of course, refer to "critical" collapse—are suddenly developed without any extension of the lesion or other apparent cause, and that under such circumstances, notwithstanding the free exhibition of cardiac tonics and stimulants, the disease almost certainly proves fatal. The observation is of the greatest practical importance. In cases of this kind, cardiac tonics and stimulants are, in my experience, of very little value once the heart has collapsed before the strain. The main object of treatment should be to prevent the cardiac failure by the steady administration of cardiac tonics and stimulants (such as oxygen inhalations, strychnine, digitalis, and strophanthus) during the earlier stages and throughout the whole course of the attack.

Again, we sometimes see death resulting from a limited croupous pneumonia in young persons whose hearts are degenerated or diseased. During the past three or four years I have seen more than one case in which a limited influenzal pneumonia in a chlorotic girl has proved fatal, notwithstanding the most vigorous and energetic treatment, solely owing, I believe, to the fatty and debilitated condition of the heart.

I repeat that the condition of the cardiac muscle and the personal equation as a whole, more particularly the state of the

arterial system and of the kidneys, are the key to cardiac therapeutics, and the only basis on which an intelligent treatment of
cases of heart disease can be satisfactorily founded; and I
emphasize the importance, on the one hand, of exact and minute
diagnosis as regards the cardiac lesion which happens to be
present, and particularly as regards the state of the heart muscle;
and on the other, the importance of taking a broad and compre-
hensive view of the individual peculiarities of each patient and of
all the factors which I include under the term, the personal
equation.

Let us now turn to the consideration of some of the individual
forms of cardiac derangement and disease.

Neurotic, Functional, and Curable Conditions.—In the
purely functional cases in which the cardiac disturbance is usually
neurotic, due to some debilitating condition (such as sexual
excess), or to a toxic cause (such as excessive tea-drinking,
excessive tobacco-smoking, etc.), and in the so-called functional
cases in which structural changes of a removable and curable
kind are present (such as the fatty degeneration of chlorosis), the
essential objects of treatment are:—

1. *To remove the cause.*—In some of the neurotic cases it is
often difficult to ascertain the cause, and in many cases it is only
by a process of therapeutic exclusion and negation (eliminating
first one thing and then another, say, from the dietary) that we
are able to obtain a satisfactory therapeutic result.

2. *To correct by appropriate treatment any deranged or abnormal
condition which appears to be present in the heart or in any of the
other organs.*—When, for example, the patient is anæmic, the
treatment of the anæmia is the first essential. When the gastro-
intestinal functions are deranged or imperfectly performed, the
correction of such derangements is necessary.

3. *To carefully regulate the whole mode of life of the individual,*
even to the most minute details of diet and regimen, fresh air,
exercise, clothing, and the like.

4. *To reassure the patient as to the functional and curable nature
of the condition, and as to the absence of organic disease.*—I attach
great importance to what I term mental therapeutics, not only in
neurotic and so-called functional cases, but in many organic
conditions affecting the heart and other organs of the body. We
are, perhaps, only too apt to forget that in many cases of organic
disease functional disturbances and structural changes of a
curable kind are present as well as the organic and incurable
lesions. In dealing with cases of organic disease of the heart,
complicated with a neurotic or functional derangement, or with a
structural change of a curable kind in the cardiac muscle, the same
measures of treatment which are appropriate for the purely
neurotic and so-called functional cases are, of course, indicated.

5. *To administer remedies calculated to soothe the irritable heart*

and to tone it up when it is in condition—as it often is, more especially in the anæmic cases—*of irritable weakness.*

The remedial measures which I chiefly employ in these functional and curable cases are:—The emphatic and confident expression of a favourable opinion; the application of a belladonna plaster to the præcordium; the internal administration of hydrobromic acid or bromide of potassium, together with strychnine or nux vomica; and the administration of iron and arsenic. In some of the cases included under this group, but rarely in the anæmic cases, I have seen decided benefit from the administration of small doses of digitalis or strophanthus in combination with or without bromide of potassium.

Organic Lesions.

(1.) **Very severe Acute Lesions.**—Passing now to the more important organic diseases, we find that in some cases the lesion is acute, or that an acute lesion is developed in the course of a pre-existing chronic disease. In the more severe and aggravated cases of this kind—but they are fortunately, comparatively speaking, rare—such as rupture of the heart itself, rupture of an aneurism of the aorta, rupture of a valve segment, cases of ulcerative endocarditis, and the most severe forms of rheumatic endo-pericarditis and myocarditis, treatment is of no avail, or of comparatively little use. I need not refer to the treatment of these cases further.

(2.) **Less severe Acute Lesions.**—In other cases in which the lesion is acute but less severe—and we may take as the type of this form of heart disease acute simple rheumatic endocarditis—I am of opinion that a great deal can be done by appropriate treatment to limit the severity of the morbid process and to prevent the development of grave permanent damage. I listened to Dr Underhill's remarks on this point with the greatest satisfaction; they are entirely in accord with my own observations, and represent my own teaching. In lecturing on acute rheumatic endocarditis, I have for many years emphasized the great importance of long-continued rest. I am in the habit of telling my students that if they would cover a page of their note-books with nothing but the word "rest," they would not be placing too much emphasis on this most important means of treatment; and that if they went away from that lecture having learned nothing more than the all-important influence of rest in the treatment of acute rheumatic endocarditis, I would be quite content.

To show the important influence which rest has on the course of acute endocarditis, I am in the habit of asking why the valves of the left heart are so much more frequently affected with endocarditis than those of the right; why the mitral valve is affected so much more frequently than the aortic; and why, when the right heart (tricuspid valve) is affected, the endocarditis so comparatively seldom leads to the production of permanent organic disease (*i.e.*, tricuspid stenosis). So far as I know, the only satisfactory answer to these questions is found in the supposition that the valves of the left heart are subjected to greater strain than those of the right heart, and that the mitral segments are subjected to greater strain than the aortic cusps.

In treating cases of acute endocarditis, our object should be to imitate Nature,—to remove, so far as possible, valvular strain; and the only method of preventing valvular strain is rest, continued not only during the acute stage of the disease and during subsequent convalescence, but in a modified form for many months or even years afterwards. The same remarks apply to the treatment of choreic and other forms of acute simple endocarditis.

But here let me say that, while recognising the great importance of rest and of removing, so far as is possible, valvular strain, it is essential to keep the heart muscle in a satisfactory and healthy state of nutrition. When the heart muscle is debilitated or fatty, a condition of irritable weakness is produced. Under such circumstances the heart is easily excited, and in consequence of the general debility and loss of nerve tone, there is in many cases also impaired nervous (vagus) control. Under such circumstances—I refer more particularly to the period of convalescence after an attack of acute rheumatism—it is not enough to keep the patient at rest in bed and to avoid all causes of bodily and mental excitement; it is essential at the same time to administer remedies which are calculated to remove the irritable weakness of the cardiac muscle, to attend to the state of the general health, and to improve the nerve tone.

The nutrition of the patient should be maintained by appropriate feeding; the condition of the gastro-intestinal, hepatic, and renal functions must be carefully regulated, and general and cardiac tonics, such as quinine, strychnine, arsenic, and iron, should be administered. Iron is especially indicated when the patient is anæmic, and when there is reason to suppose that the heart muscle is fatty in consequence of a deficiency of hæmoglobin. When the patient is a medical man or a medical student, and especially if he happens to be of a nervous and anxious temperament, I attach some importance to allaying, so far as the circumstances of the case will allow, his fears as to the subsequent development of a permanent organic lesion. I need not add that after an attack of acute rheumatism or rheumatic endocarditis, the patient should be urgently advised to protect himself so far as is possible against everything which is likely to produce a relapse of the rheumatic condition.

In those cases of acute endocarditis in which the lesion is severe and in which grave symptoms indicative of failure of the heart or of embarrassment of the circulation are developed, it is, of course, necessary to give cardiac tonics and stimulants (digitalis, strophanthus, etc.).

(3.) Cases of Chronic and Incurable Valvular Disease.—
A third group includes those cases in which the lesion is chronic and the heart permanently damaged, say, by a valvular defect which is incurable and irremovable. It is unnecessary to say that the cases included in this group present the greatest differences in detail.

In the treatment of those cases in which the compensatory changes are satisfactory, and in which there are no urgent symptoms, it is essential to endeavour to follow Nature's indications as we learn them by the observation of cases of long duration, such as those to which I have previously referred. The more important points are:—

1. *To prevent cardiac strain, and to avoid everything which is likely to embarrass the damaged heart and to aggravate or lead to fresh activity in the lesion.*

It is important to remember that cardiac strain may be due to two classes of causes, viz.—(*a*), external causes, such as muscular over-exertion; and (*b*), internal causes, such as a gouty condition with high arterial tension. One of the chief difficulties which we meet with in treating cases of cardiac disease in the labouring classes is the impossibility in many cases of their avoiding muscular strain, and in the upper classes their inability to prevent the development of the gouty condition, or their unwillingness to avoid the conditions which produce gout and high blood-pressure.

One occasionally meets with cases in which cardiac valvular lesions seem to be entirely due to muscular over-exertion, and in which the removal of the cause is attended with the happiest results. The following is a case in point:—

Some years ago a medical man, aged 40, consulted me on account of swelling of the feet, shortness of breath on exertion, and other symptoms of heart disease. A loud and long systolic murmur was present at the apex, the left ventricle was markedly enlarged, and the apex beat was well out in the axilla. The patient was perfectly healthy in other respects. He had never suffered from rheumatism. He was not gouty. He attributed his cardiac lesion to muscular overstrain; he was in the habit of riding a bicycle, and of ascending several times a day on his bicycle a long and steep hill, on the top of which his house was situated. He was advised to give up his bicycle, to avoid over-exertion of all kinds, to take strychnine and arsenic alternately with digitalis, and to attend to the condition of the bowels and kidneys. Under this treatment the symptoms gradually but slowly disappeared. When I last examined him, several years after he first consulted me, the heart was practically normal. The condition of his heart is now so satisfactory that his life has recently been accepted by one of our leading insurance companies, the premium being slightly "loaded" on account of the previous cardiac illness.

Cases such as this, which seem to show that excessive muscular exertion can produce a cardiac valvular lesion, and that the removal of the cardiac strain which muscular over-exertion causes can result in the cure of the disease, bring home to one's mind most forcibly the importance of avoiding over-exertion and cardiac strain in those cases in which the heart is organically and permanently damaged.

In this connexion I may remark, that in some cases of mitral stenosis violent palpitation and sudden and excessive action of the heart are attended with a special danger. In many cases of mitral stenosis in which the lesion appears to be well or perfectly compensated, the left auricular appendix is filled with clot. In more than one case of this kind I have known a hemiplegia developed immediately after an attack of palpitation or violent cardiac action, which presumably caused embolic plugging of the middle cerebral artery by detachment (breaking off) of a portion of the clot.

High blood-pressure and obstruction in front are, in the well-to-do classes at all events, a more important cause of cardiac strain than muscular over-exertion ; for, arising as they so often do from a gouty condition and independently of any obvious external causes, they are much more likely to escape observation, and consequently much more difficult to prevent and remove. And it must be remembered that the relief of high arterial tension is not only of importance in the treatment of cardiac disease after it is developed, but also in the prevention of cardiac degeneration and disease. The late Dr Mahomed directed attention to the fact that a condition of long-continued high blood-pressure is apt to precede the development of cirrhosis of the kidney, and that in some cases it is possible, by appropriate (anti-gouty) treatment, to prevent the development of the arterial and cardiac lesions which the high blood-pressure and continued cardiac strain would, if they continued, eventually produce.

2. *To keep the heart muscle in the highest possible state of health and efficiency.*—In order to carry out this indication it is important to attend to the condition of the digestive and excretory organs (intestines, liver, kidney, skin), and to carefully and judiciously regulate the whole mode of life of the patient. In cases of this kind attention to the minute details of every-day life (diet, exercise, clothing, sleep, alcohol, tobacco, tea, etc.) is all-essential.[1]

3. *To carefully protect the patient against everything which is likely to exert an injurious influence upon the heart,*—such, for example, as bronchitis and rheumatism.

In cases of chronic valvular disease in which the lesion is slight or stationary, in which the heart muscle is healthy and the tissues and organs sound,—in other words, in cases of valvular lesions during the stage of good compensation, the measures which have just been recommended, with, perhaps, the occasional administration

---

[1] These and some of the other points to which I have directed attention are by some considered trivial and commonplace. In my opinion they are all-important. I know from actual experience gained both in consulting and general practice,—firstly, that they are often ignored in practice ; and, secondly, that in many cases of cardiac disease the success of treatment depends far more upon minute attention to these so-called trivial details than upon anything else.

of such remedies as arsenic, strychnine, and iron, are all that are required.

I am of opinion that so long as the compensation is well maintained the administration of the more powerful cardiac tonics, such as digitalis or strophanthus, is not only unnecessary, but in many cases inadvisable and often harmful.

Temporary Breakdowns of Compensation.—But it must be remembered that in cases of this kind, in which the lesion is, under ordinary circumstances, perfectly or almost perfectly compensated, acute embarrassment and failure of the heart may be produced by undue effort, excessive strain, or the development of some intercurrent complication. In chronic mitral lesions, for example, an acute attack of bronchitis, which throws an increased strain on the right heart, is frequently attended with the rapid development of grave and serious symptoms (marked shortness of breath, œdema of the feet, etc.). Under such circumstances, the bronchitis must, of course, be treated by appropriate remedies; but an all-important point is to aid the enfeebled right heart, by the administration of cardiac tonics and stimulants (digitalis, strophanthus, strychnine, alcohol, etc.); and if it is greatly engorged, to relieve the strain by venesection. In cases of chronic valvular disease in which acute pulmonary lesions with failure of the heart are developed, I have found the greatest benefit from oxygen inhalations, subcutaneous injections of strychnine, and the internal administration of full doses of digitalis or strophanthus. As soon as the compensation is again restored, the digitalis or strophanthus may be altogether discontinued, or given in very much smaller doses, or alternated with such remedies as arsenic, strychnine, and general tonics.

The Treatment of Valvular Lesions after the Breakdown of Compensation.—In another group of valvular lesions the lesion is actively progressive, or so severe that the continued output of more and more compensation is necessitated. In cases of this kind, a time ultimately, and often speedily, arrives when more active and energetic treatment is required. It is now that digitalis and strophanthus are so valuable, in conjunction with other measures calculated to relieve the secondary results and complications which the failure of compensation and the embarrassment of the circulation produce.

Personally, I agree with those who think that there is a difference between the mitral and aortic cases; and I am glad to think, if I understood him aright, that Prof. Fraser is at one with me on this point.

The Treatment of Cardiac Cases of all kinds after the Breakdown of Compensation.—In treating cases of cardiac disease in which symptoms and signs of enfeebled and embarrassed circulation and defective compensation are developed—I refer to all forms of organic change, and not merely to the valvular·

lesions—the treatment has to be guided by the opinion which is formed as to the nature of the lesion and the condition of the heart muscle. Measures which are appropriate in one case may be prejudicial in another. This statement especially applies to rest and exercise on the one hand, and to the administration of cardiac tonics and the form of cardiac tonic on the other. I cannot agree with those who think that digitalis is suitable and equally useful in all cases.

Individual Lesions.—Let me briefly refer to the treatment of some of the forms of cardiac disease to which I have not as yet referred in detail.

Fatty Degeneration due to Deficiency of Hæmoglobin.—In those cases in which the fatty condition of the cardiac muscle is the result of anæmia, it is unnecessary to say that iron or arsenic are by far the most important remedies. In cases of this kind digitalis and strophanthus are, in my opinion, often harmful.

I need not refer to the treatment of the common chlorotic cases; but I would like to say that in older people who have long passed the age of chlorosis it is not uncommon to meet with a condition of long-continued anæmia much more allied to chlorosis than to pernicious anæmia, in which the administration of large doses of iron is attended with the most marked benefit.

A very striking case of this kind came under my notice a few months ago. The details are as follows:—

A married lady, aged 50, who had spent a large part of her life in India, and who had repeatedly suffered from dysentery and malaria, consulted me in March 1894. She had been a confirmed invalid for several years, and for twenty years had every now and again broken down with symptoms of cardiac failure. She had been treated by several physicians with the usual cardiac remedies, including digitalis, and an unfavourable prognosis had been given. She was extremely debilitated, decidedly anæmic, unable, she said, to take iron, and short of breath on exertion; she complained of palpitation and beating of the abdominal aorta on the slightest exertion, and was troubled every now and again with dysenteric diarrhœa. The heart's action was somewhat irregular, a soft systolic murmur was present at the apex, and there was marked pulsation in the epigastrium and over the course of the abdominal aorta. This pulsation was so marked that at one time it was thought she was suffering from an aneurism of the abdominal aorta,—indeed, she had been treated for that disease. The mitral lesion was thought to be organic. After careful examination, I came to the conclusion that there was not sufficient evidence to warrant the diagnosis either of an aneurism of the abdominal aorta or of organic change at the mitral valve. I did not feel so sure, however, as to the condition of the cardiac muscle; it was impossible to definitely exclude the suspicion that there might be some permanent and incurable structural change in the myocardium. Nevertheless, I determined to try more vigorous treatment by iron. Robertson's Blaud's pill capsules were prescribed, and the dose of iron was gradually increased, notwithstanding the protests of the patient that she was unable to take the remedy. An encouraging opinion was also given. Under this treatment slow but steady improvement took place. In the course of five months the patient was so much better that she was able to rejoin her husband in India, and when I last heard of her she was in every way stronger and better than she had been for many years.

p

This case is by no means a solitary one. I have met with several others of the same kind in which the patient has been dosed with digitalis—not only without benefit, but apparently with positive harm—and in which the cardiac symptoms have entirely disappeared under the administration of large doses of iron.

Fatty Degeneration due to Pernicious Anœmia.—In those cases in which fatty changes in the cardiac muscle are the result of pernicious anæmia and conditions allied to pernicious anæmia, there is no remedy in my experience at all equal to arsenic.

Fatty Degeneration due to Disease of the Coronary Arteries.—In the more serious forms of fatty heart due to disease of the coronary arteries—and it is needless to say that in these cases the diagnosis is often attended with the greatest difficulty, and is in many cases impossible—arsenic and strychnine, given either alone or in combination, are, I think, to be preferred to digitalis or strophanthus. I am disposed to think that in cases of this kind digitalis in particular is sometimes harmful.

Fatty Infiltration and Cases of Flabby Heart.—In cases of fatty infiltration and in cases of dilated flabby heart, with or without associated mitral regurgitation, careful regulation of the diet and bowels, plenty of fresh air and carefully regulated exercise, together with arsenic and strychnine, are the remedies which I chiefly employ. In cases of this kind in which there is often a sluggish condition of the circulation, an engorged condition of the peripheral vessels, including the vessels of the myocardium, imperfect action of the liver and kidneys, and it may be dropsy, systematic muscular exercise, such as is afforded by Oertel's plan of treatment,[1] often yields very satisfactory results; but it should always, I think, be carefully, gradually, and judiciously employed, and never recommended in cases in which there is reason to suspect any marked structural changes in the myocardium of a grave, permanent, or irremovable kind.

In these cases, too (dilated and flabby hearts, with resulting mitral disease, in which there are no advanced organic changes in the myocardium), Schott's plan of graduated exercise and bathing seems (from the reports of several independent observers) to be very efficacious, together with a general tonic plan of treatment and the administration of arsenic, strychnine, and, in some cases, of digitalis or strophanthus. In cases of this kind, it is always advisable to proceed cautiously and tentatively, and to watch the effect of the exercise and remedies employed; for it is often difficult or impossible to exclude organic conditions of a more serious kind, such as grave myocardial degenerations due to disease of the coronary arteries.

Cases of Senile Heart and Cases of Mitral Regurgitation with High

---

[1] I always advise patients, at all events in the first instance, to walk on the flat. Hill-climbing, as recommended by Oertel, is often, I think, even in cases of fatty infiltration, injurious or dangerous.

Arterial Tension.—In cases of senile, debilitated, and fatty hearts, and in cases of mitral regurgitation, associated with high blood-pressure and tightly constricted vessels, it is unnecessary to say that the essential objects of treatment are to relieve the cardiac strain by reducing the blood-pressure, and to tone up the feeble heart.

In the treatment of gouty conditions with high arterial tension, but without any obvious cardiac lesions, careful regulation of the diet, the avoidance of red meats and sweets, active exercise, and the internal administration of laxatives or purgatives, of plenty of pure (distilled) water and of salicylate of soda, are the measures which I find most useful.

Where the high blood-pressure of gouty patients is associated with well-marked valvular or myocardial lesions, the same means of treatment are useful, but the quantity of distilled water taken at any one time should be limited, for rapid over-filling of the vessels is to be avoided.

In the gouty cases in which the heart muscle requires stimulation, I usually rely as long as possible on arsenic and strychnine. When it is necessary to give a more powerful cardiac tonic, I prescribe strophanthus in preference to digitalis, since Prof. Fraser claims that it acts chiefly as a cardiac tonic without constricting and tightening up the peripheral arteries. I often also give iodide of potassium, and I think with advantage, in these cases. When it is necessary to administer remedies which produce more active and energetic relaxation of the bloodvessels, I chiefly rely upon nitro-glycerine.

Chronic Myocarditis and Fibroid Degeneration.—In these cases, in which the diagnosis is often attended with the greatest difficulty, rest is, I think, the first essential. Digitalis, arsenic, strychnine, and iodide of potassium are, in my experience, the most useful drug remedies. I have obtained most satisfactory results in some cases in which the blood-pressure was low and the pulse small and feeble by the long-continued administration of digitalis. I am disposed to think that digitalis is more useful in cases of fibroid than in cases of fatty degeneration of the heart. I base this opinion upon the observation of cases treated with digitalis during life and checked by post-mortem examination after death.

Cases of Advanced Valvular Disease with Defective Compensation.—In cases of advanced valvular disease, with a thorough breakdown of the compensation, large doses of digitalis or strophanthus should, of course, be employed. I was much impressed with Prof. Fraser's statement as to the relative activities of the different members of the digitalis group; and also with Prof. Sir Thomas Grainger Stewart's important statement as to the influence of strophanthus in producing rapid stimulation of the heart.

Angina Pectoris.—In the treatment of the more severe and dangerous forms of angina pectoris—*i.e.*, in cases in which there is reason to suspect that the symptom angina is associated with grave structural organic disease, though, as Dr Balfour has pointed out, the structural changes are often of such a nature that it is very difficult, and in some cases impossible to detect them by physical examination during life (disease of the coronary arteries, fatty degeneration, fibroid degeneration, small deep-seated aneurisms, etc.) —it is, of course, essential to guard the patient against sudden exertion, sudden exposure to cold, and other conditions which are likely to throw a sudden strain on the heart, either directly or indirectly, by producing sudden constriction of the peripheral vessels. In those cases of angina pectoris in which the paroxysm is the result of, or attended with, high arterial tension, it is unnecessary to say that nitrite of amyl or nitro-glycerine are the most effective means of treatment. But in those cases in which the angina attacks are not associated with excessive blood-pressure—in cases, for example, in which there is free aortic regurgitation or a soft pulse with advanced degenerative changes in the cardiac muscle—nitrite of amyl or nitro-glycerine are often useless, and in some cases not unattended with danger. In cases of this kind the free administration of diffusible stimulants and subcutaneous injections of morphia are, in my experience, the most efficient remedies.

The Treatment of Symptoms and Secondary Results.— In many of the cases of cardiac disease which I have included in the last group—all forms of cardiac lesion in which compensation is inadequate or broken down—the treatment of the secondary results and complications is, as more than one of the speakers has pointed out, an all-important point.

Secondary derangements and complications in the lungs, stomach, liver, intestinal tract, kidney, brain, subcutaneous tissues and internal cavities, all require careful or active treatment. Some of these derangements are the result of the impaired cardiac power; all of them, when developed, are apt to throw an increased strain on the heart, or to interfere (either directly or indirectly) with the nutrition of its muscular tissue. Time does not permit me to consider the treatment of these secondary results of cardiac disease and complications in detail.

Personal Experience as to the Value of Individual Remedies.—Let me now very briefly sum up my experience as to some of the individual measures and remedies which I have personally found most useful in the treatment of cardiac cases. Time does not permit me to enter into the details of diet, general hygiene, change of scene, etc., though in many cases they are of great importance.

Rest.—In many forms of cardiac disease this is, in my opinion, the most important means of treatment which we possess. Rest (more or less complete or absolute, as the special peculiarities of the different forms of disease and the individual peculiarities of each special case seem to demand) is indicated in the following affections :—Acute endocarditis ; myocardial degenerations of all forms (fatty, fibroid); in all cases in which there is reason to suspect myocarditis, whether acute, subacute, or chronic; pulmonary lesions with an engorged condition of the right heart; aortic regurgitation when the compensation begins to fail; valvular lesions with decided breakdown of compensation; cases of angina pectoris in which there is reason to suspect organic disease; aneurisms of the thoracic aorta and large bloodvessels; and all severe cases of senile degeneration of the heart.

Exercise.—This is a very valuable means of treatment in many cardiac conditions, more particularly in neurotic affections, fatty infiltration, many gouty conditions in which there are no marked degenerative changes and arterial lesions, many valvular lesions so long as the myocardium is fairly healthy, some dilated conditions of the heart in which the dilatation is associated with fatty infiltration, or the result of such conditions as excessive beer-drinking, and in which it is not associated with any marked degree of myocardial degeneration. In many cases of aortic and mitral disease, in the less severe forms of senile heart, and in the slighter forms of myocardial degeneration, judiciously regulated and moderate walking exercise is invaluable, so long as the compensation is well maintained.

By muscular exercise we are enabled to promote the condition of the general health and of the cardiac health, to hasten the circulation through the peripheral organs and through the heart itself, to prevent stasis and engorgement with all their disastrous results. So long as exercise does not produce marked shortness of breath, over-fatigue, or other untoward symptoms, it should, I think, not only be permitted but encouraged.

Graduated and systematic muscular exercise, such as is afforded by *Oertel's plan of treatment,* is chiefly, I think, useful in cases of fatty infiltration, fatty and gouty conditions unassociated with atheroma and without any marked degree of high pressure in the peripheral system of vessels.

Of *Schott's method of treatment* I have no direct personal experience, but from what I have learned from the experience of some patients I am disposed to think that it will be found to be chiefly valuable in the same group of cases (fatty infiltration, flabby hearts, etc.), and in those cases of valvular lesions in which the cardiac muscle is reasonably sound.

Mental Therapeutics.—I attach the greatest importance to sustaining the mental tone of the patient and encouraging him to hope (unless, of course, there is any good reason to the contrary) that the treatment will be attended with success. In many cases of cardiac disease there is, in my experience, no tonic which is more efficacious than a favourable opinion confidently expressed; it is especially valuable in neurotic cases and all forms of functional disease, and in the less severe forms of valvular lesion in which the valvular defects are well compensated, or in which the organic changes in the heart are associated with a nervous and irritable condition.

Iron.—This is an invaluable remedy in those forms of cardiac disease in which there is a deficiency of hæmoglobin. The form of iron which I have found most efficacious is Robertson's Blaud's pill capsules.

Arsenic.—This is a most valuable cardiac remedy. It is especially useful, I think, in cases of myocardial degeneration (fatty and fibroid conditions of the myocardium) and in neurotic cases; it is also most useful in many cases of angina pectoris. It is a most valuable cardiac tonic in many cases of valvular disease in which there has been any decided breakdown of compensation,—particularly, perhaps, in cases of aortic regurgitation.

Strychnine.—This I consider is one of the most useful cardiac remedies which we possess, both for the purpose of producing a sustained tonic effect and more active stimulation. I find it very valuable in many cases of valvular disease before there has been a decided breakdown of compensation, and during temporary breakdowns of compensation in which there are bronchial or other pulmonary complications, more particularly when given subcutaneously in frequently repeated doses, with or without inhalations of oxygen. In the same conditions I often combine it with digitalis or strophanthus.

Digitalis.—This is the cardiac tonic which I most largely use when symptoms indicative of failing compensation are developed, both with the object of producing immediate and temporary effects, tiding the patient over acute complications, and also with the object of permanently sustaining the cardiac power and preventing further breakdowns of compensation. I entirely agree with Prof. Fraser in thinking that it is most useful in mitral lesions, especially mitral regurgitation with dropsy, irregular pulse, scanty condition of the urine, etc. I agree with those who think that it should be given more cautiously and for shorter periods of time in cases of aortic regurgitation, and that in such cases it cannot be expected to produce such satisfactory results as in cases of mitral regurgitation. I need not go into further details, for Prof. Fraser's statement entirely represents my own experience on this subject. Let me, however, say that I think digitalis is not unattended with risk in fatty conditions of the cardiac muscle. I have seen at least one case of fatty degeneration of the heart in which rupture had occurred during a course of digitalis, and in which I was inclined to think that the rupture was the result of the administration of the remedy. I rarely, if ever, give it in chlorotic cases, or in cases in which I have reason to suspect that there is a decided degree of fatty degeneration due to disease of the coronary arteries; on the other hand, I have found it of great use in some cases in which grave cardiac symptoms seemed to be the result of a degenerated condition of the myocardium and in which the degeneration was, so far as I could judge, the result of chronic myocarditis or fibroid degeneration. But I speak with reserve on these points, for, as every one knows, it is often most difficult, and sometimes impossible, to form an opinion as to whether myocardial degeneration is due to fatty degeneration or interstitial changes and chronic myocarditis. Where the pulse tension is high I usually prescribe strophanthus in preference to digitalis. Under such circumstances, if digitalis is given, I agree with Dr Balfour that it should be combined with iodide of potassium, salicylate of soda, or some remedy such as nitro-glycerine, which reduces blood-pressure.

I always give digitalis in the form of tincture or infusion. I never use digitaline granules; I have over and over again seen in consultation decided poisonous symptoms produced as a result of the administration of Nativelle's granules. The more soluble liquid preparations are quite sufficiently powerful for any purpose which is required, and are much more easily handled and managed.

Strophanthus.—I have less experience with this remedy than with digitalis, but I have seen some very brilliant results produced by its use. Guided by Prof. Fraser's observations, I usually prescribe it in preference to digitalis in those cases in which the peripheral arterial pressure is increased. My experience agrees with that of Prof. Sir Grainger Stewart, that it is of great value in those cases in which it is desirable to produce a rapid tonic and stimulating effect. In such cases I often combine it with subcutaneous injections of strychnine, and, in many cases in which there are grave pulmonary and bronchial complications, with inhalations of oxygen. I also find strophanthus useful in some cases in which digitalis, owing, perhaps, to some idiosyncrasy of the patient, disagrees,—in cases, for example, in which digitalis vomiting is produced.

Alcoholic, ammoniacal, and ethereal stimulants are, it is unnecessary to say, of great use for the purpose of relieving urgent symptoms and warding off asystole. In those cases in which there is vomiting, brandy and champagne are, I think, the most useful forms.

Many persons who are suffering from chronic cardiac disease and who have all their lives been accustomed to the use of alcohol, are, in my experience, the better for a strictly moderate amount of alcoholic stimulant; in many cases of this kind alcohol seems to help digestion; as a rule I give whisky, well diluted, with meals. In functional and neurotic cases Burgundy is often a useful form of wine.

Oxygen inhalations I find of the greatest use in many very urgent conditions, especially where there is bronchitis, pneumonia, or pulmonary apoplexy.

Iodide of Potassium.—It is unnecessary to say that this is an invaluable remedy in cases of aneurism and in many cases of angina pectoris. I agree with Dr Balfour in thinking that in combination with digitalis it is a most important remedy in some of the so-called cases of senile heart. It has also seemed to me to be useful in some cases in which there appeared to be chronic myocarditis or fibroid degeneration. In some cases in which cardiac lesions or symptoms were associated with symptoms or signs of tertiary syphilis, iodide of potassium has seemed to exert a beneficial effect upon the cardiac condition.

Salicylate of soda is another remedy which I prescribe largely in gouty cases with associated cardiac symptoms, and from which I have seen the greatest benefit.

Nitro-glycerine and *nitrite of amyl* are the remedies which I chiefly use with the object of producing a rapid lowering of the blood-pressure. So far as my experience goes they are more reliable and safer drugs than nitrite of sodium.

Menthol, given in combination with aromatic spirits of ammonia and spirits of chloroform, is a most useful remedy in many cases of flatulent distention of the stomach,—a condition which is often the cause of cardiac embarrassment and sometimes of sudden, alarming, and in some cases fatal, nocturnal dyspnœa, with or without angina pectoris. I usually give a sixth or a quarter of a grain of solid menthol dissolved in half a drachm of spirits of ammonia and half a drachm of spirits of chloroform for a dose.

Purgatives are, it is needless to say, most useful in many cardiac affections, especially in mitral cases attended with dropsy, and in cases in which the right side of the heart is over-distended and embarrassed, and the organs and tissues engorged and water-logged.

Mechanical removal of Dropsical Effusions.—I agree with Professor Sir Thomas Grainger Stewart that beneficial effects can in many cases be obtained by the removal of dropsical fluids from the internal cavities. I have obtained very satisfactory results by frequently repeated tappings in some cases of ascites due to organic cardiac disease, resulting hepatic cirrhosis, and portal engorgement. In cases of hydrothorax the results have, as a rule, been merely temporary and often unsatisfactory. I rarely resort to puncturing the dropsical legs or scrotum, either by simple puncture or by means of Southey's tubes, until other measures have failed to remove or lessen the œdema. Consequently, in my experience, draining the subcutaneous tissues has comparatively rarely been attended with any marked or lasting benefit.

Massage is, I think, a more useful remedy than tapping in many cases of subcutaneous dropsy; it aids the venous and lymphatic return, and quickens the circulation in the muscular and peripheral tissues of the body. It is also of great use in many cases in which, owing to the nature of the lesion, ordinary muscular exercise is contra-indicated.

Venesection is undoubtedly valuable in many cases in which the right heart is greatly over-distended and engorged, and is particularly useful, I think, in those cases in which the engorgement depends upon temporary lung complications, superadded to mitral disease.

Dry-cupping is often most useful for the relief of congestion of the lungs and other pulmonary and kidney complications.

The *soporifics* which I find chiefly useful are chloralamid, paraldehyde, and morphia. In cardiac cases sulphonal is, in my experience, much less certain in its action than chloralamid. I have almost entirely abandoned chloral hydrate in grave cardiac cases on account of the marked depression which, in my experience, it is, under such circumstances, apt to produce. Paraldehyde is, I think, especially useful in those cases in which there is associated bronchitis,—in other words, in those cases in which morphia is contra-indicated. After the breakdown of compensation and in the ultimate restlessness of cardiac cases, small and frequently repeated doses of morphia are often invaluable. I have seen the administration of the remedy attended with marked benefit even in those cases in which the urine is albuminous. On the whole, morphia is, in my experience, by far the most reliable sedative and soporific. As Professor Fraser has pointed out, it is an invaluable remedy in some cases of angina pectoris in which nitrite of amyl fails to give relief or is contra-indicated,—cases, for example, in which the blood-pressure is low and in which there is associated free aortic regurgitation. Morphia should never, I think, be given in those cardiac cases in which there is œdema of the lungs or much bronchial secretion. I have seen very disastrous results from its administration under such circumstances.

In conclusion, I may perhaps be enabled to emphasize some of the general propositions which I consider of fundamental importance for the intelligent treatment of cardiac lesions by means of the following financial illustration :—

Financial Illustration.—Take the case of a trader with ample resources and a large balance at his bankers. He has a big reserve and is able to carry on a large business, to turn over vast sums, and to meet any ordinary demand, even when it is suddenly made, without undue strain or effort,—in fact, with advantage to his business, that is, to himself. His reserve is ample for all his requirements. A healthy heart resembles such a man ; ordinary legitimate efforts and exertions are beneficial to it ; its power is increased by exercise ; and it possesses an ample reserve of energy which enables it to meet any sudden strain which is thrown upon it,—always provided that the strain is not unduly severe nor unduly prolonged, and that after a severe or prolonged effort, time is afforded for recuperation and the restoration of its nutrition.

Now, suppose our trader enters into a big speculation which is unsuccessful and loses a lot of money. If the demand upon him is very great, his balance at his bankers may be insufficient; and if the call is very sudden he may not · have time to realise his locked-up funds, in order to meet the large demand which is suddenly made upon him. Under such circumstances bankruptcy may be the result.

This condition of matters resembles that of a heart in which a very severe lesion is *suddenly* or *rapidly* developed; the effort which the lesion demands may be so sudden that the heart cannot put forth its reserve energy : it may be paralysed, and may succumb to the lesion.

Cases of this kind, both in the financial world and in cardiac pathology, are very rare. The creditors will, in the vast majority of cases, give the trader time to realise his locked-up funds, or will take over his securities in order to meet the debt.

The same thing is seen in the case of the heart. Even grave valvular lesions which are rapidly developed are usually followed by the production of some compensatory changes. The heart gets time to put forth its reserve energy, and Nature makes an effort to produce those compensatory changes which are required to restore the balance of the circulation.

But although the trader may be able to meet a heavy loss and to stave off bankruptcy, his resources may be permanently damaged. A large part of his reserve has been exhausted. Under such circumstances he takes care, if he is a wise and prudent man, to alter his mode of trading; he restricts his operations, does a safe, non-speculative business, and, above everything else, takes every precaution to prevent a repetition of the disaster which has crippled him.

Exactly the same thing is seen in the case of the heart. A valvular defect which remains, say, after an attack of acute endocarditis, materially cripples the power of the heart. The patient is not the same man that he was before. If he is a wise man he will take care to alter his mode of life, so as to avoid throwing sudden strains on the damaged heart, and he will be particularly careful to avoid everything, such as a second attack of rheumatic fever, which is likely to reproduce the endocarditis which was the cause of the original lesion. The compensation which is in the course of time produced may be sufficient to meet ordinary efforts, but extraordinary ones cause embarrassment and failure of the circulation.

Take another case. Suppose that our trader has had a heavy loss, which has necessitated the expenditure of most of his reserve capital; and suppose that the drain does not cease with the first loss, but steadily continues, although it may be in a very slight degree. His expenditure is, perhaps, year by year a little larger than his income; he has, consequently, to make use of his remaining capital; it sooner or later becomes exhausted; and, finally, he has to live from hand to mouth. When this stage of matters is reached, a very trifling call, a demand for a sum which he previously would have regarded as a mere flea-bite, is severely felt; it may be sufficient to produce bankruptcy. In a case such as this, in which the expenditure always exceeds the income, and the capital is being constantly drawn upon, the time must sooner or later come when the reserve will be exhausted.

Exactly the same thing is seen in the case of the heart. Most chronic valvular lesions are progressive. In many cases, it is true, the progress is very slow, but there is a constant demand for the production of more and more compensation. Under such circumstances, a time will inevitably arrive when the lesion will get the upper hand, and when the amount of compensation will be insufficient to maintain the balance of the circulation. It is at this stage of the case that urgent symptoms arise and that active treatment is most required.

Further, when the reserve is almost entirely exhausted, even if the compensation is under ordinary circumstances able to maintain the balance of the circulation, comparatively trifling efforts or ailments (such, for example, as a trivial attack of bronchitis, which throws an increased strain on the right ventricle) which in conditions of health would produce little or no disturbance in the circulation, may upset the balance, and may be attended with the production of grave symptoms, such as general dropsy.

The trader whose capital is exhausted, and who is in serious straits in consequence of a comparatively trifling demand which is made upon him, may be able to meet the temporary difficulty by the assistance and help of a friend, and, after settling the demand, may again be able to resume his restricted mode of trading. So, too, the heart which is seriously crippled by a valvular lesion may, when the compensation is temporarily upset (say, by the trivial attack of bronchitis), be enabled to pull through the attack of bronchitis by the kindly assistance of digitalis or strophanthus; and, after the bronchitis has subsided, be in a position to go on, for a time at least, much in the same way that it did before.

Take another case. A trader who is overloaded with heavy liabilities and with a damaged business may arrange with his creditors, and after writing off some of his liabilities may be enabled, though crippled, to start again in a much better position than he was before. Exactly the same thing is seen in the heart. In many cases of chronic cardiac disease, by free purgation, by removing dropsical accumulations from the internal cavities, or by venesection, the heart-strain may be relieved and the organ enabled to resume its operations, and to go on for a time much more satisfactorily than it could before. Even in the gravest cases extraordinary improvement may sometimes result from active treatment. No better illustration could be given than the remarkable case which Dr Sloan recently brought before the Society at one of our recent meetings.

Again, in some cases, a trader's business is so thoroughly rotten that any extraneous help which he can obtain is useless to stave off bankruptcy. Exactly the same condition is seen in the heart. In advanced stages of myocardial degeneration, digitalis, strophanthus, and other tonics and stimulants may be totally useless to produce any improvement. Under such circumstances, the only termination which can be looked for is death.

Dr Ralph Stockman said it was not his intention to continue the discussion on the lines marked out by Prof. Fraser and Dr Balfour. With regard to the action of cardiac tonics, he might recall the condition of the heart in which they were usually administered. When the heart suffering from a valvular lesion became exhausted from any cause, it began to beat more quickly and less forcibly than before, and in consequence of this the amount of blood discharged at each pulsation was less, the arteries became depleted, and the venous system over-filled, giving rise to venous stasis and dropsy. The primary effect of a cardiac tonic like digitalis or strophanthus was simply to alter the elasticity of the muscular fibres of the heart so that they expanded more completely and contracted more completely, without, at first at least, becoming more active or putting forth greater energy. The influence of this on a hollow muscle like the heart was easily understood. It took longer to dilate, contracted more thoroughly, and in consequence filled better, and threw out at each beat a greater amount of blood into the aorta. Consequently the blood-pressure rose and the heart was better nourished. The diuretic effect was simply due to this, rather than to the rise in blood-pressure, viz., that the veins and lymphatics were enabled to absorb effused fluid, and thus the blood became more watery than it was before, and the kidneys began to discharge the extra water, the diuresis stopping as soon as the general dropsy and ascites had been disposed of. In health one got no diuretic action from digitalis, or almost none. That being the case, it was improbable, although not impossible, that one member of the same group could act better than another in producing diuresis. One got the same diuretic effect with all, so that in his opinion it was more or less nonsense to speak of one being a better diuretic than another. The action might continue longer or commence more quickly with one than with another, but the action itself was much the same. He spoke with diffidence, because he began his studies in cardiac therapeutics under Prof. Fraser, and continued them under Dr Balfour at the Chalmers Hospital. He had seen a good deal of these substances, and had also used adonis vernalis and convallaria, with much the same results from all. He was glad to hear Prof. Fraser emphasize that, and assert that the best drug to use was the drug one was best acquainted with. These drugs were often strikingly successful, but sometimes they failed. He had understood Prof. Fraser to say that strophanthus had never disappointed his reasonable expectations, and Dr Balfour had said he could get the heart to do what he liked with digitalis. He himself had been disappointed with both, where he had expected to get fairly good results. In young people the heart was more plastic, and showed a great tendency to hypertrophy and dilate. On patients up to fifteen or even nineteen, the action of these drugs was disappointing. The heart usually went on from bad to worse. In middle-aged people, especially those who were alcoholic, or who had atherosed coronary arteries from any cause, and in cases of arythmia from impaired nutrition, one got very bad results. It was very seldom that one could control arythmia with digitalis, strophanthus, or any other substance of that kind,—he did not mean aortic cases, but cases of mitral lesion where the chief symptom was breathlessness and an arythmic condition of the heart. With regard to rest, it had been a good deal spoken about. He agreed that rest was probably the most potent agent we had in the treatment of heart disease. The effect of putting an ordinary healthy person to bed was to lower the pulse-rate by ten or fifteen beats. Putting to bed had practically the same effect as giving digitalis or strophanthus,—*i.e.*, the heart slowed, filled better, and transferred the blood better from the veins to the arteries. His experience was that when one was dealing with well-to-do middle-aged people in comfortable circumstances there was no necessity for giving strophanthus, digitalis, or any other drugs. If they showed slight symptoms of breathlessness or slight swelling of the ankles, let them go to bed for a week, and take care as to diet, no special cardiac treatment being required. With regard to iodide of potassium, that was a matter about which pharmacologists differed considerably. It had been explained at last meeting that it dilated small vessels and produced a fall in blood-pressure, but that had been distinctly denied. Germain Sée said explicitly that in small doses it acted like digitalis. Later authorities held that small doses raised blood-pressure, and larger doses diminished it. Injection into the veins of an animal was not a good way to judge of its effects, because it struck the heart in too large an amount. But, apart from that, he himself had been making observations on various patients. The last was a middle-aged man with spinal sclerosis. He was treated with iodide of potassium, the dose being increased to 300 grs. per day. He could not discover any change in the pulse-rate, rhythm, or in any other respect, and the radial artery was just as compressible under the sphygmometer, being obliterated by exactly the same force as before they began the iodide. He showed absolutely no symptoms. There seemed to be little doubt that it did good in many cases of aneurism, but its *modus operandi* was very doubtful. Hale White boldly said it had no action whatever, and that it was simply rest and diet that did good. He himself was inclined to think that one got brilliant results often in syphilitic cases, and was apt to transfer that to all

cases. He had not had sufficient experience to state definitely
which view was correct. In several cases he had used barium
chloride and sparteine, but neither drug came up to expectations.
Sparteine was given up to 10 grs. three or four times a day without
the slightest effect, and barium chloride was very unsatisfactory.
With regard to the treatment of cardiac cases with a large amount
of dropsy, he was a little astonished that no one had laid any great
stress on purgative treatment, which relieved the portal system very
greatly, and allowed the kidneys to act; and if one gave mercurials,
one often produced very marked diuresis. Mercurial treatment was
a very great help to the ordinary treatment of severe cardiac cases.
With regard to tapping the pleura, which was, somewhat on the
same lines, supposed to relieve dyspnœa and dropsy, he was not
so sure about that. He had lately tapped two cases, both of which
died. One was instructive. The patient had a pretty large
accumulation of fluid. The tapping went on pretty systematically,
but the fluid always reaccumulated in a few days. It relieved the
dyspnœa, but not much more. The patient got thinner, the heart
did not compensate properly, and finally he died. At the post-
mortem the pathologist said he saw no reason why a heart like
that should not have compensated. On thinking it over, he (Dr
Stockman) saw they had been practically starving the man. It
would have been more merciful to have deprived him of food before
he had had the trouble of digesting it. In drawing off the fluid,
one drew off a great deal of albumen. There were two other cases
in which one did not get much assistance from drugs—viz., dilated
right ventricle from emphysema or other lung condition. Digitalis,
strophanthus, or any other drug gave most disappointing results.
The right ventricle did not seem to respond like the left to tonics.
The patient could be relieved by other treatment, but the results
of cardiac treatment were poor. The other cases were sudden
attacks of dyspnœa, the most terrible heart cases one had to
treat. The only things one could give were the so-called stimulants,—whisky, brandy, or some preparation of ether. But the
treatment was not satisfactory. Patients often died in the attacks,
and at best the treatment was unsatisfactory, although it occasionally pulled them through. With regard to graduated exercise, he
had paid some attention to it, but it was very difficult, here at least,
to determine what graduated exercise was obtainable. He would
think a sort of treadmill would be the most feasible thing. The
desirability of it was open to question. The object was not to
strengthen the heart as one would strengthen a blacksmith's arm by
the exercise, but to diminish the amount of fluid in the body, and
thus lessen the amount the heart had to drive on. Oertel put the
patients on a restricted diet, restricting liquids especially, and then
gave graduated exercise to make their skin act, and still further
lessen the amount of fluid in the body, and in this way the heart
responded, and had less work to do. He (Dr Stockman) questioned

if under any circumstances it were a good thing to put a damaged heart to work of that kind. It excited it just as much as alcohol or tobacco or any violent exercise would do. With the heart mechanically damaged it was not desirable. Good results seemed to be got, not so much in valvular disease as in general obesity, and there he thought such treatment invaluable; but in ordinary cardiac disease not so. With regard to arsenic and iron, he could find nothing definite in the text-books. Arsenic was said by one or two authors to relieve breathlessness consequent on cardiac dyspnœa by lessening metabolism and the amount of oxygen used; and the evidence was sufficient to justify its administration. He did not think iron was so very valuable unless there was extreme anæmia. In most cardiac cases, if one examined the blood, one found corpuscles and hæmoglobin about normal or above it. In other cases, with hæmoptysis or other bleedings, causing distinct anæmia, it was valuable; but as routine treatment it was of doubtful value. In all cases of cardiac disease one had to take individual idiosyncrasy into account. It was very difficult to lay down general rules.

Professor Greenfield said he felt in a sense compelled to say a word or two with regard to one of the most important parts of this debate, viz.,—the utility of strophanthus. He was unfortunate in not having heard all the speeches, and could only judge from the reports which had appeared in journals. But since, in this respect, he was in the same position as the great majority of the profession, it might enable him the better to appreciate the probable effect of the discussion on the minds of practitioners. He feared that the impression would be that the leaders of the profession in Edinburgh attached little importance to strophanthus, and that the tendency of the speeches had been to "damn it with faint praise." For himself, he regarded the researches of Professor Fraser as amongst the greatest modern contributions to therapeutics, for which a profound debt of gratitude was due. If the result of the discussion was to minimize the value of strophanthus, or to check its use, it would be most disastrous. He should like much to enter upon many of the points of cardiac therapeutics touched on during the discussion. Dr Bramwell had so exhaustively discussed many of these points that he thought he might leave them almost untouched, although on many points he differed from him. All were agreed as to the value of agents in different cases, that they needed to graduate and adjust the treatment to the exact condition of the patient, and that apart from the use of special cardiac tonics a large number of hygienic, pharmacopœial, and other measures,—such as regulated food, rest, and moderate exercise,—and that in many cases no special cardiac agent was required. With regard to iodide of potassium, his own experience strongly supported Dr Stockman's remarks. He had tried it in small and large doses in cardiac cases of various kinds,

and in aneurism. For the last ten years he had never once
prescribed it in either, unless in order to adjust himself to the
views of the medical attendant, or to show of how little use it
was. If he did prescribe it, he prescribed the smallest dose he
could. With regard to strophanthus, he felt very strongly that the
real point in this debate—the point of most practical importance,
and that on which the expression of opinion of the medical
thought and practice of Edinburgh would carry great weight—was
the question of the value of strophanthus as compared with
digitalis. Dr Stockman had adopted what he might call the
negative pharmacologist's view,—had, so to speak, put the two on a
level up to a certain height, whatever that height might be. He
could not agree with that view at all, nor could he agree in any
sense with the view promulgated by some hospital colleagues that
strophanthus was of use only in cases of emergency or for special
conditions. His experience of it was now of nine years' standing.
On 5th February 1886 he gave the first dose in a case of enlarged
heart with valvular disease and great failure of compensation,
with also Bright's disease, although that was not the most
prominent condition. In that case, after two or three very small
doses, the pulse became slower and slower, and in spite of all
measures he could devise to restore the circulation, the patient
died from strophanthus poisoning. He discontinued the drug as
too dangerous for him, and resolved to wait. But he consulted
his colleague Prof. Fraser, who said he had given it in such cases
with good results He tried it again, and found it succeed. He
believed he must have used it in between 400 and 500 hospital
cases, and had never once, either in or out of hospital, met with a
case of similar idiosyncrasy. He must emphasize the fact that in a
very large number of cases in which digitalis was absolutely a
failure, he had found strophanthus to act beneficially. He wished
to say one word as to objections founded on want of uniformity
of preparation. He had sometimes thought that the proper
action was not obtained, and at such times in urgent cases he had
asked Prof. Fraser for a supply of his own brand, and had made
efforts to have the stock in the Infirmary replaced with some of
the proper strength. On the whole, he could not say that these
occasional failures had been serious. They wanted a simple mode
of ensuring a proper pharmacopœial preparation of uniform
strength. The best thing, if it were possible, would be to
enforce upon pharmacists that no sample should be allowed to
be sold unless submitted to the proper pharmacological tests.
He believed this should be done with other drugs. Was
strophanthus the only drug in this condition? The same difficulty
applied to digitalis, than which there was no drug more liable
to want of uniformity in strength and in the proportion of the
various active principles. In the case of digitalis the cumulative
action was in many cases a serious drawback to its use. One

constantly met with cases in which the action of digitalis proved so risky that one could not continue its use, and was compelled to have recourse to strophanthus. He had never found, except in the single case mentioned, that there was the same risk of producing cumulative action with strophanthus as with digitalis. He had used strophanthus in a vast number of different conditions, in all forms of heart disease, prostration accompanying fevers, failure of heart's action after operations, in cases of febrile delirium, etc. His experience was that by carefully graduating the dose we might in these cases almost invariably get some beneficial effect. In pneumonia he had used strophanthus very largely. In his experience the results in pneumonia alone—in diminishing the rapid action of the heart, in increasing its force, in avoiding not only the collapse which may occur at the crisis, but the cardiac embarrassment so frequently fatal in pneumonia—his testimony and that of his residents would be emphatic that it was of inestimable value. Cases which formerly, and even now, he regarded as almost hopeless, would sometimes revive under strophanthus,—*i.e.*, strophanthus with other remedies suitable to the case; nitro-glycerine, for example, certainly often a valuable adjuvant. The action of one drug might be controlled and regulated by the action of another. He would like to mention two or three selected cases in which he owed the life of near relations and friends to strophanthus, where digitalis and other cardiac tonics had failed, and cases, apparently hopeless, of senile degeneration, sudden cardiac failure, sudden dilatation associated with rapid pneumonia and acute pericarditis. He had saved cases in which he was quite prepared to arrange for a post-mortem. He had given strophanthus in very large doses. He was afraid he would shock Prof. Fraser if he were to tell him how freely and unpharmacologically he had given it. His rule when he started with strophanthus was "not to swap horses whilst crossing the stream." He continued it with, of course, his finger on the pulse and with constant watching, *increasing* the dose when the heart showed any signs of failure. Of course he knew a serious risk might be involved if 10 or 12 minims or more of tincture of strophanthus every two hours were continued for a day or so, but with careful watching one could check it in time, and one got remarkably good results where all other measures had failed. He would feel that he had failed in his duty if he had not borne testimony to the enormous value of strophanthus,—not, however, to the exclusion of digitalis. He would certainly advise those of his colleagues who had failed with strophanthus to try it again.

Dr James Ritchie said he considered it a great privilege to have his opinions corrected, he might say his prejudices overcome, by those who had opportunities of watching the action of special drugs. At the same time he would like to take rather a wider view of the therapeutics of the heart than the mere consideration of the relative merits of drugs. He was quite ready to acknowledge that his opinions had changed very much since he left the University. He still valued drugs very highly, but as therapeutic agencies in heart affections he now valued rest and diet very much more than he had done formerly. Drugs and exercise followed at a considerable distance. He believed that perhaps the most important thing in any case of cardiac trouble was the condition of the heart muscle, next the peripheral circulation, the condition of the valves of the heart, the state of the bowels, digestion, excretory organs, and constitutional peculiarities. With reference to acute cardiac conditions, Sir Thomas Grainger Stewart had raised the question, whether in these cardiac tonics should be given? He presumed he referred to the acute stages of inflammatory conditions, viz., endo-, peri-, and myo-carditis, because in acute dilatation of the heart he presumed the majority of practitioners gave cardiac tonics from the very beginning. But he agreed that cardiac tonics should not be given in acute inflammatory cardiac conditions. Dr Ronaldson had referred to the use of salicylate in rheumatic conditions. He quite agreed with him, and would add also the use of alkalies. He had often felt constrained to discontinue the use of these when he had to do with much pericardial effusion or a considerable amount of dilatation of the heart leading to feeble action, although the condition of the joints and the amount of fever would have been benefited by their continuance. He found it a matter of great importance during recovery from acute cardiac affections to enjoin the greatest amount of care in change of posture, specially to guard against sudden strain, and to limit the amount of exercise not only for days but for months. He thought Dr Underhill's remarks with regard to children ought to be accentuated. With slight elevation of temperature and so-called "growing pains" there was very often some cardiac affection, especially mitral. In all these cases it was well to take afternoon temperature, and if it were found even a very little above normal, the patient should be kept in bed. As to valvular lesions due to acute conditions, he thought it was necessary, after the acute stage was past, and before the establishment of compensation, if it were of considerable severity, to give cardiac tonics along with exercise or rest, as might be required. After compensation had been established cardiac tonics were not necessary. So long as compensation persisted, food, exercise, and general hygienic measures were alone required. After compensation had begun to fail, then there was need of cardiac tonics and great care in diet and the amount of rest or exercise. This applied to all degenerations of the myocardium, whatever might be the nature of the degeneration. Dr Bramwell had referred to the use of tonics in fatty heart. He (Dr Ritchie) thought that in any case of feeble, rapid, irregular action of the heart one might safely give cardiac tonics. If fatty heart was suspected, he thought the most important part of the treatment was diet, and above all to regulate the use of liquids in relation to quantity and the time after meals, to regulate the amount of exercise, and to give digitalis with caution. There was a very large class of cases on the consideration of which they could hardly touch, in which there was difficulty in diagnosis. He referred to those in which there might be a small irregularity of the pulse, palpitation, or some precordial uneasiness, and on examination there might be no evidence of cardiac change. The question arose whether these were functional, or due to cardiac disease. In a large proportion of such cases there would be found evidence of overwork, worry, the excessive use of tea or tobacco, or some source of reflex irritation—most frequently in the gastro-intestinal tract. He found difficulty in dealing with reports of cases for life assurance when it was stated that there was a degree of cardiac irregularity or of palpitation, because it was often impossible to obtain information of the kind required to establish a diagnosis. In proposers who had passed middle life he thought it safe to assume that there might be some cause acting upon a heart which had commenced to undergo senile changes. He desired to express his indebtedness to Dr Balfour for his book on the Senile Heart, and for his teaching which preceded it. In functional cases Dr Ritchie found that, in addition to the removal of the cause, it was advantageous to use the bromides alone, or with digitalis. When we speak of *rest* for the heart, we use the word in a relative sense. If we diminish its rate and prolong the diastole, we increase its period of rest, but we may also diminish the amount of work it has to do in various ways. 1. By diminishing the *amount* of blood flowing through it in a definite time. When we remember the great extent of the capillary circulation through the muscles, and the extent to which exercise increases the blood-flow through these, we appreciate more fully how bodily rest diminishes the work of the heart. There is difference of opinion as to the effect on the heart of the amount of imbibed fluid. He agreed with Dr Bramwell that by limiting the fluid taken we limit the total quantity of fluid which requires to be driven by the heart, and so diminish its work. 2. By attending to the *quality* of the blood we may relieve the strain upon the heart. The food ought to be of such kind as will best nourish the heart, without overloading the blood with waste products. It must be chosen with regard to the digestive or excretory peculiarities of the patient. Dr Ritchie believed that Oertel's system of feeding all cases of cardiac degeneration with a large amount of animal food is prejudicial in some individuals. His experience was strongly against the use of stimulants, unless it were to tide over an emergency. Cardiac disease was better treated without alcohol. 3. The work of the heart may be diminished by keeping the *resistance in the capillaries* at a minimum. The capillary circulation is favoured when the surface of the body is kept at an equable warm temperature, and when the excretory organs act properly. He believed that the virtue of Nauheim in chronic cardiac cases was due to the stimulant effect on the capillary circulation. These methods of resting the heart are those which we may employ apart from the use of drugs; but two classes of drugs are useful in cardiac affections. 1st, Those which, like digitalis and strophanthus, slow its action, favour rest by prolonging the diastole; 2nd, those which dilate the capillaries, such as nitrite of ethyl, spiritus ætheris nitrosi, potassium iodide, and strychnine. In anæmic cases iron conduces to the same result by diminishing the necessity for frequent action, in order to accomplish the æration of the blood. With regard to the *relative merits* of cardiac tonics: if he wished to obtain a rapid effect he used strophanthus, but he found that a large number of patients did not tolerate it well, and that if there existed a catarrhal condition of the gastro-intestinal tract, it was more likely to produce diarrhœa and vomiting than digitalis was. When the drug was first introduced he began with doses of 5 minims, but so often was its use followed by gastric symptoms that now he began with doses of 2 minims. He was astonished to hear Prof. Greenfield say that he gave it in doses of 10 to 15 minims every two or three hours, and he could only explain the difference of experience by the supposition that they were using differently prepared tinctures. Strophanthus had the advantage that it was not cumulative. He found it more useful than digitalis in angina pectoris, and he believed that the explanation lay in the fact that it did not contract the capillaries. It was also theoretically more useful in aortic incompetence, because it did not prolong the cardiac diastole. He thought, however, that he got more lasting benefit from the use of digitalis, and that its action lasted for some time after the drug was stopped. Digitalis, by prolonging the diastole, afforded more time for the nutrition of the heart wall. Its effect on the capillaries in contracting them tended to increase the work of the heart, but this contraction could be overcome by combining it with other drugs already referred to; and in certain cases in which there was a pulse of low tension the contraction of the capillaries was an advantage in so far that by increasing the tension it increased the blood-flow through the cardiac muscle. It has been said that if cardiac tonics are required because of changes in the myocardium, they must thereafter be used continuously, and that their effect lasts only while they are being taken. Dr Ritchie was satisfied that this statement was erroneous. He had seen many cases in which the nutrition of a feeble cardiac muscle had been so improved by digitalis and strychnine that for long periods after their discontinuance the improvement was maintained. A very important question was whether cardiac tonics should be given when there was sclerosis of the arteries and impairment of the capillary circulation. His rule was to choose the less of two evils, and if danger threatened from failure of the heart, to use cardiac tonics cautiously.

Dr Russell read his contribution, remarking that some time ago there had been an enthusiasm for one drug (digitalis) to the exclusion of others. From some of the remarks just heard, he would almost say that history was repeating itself.

Dr Clouston said that in certain cases of mania and melancholia, especially in their early stages, there was a condition which tended greatly towards exhaustion, with an enormously exaggerated heart's action running up to 100, 130, or 140 per minute. The cause was, no doubt, central,—some distinct irritation or stimulation from the cortex on the cardiac vasomotor centres. He had now three cases of early melancholia : one man, wonderfully sensible if kept off his delusions, showing no restlessness, and sleeping fairly well, but with a pulse never under 100. He had a case of mania of a similar kind. He had always been in the habit of adding to the ordinary medical and mental treatment in such cases digitalis and a combination of iodide and bromide of potassium, with a view to diminishing the cardiac excitement, the continuance of which from month to month must be a source of exhaustion. There were other cases where the opposite condition existed,—*e.g.*, in stupor, where the normal resistiveness of the capillary wall to blood-pressure from within seemed entirely gone and the heart's action weak and slow, with œdema and coldness and blueness of the extremities. He was in the habit of treating these with cardiac stimulants. He had often given a mixture of strychnine to stimulate the centres, and strophanthus to act directly on the heart. There was, thirdly, a cardiac condition that actually caused a certain form of insanity, described by him as the "insanity of cyanosis," where one had a weak, senile heart with very poor action, perhaps some bronchitis, a cyanotic or deoxygenated condition of the blood, and a kind of confused delirium, which they had to treat with proper cardiac remedies. They had also the "paralytic pulse," the sharp banging pulse of the first stage of general paralysis. In general paralysis there was an unusual proportion of cases of vascular and cardiac disease. Lastly, he would say generally that, as the result of the careful examination made of patients in asylums nowadays by young physicians trained in hospitals, a very disproportionate number of their cases were found to have heart murmurs on admission, which were, no doubt, directly associated in many cases with the cortical condition that had caused the insanity.

Meeting VII.—February 26, 1895.

Dr CLOUSTON, *President, in the Chair.*

DISCUSSION ON CARDIAC THERAPEUTICS—*Continued.*

Dr G. A. Gibson could not avoid stating his opinion that there had been a lack of guiding principles throughout much of the discussion. There had been too great a tendency to reduce the debate to the level of a duel between the advocates of two substances which might be regarded as friendly rivals. Dr Byrom Bramwell, however, had done a real service to the Society by laying down some principles of cardiac therapeutics. He (Dr Gibson) thought a good many of the discrepancies between the views on digitalis and strophanthus could be easily explained as being due to extrinsic circumstances. The different qualities of strophanthus, for example, might depend on the different districts in which it grew. There were many different qualities among Havanna cigars, depending on the parts of the island in which the plant grew. In the same way it was well known that digitalis presented great differences according to climate and soil. It could not be doubted that in the case of strophanthus the same differences must exist. With a substance, moreover, like digitalis, containing so many active principles, the special preparations employed must have a great deal of influence on the results obtained. The infusion of digitalis was better as a diuretic than the tincture; the media of different preparations taking up different active principles to a greater or less extent. He thought the Society might have heard a little more about blood-letting, by means of which imminent death was often averted. In his own experience he had frequently required to have recourse to this remedy, and usually with success. Exercise must be used for individual cases on their own merits. So also with rest. It was useless to make a patient rest in a dull room with a northerly aspect; there must be plenty of oxygen— plenty of sunlight. His intention was, however, not to pass in review the observations of previous speakers, but to make a very few remarks on the relief of cardiac pain,—a subject of the greatest importance, especially in the senile heart. We could not draw the line between what is called cardialgia and true angina pectoris. The position of the pain did not help us, and there was a perfect gradation in its character from the slightest to the gravest. He could not in this relation pass over the recent work of Dr Mackenzie and of Dr Head as regards the position of pain. In accordance with the views of the late Dr Ross of Manchester on the segmental distribution of sensory disturbances, the pain associated with the heart was always connected with the 8th cervical and 1st, 2nd, 3rd, and 4th dorsal nerves, and the portion of the cord from which those nerves took origin.

In this way it was possible to distinguish the proximal centres connected with the pain. Pain was here, as it always was, a central discharging lesion. The pain in cardiac lesions was usually connected with hyperæsthesia, and this might guide us, as Dr Mackenzie had shown, in regard to the site of the lesion. The powerful depression which had been called the impending sense of dissolution was not a sensation *sui generis*, or entirely confined to cardiac affections, but was found in different degrees in many visceral troubles. He agreed with Dr Balfour when he said there was no angina without cardiac failure of some sort. Increased pressure was simply a consequence of the pain, as well seen in peritonitis, and could not be regarded in any way as a cause. The various forms of cardiac pain were more common in degenerative than rheumatic conditions. The coronary arteries were then involved, and we had a condition of ischæmia of the cardiac muscle, as well as of structural changes in its fibres. To relieve the pain it was necessary to raise the nutrition of the whole circulatory apparatus, and primarily that of the heart. As drugs we must give the first place to the iodides, which were *facile princeps*. Nourry's iodated wine, or the syrup of hydriodic acid, might be used, or one of the salts, of which iodide of potassium was the best. Under the continuous use of such remedies much greater benefit could be obtained than by the employment of any other drugs. For the rapid relief of angina iodide of ethyl was considerably more active, and more certain in its effects than nitrite of amyl. Nitro-glycerine or nitrite of sodium might be used in cases where a prolonged effect was desired; he only employed the latter, however, as a rule, in asthmatic conditions. There were disadvantages attending its use in cardiac cases. Of other drugs, opium, as Professor Fraser had said, was a sheet-anchor in painful cases in old people. There was really no risk in its use with proper care. The diathesis of the patient must be considered. In the anginous attacks of gouty people alkalies and colchicum were of great use. And as all of the pains were associated with cardiac failure, it was, as he had already remarked, necessary to improve nutrition. He doubted if simple anæmia of the healthy cardiac muscle could produce them, and he was also sceptical as to neuralgia or neuritis being a valid cause. Probably they were due to local irritation of sensory nerves. We should surely have some means of averting the predisposing causes of these degenerative conditions with their attendant cardiac pains. Dr Balfour had on the title-page of his work on the Senile Heart, for which he was glad to have an opportunity of publicly expressing his admiration, quoted the words of Manilius, "Nascentes morimur." We could, however, ward off the tendency to degeneration by systematizing the habits of the patient and by arranging his diet. He had a great belief in distilled water as an invaluable agent in causing an increased tissue change, and thus lessening degenerative tendencies. It was an insipid drink, but might be

rendered palatable by being aërated, as well as by the addition
of different substances; and patients did not seem to have any
rooted objection to it given in this way. Its use could not be
too highly estimated in lessening the causes of senile degeneration.

Dr James said that he was not going to enter into a long disquisi-
tion on the treatment of heart diseases, because he felt that if he
did so he should merely be repeating, not only what they had all
heard again and again in this discussion, but what they had all
heard again and again ever since they had begun the study of
medicine. In the treatment of the heart and circulatory system,
they knew they had to look to the condition of every system in
the body. He was not going to enter into this; and if, in his
anxiety to avoid repeating platitudes, he found himself able to
express the results of his own observations and experience mainly
as doubts and perplexities, he was sorry; but he could not help it.
He would, at any rate, be brief. His first perplexity he could best
illustrate in connexion with the treatment of the cardiac condition
in an acute disease like pneumonia. They all knew that if in a
case of pneumonia the pulse continued not too rapid, and of fair
strength, the patient was safe, for the heart was equal to the work
which it had to perform until the crisis was over. All that was
required was rest and feeding. But if, in the course of a few days
of the disease, the pulse began to get rapid and feeble, they knew
that the routine treatment was the administration of digitalis,
strophanthus, or strychnia. Now, in the first place, they had to
remember that the normal rate and tension of pulse differed much
in different individuals. Hence a pulse of 110 in one individual
might be quite as serious as a pulse of 140 in another, so that one
had difficulty in knowing when a drug like strophanthus was really
indicated. But the most important question seemed to him to be
to explain why digitalis, strophanthus, or strychnia should do good.
Of course, they were told that those drugs slowed the pulse by
increasing the length of the pauses, and so gave the heart a longer
time in which to rest and nourish itself. But did such treatment
really aid the heart? Supposing, for instance, they had a patient
on the third or fourth day of a pneumonia with a pulse of 140,
and a tension, as ascertained by the sphygmomanometer, of $2\frac{1}{4}$; if
they injected hypodermically the twentieth of a grain of strychnia,
they might find within a few minutes that the pulse-rate was
reduced to 120, and the tension increased to 3. But was the heart
the better for this? It had certainly longer pauses and a longer
time to nourish itself, but the increased tension meant that it was
doing more work. Stimulation of the vagus nerve in animals, we
believe, promotes the nutrition (anabolism) of the heart; but we
have to remember that whilst stimulation of this nerve slows the
heart, it at the same time has a lowering and not an increasing
effect on the blood-pressure. Of course, we all know that in pneumonia there are times when strychnia, digitalis, or strophanthus

are indicated and do good. But one cannot shut one's eyes to the possibility that a low tension with some rapidity of pulse may be, on the whole, salutary. Further, it may be that if in a case of pneumonia, instead of simply waiting and giving strychnine, digitalis, or strophanthus, when in the later stages the pulse is failing, we, as our forefathers would have advised, had given a drug like tartar emetic in the earlier stages, the strength of the heart required at the period of the crisis might have been better husbanded. In his own experience the procuring of sleep was of the greatest importance in keeping up the strength of the heart in pneumonia. Whilst a patient is sleeping his pulse-rate is slowed, and the tension is not markedly increased, so that the heart is in the condition in which its nutrition can best be kept up. He next wished to say a little as regards the value in heart diseases of the so-called dry diet. Every one knew the great value of such dieting in those cases; but what was the explanation of this? It had been stated that by dry diet the bulk of the blood was diminished, and hence the heart had less difficulty in driving it on. But this explanation seemed to him not quite satisfactory. All observations showed that, although great variations might exist as regards the quantity of blood in the body, yet the quantity of blood driven out by each ventricular contraction remained the same, and the well-known experiments of Worm Müller showed that with great augmentation of the quantity of blood in the vessels the arterial pressure remained the same. It was, of course, evident that the smaller the total quantity of blood the more would tissue metabolism be favoured. But he was of opinion that the dry diet owed its efficacy for the most part to improving digestion and diminishing the weight of the body. Lastly, as regards the use of strophanthus and digitalis in heart diseases, he had to express perplexities. Like other observers, he had had cases of double aortic disease in which digitalis did not suit, and in which strophanthus had done good; and he knew that the explanation of such a result given was that digitalis, by increasing the blood-pressure and prolonging the diastole, tended to increase the distension of the left ventricle. But, on the other hand, he had seen many cases of double aortic mischief in which digitalis proved useful when strophanthus had failed. Similarly, in mitral stenosis, he had seen some examples of this valvular lesion in which digitalis did not suit, but he had seen others in which it had suited most admirably. In this affection, too, they had to remember that any drug which slowed the heart's action would, in acting beneficially on the left ventricle, be as likely to act injuriously on the right, for, in giving the left ventricle plenty of time to fill itself, it would give the right ventricle the same time in which to become over-distended. In his opinion, no general law as regards the use of those drugs could be stated, and in working with them he was often reminded of the following statement of Copland :—" It must be manifest that if a mode of treatment be empirically followed in all cases said to be typically the same, although different or even opposite as respects vital power, complication, and stage of advancement, it must be injurious about as frequently as beneficial." So with strophanthus and digitalis. In some cases the one did good and the other harm; in other cases the opposite occurred. In other cases they both seemed to do good; in others, again, neither did good. We could, in his opinion, formulate no law for their application; we could only treat each case individually; but it was a satisfaction to think that the same conditions which would render them unsuitable in one instance would render them as suitable in another.

Dr George W. Balfour read his supplementary contribution on CARDIAC THERAPEUTICS:—

MR PRESIDENT AND GENTLEMEN,—Feeling that the discussion has not altogether proceeded on the lines originally intended, but has diverged from cardiac therapeutics generally with indications for their use into a controversy as to the merits of two special drugs, I have asked permission of the President to give a few supplementary remarks on the general question, even at the risk of repeating much of what I have already said.

The course of discussion during the past two evenings must, I think, have convinced every one that cardiac therapeutics and their indications is too wide a subject to be dealt with in so limited a time.

Remembering this, in the few words I have now to say, I intend to be merely suggestive, and shall not in any wise attempt to treat the subject exhaustively.

When a case of probable cardiac disease presents itself for treatment, we must first of all make a careful investigation of the whole case, and of every organ, especially those—as the lungs, liver, and kidneys—which are so closely connected with the heart, and whose condition has a most important bearing upon the past and on the future history of the case; and upon the results obtained we base our diagnosis. The prominent symptom complained of is very often a guide to the nature of the case, and also an indication of the character of the treatment required. But to make any symptom useful in this way we must clearly understand what the patient means by his complaint, and we must endeavour also to understand what the symptom means to us, and what are its connexions with the other phenomena present.

1. Palpitation, for instance, is a very common complaint, but to the ordinary observer palpitation usually means anything abnormal in either the rate or the rhythm of the heart's action. It is, therefore, a symptom with many meanings, each one of them indicating a different line of therapeutics. Ordinary true palpitation is indicated by a forcible beating of the heart and larger arteries, the smaller arteries taking no share in the

phenomenon in regard to force of beat, at all events. It is brought on by reflexes of emotional or gastric origin, never by exercise. Such patients are feeble and more or less anæmic, and it is their general health that wants improvement, a general tonic regimen that is required, and not any special cardiac treatment.

2. Then we have the forcible augmentor action that follows exertion in anæmic individuals. In such cases the heart's action is not so violent and throbbing, and the radials, as well as the larger arteries, beat fully and forcibly, all the phenomena ceasing at once when the patient becomes quiescent. In such cases absolute rest is required, the general tonic regimen, with such special tonics as may be required,—probably iron and arsenic, possibly various others. In such cases we must see that there is no special cause for hæmolysis, and no interference with hæmogenesis. Very frequently such cases are benefited by cardiac tonics, but these are not always required. Each case must be individualised and treated on its own merits.

3. Next we have the violent palpitation of Graves' disease, which so often long precedes either the goitre or the prominent eyeballs, and which may be and may remain the solitary symptom of the disease. In such a case the action of the heart is not only violent but noisy, and the whole arterial system, to its minutest branch, throbs disagreeably. This affection is seldom much benefited by remedies directed to the heart, and is most successfully treated by special treatment adapted to remove its cause.

4. We may have rapid heart action set up by the initiative action of an acute over-strain, and this often terminates in valvulitis and in stenosis, especially of the mitral valve. Such cases, if seen early enough, are often much benefited by pushing belladonna or atropine till the system is fully affected. At a later period a different treatment is usually more successful.

5. The rapid, irregular pulsation due to interference with the metabolism of the cardiac muscle from an imperfect blood-supply due to mitral stenosis, or some less obvious cause, is not always amenable to treatment. Perfect rest in bed, with moderate doses of digitalis, have been occasionally attended with remarkable success.

6. True tachycardia, rapid feeble pulse with embryocardiac heart sounds, arises from a multitude of causes, and thus each case requires to be specially treated from its own standpoint.

7. Lastly, we have that remarkable phenomenon tremor cordis, which seems always to be produced by some gastric reflex, and never either by exercise or emotion. This is best treated by attention to the general health, and by moderate open-air exercise.

But it is not only cases of palpitation that require to be differentiated, and each relegated to its own peculiar category for the purpose of treatment; every other symptom usually complained of in connexion with the heart must be investigated in a similar manner.

Thus breathlessness may be due to simple anæmia, deficient supply of oxygen carriers in the blood, or to backward pressure congesting the lungs and interfering with the aëration of the blood, or it may be due to limitations of the air space from œdema of the lungs or effusion into the pleura, without any marked indication of venous remora. Or, lastly, in the form of cardiac asthma, the aëration of the blood may be prevented by vascular spasm due to reflex action of various origins.

Even œdema is not always so much due to cardiac debility as to the influence of position, of accidental compression of the veins, or of an imperfect constitution of the blood.

The condition of the heart itself must also be carefully investigated. First, in regard to the age of the patient, in early life simple dilatation is probably due to anæmia, a so-called functional murmur is simply a curable regurgitation, and if we get them early enough we can cure them, while if we leave them alone the heart may become permanently dilated, and the unfortunate patient is handicapped for life. After middle life simple dilatation is usually associated with the other phenomena connected with the senile heart, a condition which is not curable, but the symptoms of which may be much relieved by treatment, by which we may so effectually apply the drag as to arrest or, at all events, restrain the inevitable downward progress. An old heart may be fibroid or rheumatic as well as old, but under the term Senile Heart I have described a condition which has a distinct pathology of its own,—a pathology of the highest importance in the economy of life, and through which, when thoroughly understood, we may, by judicious treatment, add much to the comfort and prolongation of life.

For the present Professor of Pathology to call the senile heart only a "well-turned phrase," is only a proof that it is a mistaken idea to suppose that it is only Scotsmen who confound morbid anatomy with pathology.

Next we endeavour to expiscate the condition of the valves and openings of the heart to which any murmur may be due, whether these murmurs are simply due to want of coaptation of the valves, or to serious alteration in their structure or in that of the orifices from rheumatic or atheromatous degeneration. All of these matters have a distinct bearing on the treatment of the case and on the future of the patient; and we can understand how important it is to make a careful and exact diagnosis of the nature of the case before we undertake the treatment.

We need not trouble much about whether the coronaries are atheromatous, because it is impossible to ascertain this during life; nor need we consider whether the heart is fatty or not, because this also is impossible of ascertainment, and to hold our hand from appropriate treatment for a mere surmise is to throw away for a chimera all our prospect of benefiting the patient. Moreover, of all the fatty hearts I have seen post-mortem, not one has ever been injured by any treatment, however energetically it has been pursued.

When a patient comes to you complaining, he is suffering, and must, if possible, be put right; but when you accidentally discover a murmur in a person apparently healthy, there is not usually any call for treatment; the only exception is a young spanæmic person, girl or boy, with a so-called functional murmur. The hearts of such patients must be attended to, whether they complain or not, otherwise they may find themselves later in life seriously handicapped.

It is an unwise error always to suppose that recovery or improvement has been due to the use of this or of that drug. In past ages many cardiac patients recovered from ruptured compensation without any material aid from drugs. In the present day, especially among hospital patients, many recover, even after dropsy has set in, under the influence of diet and rest alone, and this helps to account for many recoveries under the use of drugs of no great activity. Powerful drugs are always powerful for evil as well as for good, and in the hands of the less skilful a less active drug may be more useful than one which is more so, but with the management of which the medical man is less acquainted.

In the treatment of cardiac disease it is, before all things, needful to keep the patient cheerful and free from anxiety. If there is cause for anxiety,—and heart cases are never free from this,—it is well to inform the friends; and when these are injudicious, it is better to run some risk of being misunderstood yourself rather than disturb the peace of the invalid.

Whenever the cardiac compensation is incomplete, when exertion brings on dyspnœa, even although there be no evident soakage of the tissues, rest is paramount. Rest, diet, and heart tonics will speedily restore the patient to comfort; while exercise, however carefully graduated, only tends to make the breakdown of compensation complete. Only in the early stage of a gouty heart is exercise likely to be of much benefit, and then it must be carefully carried out. Regular, moderate exertion helps to keep the myocardium well nourished; whatever goes beyond tends to promote hypertrophy; and as the coronary arteries have only a limited feeding-power, excessive exercise tends to promote irremediable failure of the heart. Moreover, exertion too long continued, although not excessive in character, promotes muscular collapse, and we can easily understand what this may mean to a patient with a weak myocardium. In all patients, but especially in young patients, though we may insist on the avoidance of active exertion of any kind, it is well to promote the nutrition of the skeletal muscles by carefully conducted massage; in this way all the benefits of exercise may be obtained without any of its risks, and the patient is kept well nourished, instead of wasting to a neurotic skeleton. The diet in cardiac cases is always a matter of paramount import-

ance, but its principles are easily comprehended.   A cardiac patient
has a feeble digestion, therefore he must avoid everything known
to be indigestible, either generally so or specially, as to his own
idiosyncrasy.   He must take but a limited quantity at each meal,
because his gastric juice is poor in quality; and to avoid diluting
this poor gastric juice, as well as because liquids are digested and
absorbed with difficulty in such cases, the meals must be as dry as
possible, and any fluid required should be taken about four hours
after the last meal, when the digestion is completed, or nearly so.
Then the fluid quenches any thirst that may exist, and washes all
the refuse acids and débris out of the stomach, which is thus prepared for its needful rest.   Taken in this way, fluid, unless in
excessive quantity, produces no discomfort, and passes at once out
of the system.   A sufficient time should elapse between each meal,
to allow of the completion of the digestion and the needful rest of
the stomach.   The principal meal should be taken in the middle
of the day, and the evening meal should always be light.   A special
dietary must be arranged for each case, to provide not only for
his necessities, but also for his idiosyncrasies; we must rather
consult with our patient as to what he can take than dogmatically
lay down the law as to what he ought to take; in this way
we shall establish a mutual confidence which will be greatly
conducive to the patient's obedience and to the satisfaction of
both.   Alcohol is only to be prescribed when specially required,
and permission to use tobacco must be given with some caution,
though it need not be absolutely forbidden.

The drug remedies employed in cardiac disease are not numerous,
but they are of extreme value.   Nux vomica, usually employed in
the form of the liquor strychninæ for the convenience of accurate
dosage, is a most valuable remedy in all cases where the cardiac
energy is defective without any evident structural lesion, and may
be continued for a long time—many years even—with only a
gradually increasing benefit, provided we keep the dose short of a
cumulative one.   Five minims of the liquor strychninæ every
twelve hours I have found to be such a dose; five minims every
eight hours may be taken by some, but you cannot be sure that such
alarming symptoms of saturation as snapping of the jaws shall
not ere long develop.   Five minims every twelve hours is the
largest safe dose for the majority of mankind, and will be found
never to give rise to any troublous symptoms, but only to a marked
and steady improvement, due to energizing of the heart muscle,
the cardiac ganglia, as well as the vasomotor centre.   Strychnine
is also an admirable tonic for the stomach, especially in the
catarrhal condition accompanied by venous congestion, which is so
constant an accompaniment of a weak heart.   Strychnine is not only
an admirable tonic for energizing a weak heart without evident
lesion, but is a most useful adjunct to other more powerful cardiac
tonics when such are required.

Arsenic is also a most valuable heart tonic ; there is the greatest difficulty in understanding how it acts ; there can be no dispute as to the reality of its action. A friend once said to me, "I don't know what you expected from the arsenic, but I know the benefit I have received ; I can now go upstairs much easier than formerly." This is the benefit the Styrian mountaineers receive,—they climb their hills with less effort; it produces, as Trousseau has said, a " très grande aptitude à la marche." Arsenic has a powerful tonic effect on the nervous system in relieving even the pain of angina ; it improves the whole tone of the system, and gives even to old people a healthy complexion. It is seldom advisable in any case even of slight cardiac failure to trust to arsenic alone, but it makes a most useful adjuvant to strychnine or other cardiac tonics.

Iron is too well known as a necessary drug in the cardiac failures of young people, especially of chlorotic females, to require more than a passing notice here.

But of all cardiac tonics there is only one of paramount importance, and that is digitalis, an indigenous drug of the very highest value, which gives its name to a whole group of remedies of similar action, of which only one comes within a measurable distance of itself in the possession of reliable properties, and that is strophanthus.

Upon each of the last two meetings of this Society we have had a professor singing the praises of strophanthus. But, sir, early in my life I learned that professors were not infallible, and I have seen no reason to change this opinion. One of the ablest and most esteemed of my professorial teachers taught me that in the treatment of pneumonia " the utmost confidence may be placed in general blood-letting, which should always be large," and that " the only essential action of the prognosis is the day when the treatment is commenced ; the remedy being often ineffectual when delayed more than two or three days from the decided commencement of the disease." Another professor, celebrated for his skill in therapeutics and dietetics, told me that the most certain treatment for aortic regurgitation was starvation, and its only drawback was that so soon as you began to feed the patient the murmurs all returned. A third well-known professor used often to send to my ward at the end of the summer session cases of cardiac disease complicated with dropsy, which he had been for weeks treating with what he believed to be the most useful remedy for such cases—aconite. I need not describe the condition in which such cases were when I received them. Strophanthus has one great advantage over its congeners in action—its active principle is soluble in water, and so can be readily employed hypodermically ; it also acts with great rapidity, and may therefore be occasionally employed hopefully in circumstances where no other drug would be likely to be useful. I do not specially refer in this to cases of pre-critical collapse in pneumonia, because I believe that properly treated pneumonia never presents this phenomenon, but to sudden cases of cardiac collapse which occasionally occur in certain neglected cases of heart affection. Prof. Fraser has placed the profession greatly in debt, as well as built himself an enduring reputation, by the care and skill with which he has investigated the properties of strophanthus, but our acknowledgment of indebtedness does not lessen our duty to our patients, nor shut our eyes to the one great defect in its action. As I have said, strophanthus in a sufficient dose contracts the heart rapidly and certainly; whether by this action it also acts as a diuretic I scarcely know, because in both hospital and private practice I have found it to be uncertain in all doses, and also because we know that rest, warmth, and diet effectively suffice to restore ruptured compensation in both hospital and private patients, and in this way act as efficient diuretics. The defect which I have found in connexion with strophanthus is that though it forces the heart to contract it seems to have no tonic action on it; it does not appear to promote the nutrition of the heart muscle so necessary to its restoration to a healthy tone, which is so characteristic of true digitalis action. Whether this is due to some defect in the constitution of the drug, or, as seems probable, is only due to its inefficient action on the arterioles, it is a drawback which I have distinctly noted, not only in my own practice, but also in the practice of others whose patients have happened to come through my hands, some of whom had taken strophanthus for many months. This drawback is a very serious one, especially in the treatment of that large and important group of heart cases which I include under the term Senile Heart, a group of cases of the very highest importance and of constant occurrence in private practice, but which are comparatively uncommon among the crowds of heart patients who throng our hospital wards.

In digitalis itself we have a most valuable indigenous drug, which, skilfully employed, is capable of producing precisely that action on the heart which we desire, certainly and without risk. For more than 120 years digitalis has been employed as a sovereign remedy for dropsy, but it is only during the last thirty years—if so long—that its valuable properties as a heart tonic have been duly recognised. When I hear people talk of the dangers of its use, I well remember the first information I received as to its use in heroic doses. A professional brother told me that a friend of his own in Aberdeen, who attended the navvies building the railway to that city, used to treat his pneumonic patients by one large blood-letting followed by half an ounce of tincture of digitalis, and he added he never saw them again. My reply was, I was not surprised. Oh, but, he said, they all recovered and came to see him. Again, I remember another professional brother who carried on a large and arduous practice for more than fifty years, notwithstanding a bad heart from which he suffered. Many years ago he consulted me, and I had to tell him that compensation was failing and that he ought to take digitalis. "Not if I know it," was his reply; "I remember, when I was resident in the Infirmary, a poor man who died suddenly from the cumulative effects of three drops of the tincture of digitalis given three times a day." I am glad to say that my friend ultimately became a convert to the utility and innocuousness of digitalis skilfully employed. He owed many years of active life to the drug, and he was a most skilful adept in its use. In contradistinction to this, it is exactly twenty-five years this month since an eminent professor declared in this Society his adhesion to the old doctrine that digitalis was a powerful and dangerous sedative to the heart, depressing and enfeebling its action, and not to be administered in sensible doses, but with extreme caution, and this view he illustrated by sphygmographic tracings from a patient in the Infirmary treated by himself. Cases of heart complaints, such as those commonly treated with digitalis, are liable enough to sudden death from various causes, but we may acquit the drug of all share in the fatal issue. I know very well that excessive doses often produce great uneasiness and discomfort, but Withering has recorded cases in which enormous doses of digitalis have been successfully employed in the removal of dropsy, and I myself have known a cardiac patient swallow a whole ounce of tincture of digitalis with no more untoward result than that the pulse for a whole week was never over 40 per minute.

Digitalis may be given with three objects in view,—1st, to improve the nutrition of the myocardium, and so augment the force of its contractions as well as the energy of the cardiac ganglia; 2nd, to contract dilated ventricles; and, 3rd, to remove dropsy.

The tonic action of digitalis is certainly attained by administering the drug in such a dose and at such an interval that the quantity of the drug ingested is balanced by that excreted before a second dose is administered. What remains is improved nutrition of the myocardium, due to the action of the drug while being slowly excreted; this remains, and is added to by each dose, so that the heart gains strength and tone; the energy both of the muscle and the ganglia being slowly improved, without the slightest risk of any cumulative action from the drug. The dose ordinarily best fitted for this end is a grain of powdered digitalis leaves, or its equivalent in any of the other preparations, every twenty-four or twelve hours, but not oftener. Such a dose may be continued for months or years, with nothing but increasing benefit. Bulky and plethoric individuals may be the better of a larger dose; meagre and anæmic persons may demand a slightly smaller one. I am not aware of any other reason for varying the dose, especially I have not met with any cases of special idiosyncrasy in regard to this drug. The various preparations of digitalin—especially Nativelle's granules, and Merk's in doses of $\frac{1}{100}$ of a grain—are very

t

well adapted for producing this tonic action, though very unsuited for any other use, as in larger doses they are extremely apt to produce sickness and discomfort.

Flabby dilated hearts, if not much hypertrophied, and especially if young, may often be very well contracted by larger doses administered more frequently—as 1½ gr. or more every eight or every four hours. Such doses, however, require to be carefully watched, as the primary slowing of the pulse always induced is apt to pass somewhat suddenly into the allorhythmic pulse of digitalis poisoning—a condition sufficiently distressing, though not dangerous if the recumbent position be maintained. In aortic regurgitation, when the left ventricle begins to fail—whether the mitral valve has been opened up or not—digitalis in large doses, but at some considerable interval between, is imperatively required, and is often of the utmost benefit. These large doses keep the ventricle somewhat contracted, and by improving the tone of the myocardium they enable it to withstand the dilating hydraulic pressure of the column of blood. The idea that a prolongation of the diastole favours further dilatation is a mere myth. The lengthening of the diastole is more than compensated for by the increased tone of the ventricle, which slowly regains its compensation. For the removal of dropsy some degree of saturation is necessary. For this purpose our predecessors used digitalis pretty freely, as much as from 3 to 12 grains every eight hours; but whatever the dose given, we must remember that the equivalent of about 40 grains may usually be given before symptoms of saturation appear; that the more rapidly the drug is ingested the more certainly the diuretic action is attained; while once diuresis has set in, the drug may be stopped for a day or two, and the effect subsequently kept up by smaller doses continued for a longer time. Digitalis is chiefly of use, as Withering has pointed out, in those with feeble intermitting pulses, soft and readily pitting limbs. When the pulse is hard and cordy, the limbs tense and brawny, digitalis is of no use; we must in such cases lower the blood-pressure by free purgation, and get some of the fluid away before the drug will act; or we may drain the limbs by incision or Southey's tubes; or we may use diuretin, which is occasionally of great service. But cases of this character are always tedious in treatment, and generally unsatisfactory in result. Digitalis is of no ultimate benefit in the slow ingravescent asystole which often sets in at the end of a cardiac affection—that is equivalent to saying it cannot cure death. In other cases digitalis will always be found to do yeoman service—though, unfortunately, death only too frequently occurs during the process of treatment, from embolism or other unpreventible causes. In the removal of dropsy, other diuretics, as squill, broomtops, and electuary of bitartrate of potass, are often of great service in combination with digitalis. Tapping is occasionally a necessity, but it is not to be undertaken without careful consideration, as we may unduly reduce the strength of the patient by inconsiderate tapping. The removal of a few ounces of fluid from a pleura is a very simple piece of braggadocio, but often repeated it may do harm, and is never of any use. Fluid in the tissues is chiefly of consequence as an indication of heart failure, and it is the recuperation of the heart, and not the removal of the fluid, which we must chiefly consider, with this exception, that we must never forget that considerable anasarca of the limbs acts mechanically in compressing the capillaries and venous radicles, and thus raises the blood-pressure, and embarrasses the heart's action. With a feeble heart it is thus often of the greatest importance to drain the limbs; but a few ounces in the pleura can do no harm in this way, and are best left alone. Purgatives, especially cholagogue purgatives, are often of great use in lowering blood-pressure, and in removing sources of injurious reflex action from the primæ viæ, and are thus frequently of great service in restoring harmony to the movements of an irritable, irregular heart. Even emetics may be of service in hearts of moderate strength, when an undigested meal has induced one of those horrible attacks of tachycardia. I have seen so simple a meal as fish and potatoes in no excess start a pulse-rate of 150, with a wobbling ventricle. In these cases there is flatulence, but this, when removed, is speedily reproduced, and no permanent relief is obtained till the stomach is emptied, which, if not done artificially, may in these circumstances take fully twelve hours. Colchicum, in various preparations, is very useful in the irregularity of gouty hearts, and considerable doses are often required.

Next we have the use of nitrites and their allies nitro-glycerine and iodide of potassium in lowering blood-pressure, and thus enabling digitalis to act beneficially in certain conditions, where otherwise it does harm. Nitrite of amyl flushes the face, produces fulness of the head and a rapid pulse-rate, all of which are disagreeable, and limit its usefulness. It may be used very freely; one medical friend used to go to sleep with a handkerchief soaked in amyl lying on his face. It is always best freshly prepared, and if kept does not seem to relieve the pain, though it continues to flush the face. Spirit of nitrous ether and nitrite of sodium may be used, but are inferior in action to amyl, though more permanent. Nitroglycerine in tablet, or 1 per cent. solution, is more generally useful; its action is more certain and more prolonged, lasting from one to four hours; the dose may be increased as occasion requires up even to eight or ten minims. For immediate action in anginous seizures nitrite of amyl or nitro-glycerine are best calculated to give immediate relief. But for a lasting effect iodide of potass certainly lowers the blood-pressure for a longer period continuously without bad effect, and is therefore most useful in combination with digitalis to prevent that irritability and increase of dilatation apt to follow its use in cases of high blood-pressure. I am told—I believe on the authority of experiments on animals—that iodide of potassium does not unlock the arterioles, and cannot lower blood-pressure. To this my reply is, that I find it does so in man. I also find that a dog will be killed by a dose of calomel which any old woman could take with impunity, while he will take as much aloes as will kill two men; and I prefer to trust my own experience to that which is gained from so uncertain a source. I am also told that there is no high blood-pressure, or, at all events, not always high blood-pressure, in angina. I once thought so myself; but I am satisfied that in every case of angina there is an initial rise of blood-pressure, though it rapidly drops, as we can readily understand, from failure of the heart to keep it up.

Flatulence is most successfully treated by careful dietary and galbanum pills, though it may be temporarily relieved by carminatives of various kinds, from Dalby's upwards.

Sedatives, such as the bromides, are often of the greatest service in soothing irritable hearts, even in the palpitation of young people.

Morphia is the chief narcotic, and is of the greatest service in relieving the pain of angina where it persists after relief to the blood-pressure has been secured by nitro-glycerine; it is also the only certain relief to the distressing symptoms of cardiac asthma. But we must give enough; if we use it at all we must use it efficiently, beginning with $\frac{1}{4}$ or $\frac{1}{2}$ gr., and giving even more if requisite, running every risk for the sake of giving relief to suffering where that is imperatively required.

Paraldehyde is a good hypnotic, disagreeable to take. Chloralamide lowers blood-pressure and quickens heart-beat, but is a very good and useful narcotic, though, I think, inferior to Chloralose, which lowers the blood-pressure but does not excite the heart, seeming rather to steady and regulate its action. Patients using it fall asleep readily, waken easily and refreshed, and have neither headache nor gastric disturbances,—4 grs. in cachet at bedtime, repeated should the patient wake after only an hour or two's sleep. Given in this way chloralose seldom fails to ensure a good night's rest, and it never produces any cardiac or gastric discomfort. Chloroform and chloral are powerful remedies, not to be recommended except in special circumstances, on account of their powerful anæsthetic properties. But otherwise they are safe enough; they slow the pulse, but do not apparently depress the heart's action. I have given chloroform to many anginous patients, and to some cardiac patients who were actually moribund, with nothing but good effect. Chloral has the same danger as chloroform, but is otherwise safe, and may occasionally be of value.

Prof. Fraser, replying, said he did not think that he could claim the same latitude as Dr Balfour had taken in opening up the whole subject of cardiac therapeutics again. He had mainly to reply to the remarks made by previous speakers during the three nights over which the discussion had extended, and so he could not much extend his opening remarks. In the first place, however, he must remove a misapprehension. It had not been his intention in the remarks with which he had opened the discussion to specially emphasize the merits of any one remedy; for, as he then stated, his intention was to demonstrate the remarkable therapeutic value of a pharmacological group of remedies, which he would illustrate in connexion with one member only of the group, merely because his experience with it had been greater than with any other member. His illustrations had been taken from the worst forms and conditions of cardiac disease, so as the more emphatically to illustrate the great therapeutic value of this group of substances, the members of which, by a direct action on the muscle of the heart, increase the strength and efficiency of the cardiac contractions with a power unequalled by other remedies. In a secondary position, in a sense, came all other measures and remedies, such as rest, diet, arsenic, nitrites, morphine, strychnine, measures for removing fluids and increasing eliminations, etc. He had referred to these, but merely referred, for detail was impossible. To have dwelt on them all with detail would have occupied a whole meeting of the Society, and in that case he might have prevented the Society from hearing the very interesting statements, founded in most cases on long experience, and in all cases on intelligent observation, which had been made in the course of the discussion by those who had discussed the topics which he had purposely refrained from dwelling upon. To only a few of these secondary measures and remedies could he now refer. He termed them secondary, and he must adhere to the opinion implied in this designation, even although Dr James Ritchie had said that rest and diet occupied the first position in the treatment of cardiac diseases, and that remedial substances occupied a very secondary position. If so, by what amount or kind of rest and diet would Dr Ritchie prevent death in a patient with intense orthopnœa, general and pulmonary œdema, regurgitation through the auriculo-ventricular orifices, scanty and albuminous urine, and the other evidences of grave cardiac disease? Hygiene, diet, and all the other accessory methods of treatment had their proper place, but not the first place in the treatment of a patient suffering from the effects of a grave cardiac lesion. He had been glad to hear Dr Affleck place so much value on morphine, paraldehyde, etc., in the treatment of the sleeplessness and pain of aortic disease. He agreed with Dr Gibson in his remarks on angina. Some reference had been made to the use of the nitrite group of substances. Nitrite of sodium was one of the most valuable. It was crystalline, soluble, stable, non-volatile, and so possessed pharmaceutical advantages over other members of the group. It did not so readily produce headache as nitro-glycerine. If used in proper doses ($\frac{1}{2}$ to

2 grains) there was no difficulty in maintaining the action of the nitrite group by its administration. The effects were more permanent than those of nitrite of amyl or of ethyl. The action of all the members of the group, however, became less after several administrations, and therefore subsequent doses must be increased. Prof. Fraser agreed with Dr Stockman that the indications for the use of iron in cardiac cases were rare, and therefore, as a rule, its administration was unnecessary. For some years he had had the blood examined and the corpuscles and hæmoglobin estimated in cardiac cases in the hospital, and it was surprising in how few any important degree of anæmia was present. Sometimes the administration of iron did harm, as in cases of auriculo-ventricular disease, when it increased visceral congestion, for example, in the liver and kidneys. He thought that the routine use of it without an actual examination of the blood was pernicious, and had probably arisen from conclusions drawn from the pallid appearance of some cardiac cases,—*e.g.*, aortic disease, and not from actual examination of the blood. He had been interested in Dr Russell's account of the successful treatment of certain weak and slow heart conditions by the use of belladonna, when digitalis had not been successful. He thought these cases were rare ; but he had now under his care a patient who exemplified this condition, whose cardiac insufficiency was so great that he could not sit up in bed without suffering from syncope. Digitalis, strophanthus, caffeine, convallaria,—each failed in turn to give relief, but belladonna soon did so. It was, however, a mistake to say that belladonna acted by relieving spasm of bloodvessels, as Dr Russell had suggested. It only relieved spasm of bloodvessels in lethal or large toxic doses. In medicinal doses it contracted bloodvessels, but it also paralysed the cardio-inhibitory fibres of the vagus and stimulated the heart through its vasomotor ganglia, and so increased blood tension. Remarks had been made by Dr James on the treatment of the heart weakness of pneumonia. He spoke of digitalis, strychnine, and strophanthus, and grouped them together, as if they all acted in the same manner. He (Prof. Fraser) must object to that. Strychnine did not act on the cardiac muscle, but on the bloodvessels, which it contracted through the vasomotor centres, and so it was impossible to compare the relative values of these remedies in any single condition of disease. Contrary to the opinion of Dr Bramwell, he placed little value upon the inhalation of oxygen in cardiac feebleness or cardiac dyspnœa ; and he was unable to understand, as Sir Thomas Grainger Stewart had urged, how the removal of only a few ounces of fluid from the pleural cavity could appreciably assist the contractions of a labouring heart or produce any benefit commensurate with the inconveniences and uncertainties of the operative procedure. It was of practical value, however, that the many remedies and remedial measures used in the treatment of heart affections which belonged to this secondary group

had been discussed by the various speakers, for it emphasized the fact that many cases of cardiac insufficiency could be successfully treated without the use of the more powerful remedies, and that the more powerful remedies should only be used when their exhibition was absolutely necessary. Dr Russell had referred to cases where cardiac murmurs were associated with digestive troubles and in which digitalis proved unsuccessful, but where not only the symptoms of indigestion, but also those of cardiac disorder, disappeared under successful treatment of the former symptoms. Dr Russell did not say that the heart murmurs were associated with evidences of cardiac insufficiency; and if they were not, in accordance with what was stated when opening the discussion, he (Prof. Fraser) agreed that the administration of digitalis is "bad practice." In such cases there is often anæmia with the dyspepsia, and the best remedy is iron; but when the anæmia and slight cardiac disorder are secondary to dyspepsia, and especially if there be epigastric pain and tenderness, the best success is obtained by first removing dyspepsia by the administration of small doses of bichromate of potassium, and then, if anæmia is shown to be present by an estimation of the blood-constituents, iron should be given in rather large doses. Sir Thomas Grainger Stewart had laid it down as a principle that during active changes in the heart cardiac tonics should not be administered. He (Prof. Fraser) would like to learn what was meant by active changes. If this meant arteritis, myocarditis, laceration of a cusp, endocarditis, he did not see why these tonics should not be used, provided cardiac failure were present. Even in acute myocarditis he could not admit that any injury could be done by administering them, although, no doubt, in extreme disorganisation of the myocardium it might be difficult to produce the action of these substances upon the heart muscle. But then acute myocarditis is so rare, and so difficult to diagnose with certainty, that he could not understand how any practical application was to be made of this theoretical contra-indication. Muscle degeneration might be so advanced that a healthy circulation could not be brought about; but even in extensive myocardial degeneration life might be saved by the administration of strophanthus. A heart was exhibited of a man, aged 51, with advanced cardiac insufficiency and œdema of the lungs and extremities. The heart's action was so rapid and feeble that the rate could only be estimated by auscultation over the precordia. Under the administration of strophanthus the pulse-rate was reduced on the first day from 130 to 120, and on the second to 98; and the strength and amplitude of movement of the pulse were correspondingly improved, so that it could be readily counted within a few hours, and had assumed normal characters on the second day. In this case it was demonstrated that by the action of a cardiac tonic a heart which was rapidly dying could be restored to an almost normal condition of functional sufficiency in a few hours, even when the muscular wall was extremely degenerated ; for, although the heart continued to act effectively, the pulmonary œdema increased and caused death, and at the post-mortem examination it was found that a great part of the muscle of both ventricles was replaced by fibroid tissue. These substances failed only when the heart muscle had undergone too great a degree of degenerative change. He could not, therefore, agree with Sir Thomas Grainger Stewart and Dr Ritchie in not using them in cases of acute disease. The existence of cardiac failure was the great and only indication for their use. If this does not exist, it would be improper to use them ; but it would equally be improper to refrain from using them in the existence of cardiac failure merely because of there being a possibility—always impossible to anticipate—of some injurious consequence resulting. Dr Balfour had remarked that, as the result of rest and diet, several of the symptoms of cardiac disorders occasionally disappeared. He had also observed this, and there-fore, in making observations on any cardiac remedy, he had not administered it till the patient had been several days under obser-vation. The discussion had, in the remarks of several speakers, diverged into the side issue of the relative advantages of one or other of the more important cardiac remedies. The disadvantage of digitalis was its cumulative action. As to the advantage of iodide of potassium in aneurism, in some cases it did good, but in others it was disappointing. Every one, however, who had seen many cases of aneurism must admit that it occupied the first place in the treatment of this disease. It did not, however, dilate the bloodvessels. If dilatation of the bloodvessels were an advan-tage in the treatment of aneurism, why did not nitrites do good ? for by their administration it was possible to dilate bloodvessels efficiently. He could not reconcile this explanation with the fact that Dr Balfour now allowed his patients to take exercise, which must inevitably raise blood-pressure. Iodide of potassium in large doses no doubt weakened the heart ; but Dr Balfour did not now give large doses, but small doses, which neither weakened the heart nor dilated the bloodvessels. We had merely Dr Balfour's opinion that the bloodvessels were dilated, but we would like to know the facts on which this opinion was based. The explanation of the therapeutic value of iodide of potassium was more probably to be found in the changes which it produced upon the structure of the diseased artery, whereby some degree of its normal elasticity was restored. Sir Thomas Grainger Stewart had praised stro-phanthus because it was rapid in its action. This was due to the facts that it was soluble, crystalline, and easily diffusible, and so did not accumulate in the stomach or blood. For the same reasons it was easily eliminated, and could be administered over a long period of time. Dr Ritchie had said that its action did not last so long as that of digitalis ; but how did Dr Ritchie ascertain this, and to what part of its action did he refer, and from how many comparable cases did he derive this opinion? Dr Balfour stated that strophanthus did not "feed" the heart, whereas digitalis did. Trustworthy data must be very difficult to be obtained for this opinion. It was not clear what was meant. It cannot be that the minute doses of the non-nitrogenous digitalin actually supply nutriment to the heart. It may have been meant that the nutrition of the heart was specially favoured by some peculiarity in the action of digitalis; but, in equal doses, strophanthus increases the movements of the heart more than digitalis does, and digitalis, by its contracting influence on bloodvessels, should be less effective than strophanthus in supplying the heart with its normal nutriment through the bloodvessels. One speaker had said that there was no practical difference between the members of this group of substances, but in his opening paper he (Prof. Fraser) had shown that there were differences. Except on historical grounds, the group was more a strophanthus one than a digitalis one. Strophanthus possessed the essential action in a more perfect form, and without the complications of digitalis. It was a disadvantage in many cases of mere cardiac weakness and insufficiency to constrict the vessels, and so put extra strain on the heart. Dr Balfour had expressed a preference for digitalis because it was indigenous, and he had had the courage to repeat the remark to-night. He might for the same reason prefer gooseberry wine to champagne, or deprecate the use of good Scotch whisky in India when crude arrack is indigenous. He must, however, admit that strophanthus had suffered because it was the product of a distant country. There were several species of the genus, and while its therapeutic effects had been determined with only one of these species, the seeds of several of the others had indiscriminately been substituted. The whole fruit, and not the seeds only, and immature seeds, poor in the active principle and rich in irritating resin, had been used to prepare the tincture; seeds already exhausted with alcohol had been re-sold in the market; and, further, even when good seeds were used, petroleum ether had been substituted for ethylic ether, preparatory to percolation with rectified spirit, with the result that the tincture contained much resin, which produces stomach and intestinal disorder. He expressed his great gratification on account of the interest taken in the discussion of this question. It should lead to good results in the treatment of a most important class of diseases. He thought the Society was much indebted to the Council for having originated the discussion, and for having carried out the arrangements so satisfactorily.

Meeting VIII.—March 6, 1895.

Mr JOSEPH BELL, *Ex-President, in the Chair.*

I. ELECTION OF MEMBERS.

The following gentlemen were elected Ordinary Members of the Society:—James Scott, M.B. C.M., 32 St Patrick Square; John Hardie, M.B., F.R.C.S. Ed., 12 Newington Road; John Orr, M.B., M.R.C.P. Ed., 52 Grange Road; Jno. Hosack Fraser, M.B. C.M., Bellfield, Bridge of Allan; John Struthers, M.B. C.M. Ed., South Africa.

II. EXHIBITION OF PATIENTS.

1. *Dr A. Lockhart Gillespie* showed—(*a.*) A young man with DEFORMITY OF BOTH HANDS, only the thumb and two fingers being present, the other fingers with corresponding metacarpal bones being deficient. (*b.*) Two children, both deaf-mutes, sisters, with GOITRE AND RAPID PULSE. There were four sisters and one brother in the family. All the sisters were deaf-mutes and had suffered from goitre, but the brother was healthy and could hear and speak. No history of deaf-mutism among relations. About a year ago he found the eldest girl suffering from breathlessness, and found a considerable goitre, neck being 12½ inches in circumference, pulse 92 when she was at rest, 140 when she ran round the room. No other symptoms. She was given bromide and iodide of strontium, and in a very short time (March 6) pulse at rest 90, and on running round room 130. After a month of treatment, neck was 11½ inches, pulse at rest 80, quite regular, and after exercise 100. The good effect had been permanent, neck about the same, but pulse lower. The younger girl, also with slight goitre and irregular pulse, had been put on the same treatment with success. Another of the sisters had suffered from what he thought was pachymeningitis cervicalis hypertrophica, from which she did not quite recover, having still a stiff neck. In answer to Mr Bell, he stated that the father and mother were not related. (*c.*) A girl from Donaldson's Hospital with a PATENT ANTERIOR FONTANELLE. The forehead had been pushed forward by the growth of the brain, so that the upper part overhung the lower, the upper part of the frontal bone being open in the middle line for about ¾ inch. (*d.*) A demonstration in LIP-READING was given by one of the teachers in Donaldson's Hospital on two young boys, both deaf-mutes. They repeated after the teacher vowels, initial consonants, and terminal consonants, and answered such questions as: Do you want to go home? Where do you live? What is your name? Do you

know any of these gentlemen? Also answering correctly a few questions on history.

Mr Bell thanked Dr Gillespie for his interesting cases.

2. *Dr Norman Walker* showed a case of a PECULIAR LINEAR ERUPTION in a little girl, which commenced on the wrist, ran up the arm, and down over the chest. The only cases at all like this which he could find were two cases shown by Dr Lee to the Clinical Society. For these cases Dr Crocker suggested the name "larva migrans." Also a case of KERATOSIS PILARIS or LICHEN SPINULOSUS. The patient was 11 years old, and the disease had lasted for six months. The spikes were very prominent, and the distribution was the usual one.

Mr Bell said he had been puzzled over a case similar to the former in the form of a pattern on the legs of a stalwart young fellow from the country, until he found an arabesque pattern in aniline dyes on his stockings.

III. EXHIBITION OF SPECIMENS.

1. *Dr Wm. Russell* showed—(*a.*) An OVARIAN TUMOUR which had been diagnosed as a fibroid. The patient died of infiltrating encephaloid cancer of the liver. (*b.*) LUNGS of two patients, æt. 80 and 86, who died of influenzal pneumonia. (*c.*) An ANEURISM of the ABDOMINAL AORTA. (*d.*) An IMPACTED GALL-STONE, the gall-bladder being tacked to hepatic flexure of colon and abdominal wall, and thus rendered functionless.

2. *Dr Leith* showed a PANCREAS with ABSCESSES in head, tail, and body. No abscesses elsewhere. Cystic duct and common bile-duct were both distended, owing to impaction of gall-stones, of which he had left one in position fixed near the papilla. Both hepatic ducts, and for a considerable area the branches of the left duct, were filled with gall-stones. The patient was a woman 63 years of age. There were two or three points of interest about the case. First, the rarity of abscesses in the pancreas in connexion with gall-stones. They were comparatively common in the liver. Gall-stones and biliary sand had existed for a long time in this case. She died a fortnight after admission to hospital with a fractured femur, cause of death being somewhat obscure until disclosed by the post-mortem examination; but he had no doubt it was related to this suppurative pancreatitis. Her own doctor, although frequently called to consult about asthmatic or bronchial attacks, never had any suspicion of gall-stones. It was interesting to find a case of passage of gall-stones without pain, but when 19 she had begun to take morphia, and had taken it in repeated doses since then,—*i.e.*, for forty-three years,—and practically during the last twenty years she had taken over 73,000 grains of morphia, and had spent £400 on it, according to her doctor's computation.

Probably the microbes passed through the patent terminal part of the common bile-duct into the pancreatic duct.

IV. EXHIBITION OF PHOTOGRAPHS.

Dr Leith showed Photos. of an ANEURISM opening into the superior vena cava. It had occurred within a month of Dr Bruce's case. It was diagnosed during life. The photos. showed anterior and posterior views. The sac was about the size of a fœtal head. The opening was into the posterior part of the right side of the superior vena cava, about ½-inch below its commencement. The right and left innominate veins were both largely blocked with pretty firm clot, thus further hindering venous return from upper part of body, so that the collateral veins of thorax and abdomen were greatly distended, especially on one side. Another interesting feature was that the right side of the heart was greatly dilated and somewhat hypertrophied, while the left side was pretty nearly normal. The patient was a man æt. 50.

Mr Bell said he hoped this case would be recorded along with Dr Bruce's.

V. ORIGINAL COMMUNICATION.

SOME QUESTIONS WITH REGARD TO THE DIAGNOSIS, PROGNOSIS, AND TREATMENT OF SUPPURATION IN CERTAIN OSSEOUS CAVITIES.

By P. M'BRIDE, M.D., F.R.C.P. Ed., F.R.S.E., Surgeon Ear and Throat Department, Edinburgh Royal Infirmary.

THE cavities referred to in the title of this paper are those connected with the ear and nose. Aural and nasal specialists have of late years striven to extend the operative domains of their respective specialities. Some of the surgical measures proposed have, however, not been of unmixed advantage to their patients; but in the case of suppurative diseases, where most of the progress has been made along well-recognised and scientific lines, common alike to the specialist and general surgeon, much good has resulted from an increase of operative activity.

Were I to endeavour to treat fully of suppurative ear disease alone, I should require many hours, if not days; while empyema of the accessory cavities of the nose would require as much time for its discussion. My object to-night must, therefore, be merely to raise some points which have seemed to me worthy of discussion, and, if possible, to receive some light drawn from general surgery upon matters which I have had difficulty in elucidating.

With these objects in view, I shall divide my subject into two headings, viz.,—1, Suppuration of the Middle Ear; 2, Suppuration of the Nasal Accessory Cavities.

SUPPURATION OF THE MIDDLE EAR.

It is, of course, now well known that in suppurative ear disease —more particularly when it has become chronic—the great desideratum is free drainage. This may often be obtained in acute cases by simple incision of the drum membrane, and sometimes in chronic suppuration by excision of the membrane and malleus, with or without the incus.

I will not dwell, however, upon these operations, which will probably remain confined to the practice of the specialist. My experience of excision of the membrane and malleus has been limited, but in one instance I achieved not only complete cure of the suppuration, but also marked improvement in hearing. Of common interest alike to surgeons and to aurists are the various operations for gaining more or less free access to the middle-ear cavities—viz., tympanum and mastoid antrum—from without.

I do not wish to put off time by entering into the history of the methods which have been adopted. Schwartze may be said to have first introduced drainage through the mastoid as a generally practicable and useful operation. His method was to chisel or gouge a canal into the antrum, and thus secure free drainage. Küster, and, following in his footsteps, Von Bergmann, pointed out that an attempt should be made to reach the whole diseased area, and these operators endeavoured to attain this end by removing the posterior and upper walls of the osseous meatus. After Küster's first communication, Zaufal practised an operation which, in uncomplicated cases, may shortly be described as follows:—An incision is made from below the centre of the mastoid upwards until the temporal line is reached, at right angles to its upper extremity another cut is carried forwards, and the whole flap, including periosteum, is reflected. The membranous meatus is either incised in its upper and posterior parts, or the whole is dissected out as deeply as possible, cut through, and reflected forwards, as in Stacke's operation. In the former case the upper and posterior parts of the membranous covering of the osseous meatus are removed as nearly down to the membrane as possible. It is then advised to chisel away layer after layer of bone, beginning 1 cm. behind the meatus, and driving the instrument into it. If after the removal of several wedges a cavity is not reached, a smaller gouge is used, which is worked in the upper and posterior part of the newly-formed wound until the antrum is arrived at. Then the posterior wall, in so far as it remains, and the outer wall of the tympanic attic, are snipped away with bone forceps (Luer's specially modified). I have thus merely sketched this method, because it seems to me to fulfil surgical principles. Stacke afterwards proposed throwing forward the auricle, together with the dissected-out membranous meatus, gouging off the upper and outer osseous wall of the tympanum, and removing diseased ossicles, etc. He soon found it necessary to extend his method, and, so far as I understand the position, to advise opening the mastoid according to Schwartze's method, then following it up by his own operation, and finally taking away the intermediate portion of bone,—a proceeding very similar in its effects to Zaufal's previously practised operation.   As before stated, I have no intention of entering fully either into the various methods of operating, nor into the claims of individual authors to priority.   I therefore pass over the many modifications of the above methods which have been suggested, such as transplantation of skin flaps into the mastoid wound with a view to establishing a permanent opening, or lining the cavities with healthy skin.   Nor does the actual instrument used seem to me of sufficient importance to justify very serious discussion.   The suggestion that a dental burr should be employed instead of a gouge has certainly one justification, in that a polished surface is more easily inspected than one in which inequalities are present.   I have performed a considerable number of these operations, and have always found that they read much easier than they are in reality, for authors do not very vividly describe the more or less constant presence of oozing which is liable to obscure the surface of the bone in the deeper parts, no matter whether it be roughened by the gouge or polished by the burr.

This paper would pass far beyond its legitimate dimensions were I to attempt to define closely the indications for the various methods which have been sketched.   I should, however, like to make a few remarks in this direction, and for the purpose I may perhaps be permitted to divide the class of cases for which such operations are justifiable into—1, Recent; 2, those of long standing.

(1.) *Recent Cases.*

Cases of middle-ear suppuration of recent origin, and in which no great amount of destruction of the drum membrane has taken place, are, in my opinion, usually curable by means of Schwartze's operation alone.   By recent I mean those of but a few months' standing, and by the term curable I intend to convey that the hearing becomes normal, or nearly so, and that the perforation of the membrane heals.   Now, as this has been my experience, it has naturally given rise to the question, whether in cases of subacute suppuration threatening to become chronic we ought not to open into the mastoid antrum more frequently than we are now inclined to do.   Given a small perforation of the tympanic membrane with persistent discharge, ought we not to drain through the only available channel—the mastoid—at an early stage, so that we may restore the hearing and prevent the risks of subsequent chronicity?   On the one side we must weigh the fact that opening the antrum is not quite devoid of danger, and on the other the risks to hearing, and, in a minor degree, to life, associated with chronic suppuration.   I admit that on this point I am still somewhat in doubt.   I am not at all prepared to say that the patient who shows early evidences of mastoid complication, or at least suffers from deep-seated pain in the ear—indications of defective drainage—and who has his mastoid antrum opened, does not in the end come off best, recovering, as he usually does, completely. In the after-treatment of these cases, it has seemed to me that it is very desirable to keep them, as far as possible, dry. After the antrum is opened and scraped out in such a way as to avoid injuring the intra-tympanic structures, a stream of antiseptic fluid is usually employed, both to clear out débris and pus, and to show that a through drain has been established. The parts should, however, thereafter be most carefully dried with sterilised iodoform gauze, then thickly dusted with the powder recommended by MacEwen (iodoform 1, boracic 4), and finally packed with sterilised iodoform gauze. In these recent cases the parts are generally quite sweet after five or six days.

(2.) *Chronic Cases.*

In chronic cases I have comparatively rarely found anything approaching a cure. By a cure in these cases I do not imply restoration of good hearing, but only absolute cessation of suppuration. It has been recommended by surgeons to drain through the mastoid in cases of chronic suppuration which have resisted treatment for a year. My own experience has made me an opponent of this view, for the following reason :—We ought before proposing a serious operation to be able to hold out to our patients a probability of success greater than can be achieved by more simple methods. Now, experience with regard both of my own cases and of those which have come under my care after treatment by others, has by no means convinced me that we can fulfil this postulate. In most cases of chronic suppuration we can, with the co-operation of the patient, reduce the discharge to a minimum, by treatment applied through the external meatus. The actual method adopted must, of course, vary with each case ; but I may here merely indicate such simple remedies as cleanliness, caustics, removal of granulations and polypi, etc.

Again, we may in cases of disease of the attic with perforation of Shrapnell's membrane, gain much by removal of the membrane and malleus. In a few instances we can by these methods make no impression upon the discharge, and in such cases where the flow of pus is large and continuous, we may, I believe, generally take for granted more or less extensive disease of bone.

In the class of case I wish to discuss now there is a certain amount of purulent discharge, which, however, is by no means copious, and we have no other indication for external operation. I question very much whether under these circumstances we can ever hold out a probability of permanent cessation of the discharge after opening up the middle-ear cavities by any of the external operations which have been advocated, and which would

be, under the circumstances, justifiable. I have now operated by
different methods on numerous chronic cases in which operation
was urgently indicated on general grounds, and only in a small
proportion have I been able to obtain what could justly be termed
a cure. What has misled many is dependence on the statements
of patients. An individual has a running ear; the mastoid is
opened, he is dismissed with "no running from the ear."

In most of these cases, however, I venture to say that at some
period within six months after healing of the wound, a small
amount of fœtid discharge can be detected in the meatus or middle
ear; and if no precautions be taken, the case will soon be as bad
as ever. If it be kept clean and treated on otological lines, it may
altogether cease for a period, or even permanently. In a few cases
a more or less permanent result is attained, but it does not seem
that in chronic cases we are yet in a position to advise draining
through the mastoid where the only symptom is a moderate
amount of purulent discharge.

The actual method of operating is another point of considerable
interest, but time does not permit to discuss each method in detail.
I will only say that it appears to me that the operator should not
slavishly follow any man or method, but set out with the object
of removing so much of the bone as is diseased, and then exposing
the middle-ear cavities as completely as possible without involving
the patient in undue risks. These risks may be briefly sum-
marised under the following headings :—1, Hearing; 2, Facial
nerve ; 3, Life.

In many cases the auditory function is already so far injured
that any danger of making it worse may be ignored. The facial
nerve may be injured in any mastoid operation, but it runs most
risk of suffering when the bridge of bone left after the posterior
wall has been removed and the mastoid antrum exposed, is
attacked. I have more than once been compelled to leave it
because of twitching of the face having occurred during attempts
at its removal. Again, it must also be remembered that in these
cases we are dealing with intensely septic cavities, and we must
not—unless we have reason to believe in the existence of intra-
cranial suppuration—do anything by the removal of healthy bone
to bring them into communication with the cerebral structures.
Diseased bone is, of course, septic, and we may freely remove it.
Thus I have twice opened up extra-dural abscesses by acting on
these lines, and once freely exposed the lateral sinus. Two of
these cases were of considerable interest, and deserve a passing
reference.

1. J. N., æt. 30, gave a history of purulent discharge from the
left ear of only three weeks' duration; but this was probably a
recrudescence of old middle-ear suppuration, as examination of
the ear showed a quantity of granulation tissue. The history he
gave was pain behind the ear lasting for ten days, but he stated

that this had somewhat abated within the last two days. He nevertheless looked extremely ill when he was admitted to my ward on the 12th of June 1894. His temperature went up to 101°, but his pulse did not at any time exceed 80. The case seemed urgent, and I did not delay operation in order to inves· tigate the symptoms further. I, however, ventured to express the opinion before operating, that probably a mastoid suppuration had relieved itself by breaking through the bone inwards. My reasons for this were—(1), The history of prolonged pain; (2), the relief of pain during the past two days; (3), the temperature rising to 101°, and pulse not exceeding 80 as a maximum; (4), the fact that notwithstanding the relief of pain he looked like a cerebral case. I operated on the 13th of June, and came upon a quantity of cholesteatomatous matter in the mastoid, and also upon pus welling up from between the bone and dura mater, which latter was freely exposed. Next day, when dressing the wound, a good deal more of the cholesteatomatous material was removed. The patient, apart from a tendency to slight suppuration of the ear, made an uninterrupted recovery. Whenever he was well enough I had his eyes examined, and Dr Mackay was good enough to report with regard to the left eye, "Distinct optic neuritis, also a patch of opaque nerve fibres; the neuritis is in an early stage; no interference with vision." On July 4th Dr Mackay reported, "Still shows a considerable amount of optic neuritis in each fundus. His right eye has full vision; his left about half for distances." On the 12th February 1895 Dr Mackay reported, "Fundi still show traces of the optic neuritis through which he has passed. The vessels still unnaturally tortuous, and the retina about each disc has not regained complete transparency. He has full vision with each eye."

2. N. G., like the last patient, was admitted one afternoon and operated upon next day. He had on admission great pain in the left ear, and fever, the temperature varying between 102°·4 and 106°·2. He also had rigors and sweats. After a consultation with Mr Duncan I resolved to operate on the mastoid at once, as there was probably thrombosis of the lateral sinus. I accordingly opened into the mastoid process, beginning rather further back than usual. The bone was sclerosed, but after proceeding with the operation I found a small collection of cheesy and fœtid pus. In clearing away the bone around it I came upon the sigmoid sinus. This was seen to be healthy, so far as could be judged. The wound in the bone was then carried forwards into the middle ear. This patient also made a very satisfactory recovery.

The next question which I should like to discuss is—Assuming the middle-ear structures to have been opened up from behind, what is the best after-treatment? My own practice is to syringe thoroughly with 1-2000 perchloride solution at the time of operation, then dry out carefully and fill the cavities with a mixture of boracic acid and iodoform. The wound and the meatus are then plugged with sterilised iodoform gauze ; and if the posterior wall of the meatus has been removed, it is of very great importance to plug the meatus first, lest stenosis should result. There is often a good deal of oozing within the first twenty-four hours after the operation, so that it may be necessary to change the dressings on the following day. After this the frequency of the dressing must depend upon the time the parts remain sweet. It has appeared to me that irrigation is better avoided so long as there is no smell from the dressings. As I have said, my experience has usually been that a complete cure of the suppuration is the exception rather than the rule, although the discharge may be reduced to a minimum, and thus lead a casual observer to infer a cure. For this reason I am inclined to make free use of the lead nail, which can be worn without discomfort, and which permits of thorough cleansing with antiseptic liquids in those cases which have failed to be cured by the dry method of dressing. Now, if the lead nail requires to be employed after such operations, I am by no means sure that the simple opening of the antrum according to Schwartze's method is not in many cases preferable to the more modern operations which include removal of the posterior wall of the meatus. I have not so far practised Zaufal's operation exactly as he describes it, and I can quite imagine that it may give a larger proportion of absolute cures than other less energetic methods; but extensive operations in this region must of necessity involve the risks which have been already indicated. Much more could be said as to these mastoid operations did time permit, but my desire has been merely to bring forward certain points for discussion, viz.:—

(1.) In subacute cases of middle-ear suppuration threatening to become chronic, ought we not to open the mastoid early, even without the presence of the usual indications ?

(2.) In what proportion of chronic cases can a cure of the middle-ear suppuration be obtained by mastoid operation? In my own experience, definite cure of the suppuration very often does not result.

(3.) If this be so, is there any justification for the proposal to drain through the mastoid in a case of chronic middle-ear suppuration in which the discharge is not very copious and no other definite indications exist ?

(4.) Is it desirable to operate by Zaufal's or some analogous method in every chronic case in which we feel justified in opening the mastoid ? Of course all diseased bone should be removed wherever found, but Zaufal's method implies very free removal of healthy bone as well.

SUPPURATION OF THE NASAL ACCESSORY CAVITIES.

I have spent so much time over my remarks upon ear disease that I shall make what is to follow as short as possible.

It is unnecessary to go over in detail the semeiology and

diagnosis of suppuration of the different accessory cavities. It is now generally accepted that a purulent discharge from the nose, more especially if confined to one nostril, is a probable indication of empyema of one or more of the accessory cavities—provided such gross lesions as ulceration, caries, rhinolith, or foreign body can be excluded. The discharge, when coming in any quantity from the nostril, will in all probability be found to originate in the antrum, the frontal sinus, or the anterior ethmoidal cells, and in that case examination will show that it tends to appear in the anterior part of the middle meatus. Disease of the sphenoidal sinus or posterior ethmoid cells will usually be associated with the presence of discharge in the posterior part of the nostril or naso-pharynx. I may, however, state in passing that this also sometimes occurs in uncomplicated antral cases. If, then, in a patient we have arrived at the conclusion that the antrum, anterior ethmoid cells, or frontal sinus are at fault, we usually suspect the antrum first. By various methods—*e.g.*, posture test, transillumination, introduction of a tube into the natural opening, and eventually exploratory puncture, followed, if necessary, by washing out—we can usually determine whether or not it contains pus. We can thus eliminate any doubt with regard to this particular cavity. Sometimes we find that it is healthy ; or, again, we may, after washing it perfectly clean, ascertain that pus still finds its way into the middle meatus of the nose. If this be so, we are driven to the conclusion that either the anterior ethmoidal cells or frontal sinus are giving rise to the discharge. Here we come upon a very weak spot in our diagnosis, and I am not by any means sure that even the most skilled rhinologist can ever do more than express a pious opinion or explore. I shall presently refer further to the connexion between polypus and empyema of the accessory cavities. At present I shall content myself by saying that suppuration of any of these cavities may give rise to the presence of polypoid growths. In such cases pus comes from the affected part or parts, while bare bone may usually be detected by pressing a probe against the œdematous granulation tissue. Here we have at once the picture described by some authors as indicating disease of the ethmoidal cells. No doubt, in many of these cases they are affected sometimes alone, oftener in association with the frontal sinus and maxillary antrum. Sometimes we can venture to say that probably the disease is chiefly in the ethmoid, but rarely can we certainly eliminate the frontal sinus. In such cases, fortunately, the indication for treatment is to remove with a snare, small cutting forceps, or a sharp spoon, all granulation tissue, and it is often desirable to take away also part of the middle turbinated bone. The free drainage thus effected may relieve the flow of pus from the nose. Are we, however, to say that therefore the condition was confined to the middle turbinated body and ethmoid ? May it not have been that by these means a free drain from the frontal sinus was permitted which resulted in cure? I have found it extremely difficult to diagnose suppuration of the last-named cavity to my own satisfaction, and I have found it equally difficult to decide what method of treatment to adopt when it has appeared that probabilities were in favour of latent empyema of the frontal sinus. I may mention that pain about the frontal region may be due to empyema of the antrum or ethmoid cells, or to neuralgia alone. A moderate flow of pus from the nose is not a very dreadful evil, and we do not often hear of brain mischief as a result of extension from the frontal sinus. Taking these facts into consideration, one is often placed in doubt as to whether exploratory opening is justifiable, considering the possibility of permanent deformity which it carries with it. Other methods of treatment suggested are—1, Washing out by the natural orifice, which can only occasionally succeed ; 2, an attempt to penetrate the floor through the nose, as recommended by Schäffer. The one is rarely successful, and the other is generally regarded as dangerous unless the bone is softened by disease.

I have, I think, said enough to indicate the difficulties which beset us in arriving at a correct conclusion with regard to what I may term the anterior accessory cavities. In empyema of the posterior ethmoidal cells and sphenoidal sinus diagnosis becomes still more difficult. When posterior rhinoscopy reveals the presence of pus above the middle turbinated, one of these cavities may be suspected. Again, matter trickling down and tending to form a crust along the septum posteriorly is believed to indicate suppuration of the sphenoidal sinus. A probe passed along the middle turbinated and upwards may detect caries of the anterior wall of this cavity, or pass into it. Sometimes the orifice may actually be seen after reduction of the middle turbinated or in atrophic catarrh. However, affections of the posterior ethmoidal cells and sphenoidal sinus are matters which are, perhaps, not quite so clear to specialists as might be inferred from the somewhat too definite and dogmatic tone of some writers.

The connexion between suppuration of the nasal accessory cavities and polypi is a matter of interest alike to specialists and surgeons. Various attempts have been made to show that polypi are commonly associated with either disease of bone or affections of the accessory cavities. Where reliance is placed upon the probe mistakes are very apt to occur, for in all forms of polypoid conditions the delicate muco-periosteum goes, I believe, to form part of the soft œdematous growth. Thus a probe will easily pass through it and impinge upon bone. From experience I should say that so-called nasal polypus may—

(1.) Exist as a condition the etiology of which is not very clear.

(2.) Be caused by suppuration of the antrum or one of the other accessory cavities.

In the first case, while there is often a great complaint of nasal discharge, it is usually found to be serous and not purulent, while it is perfectly odourless, nor does the patient complain of a bad smell or taste. The growths themselves are of that greyish-blue which is so well known to us all.

Where polypus depends upon suppuration of the accessory cavities the tumours often have a more red and fleshy look; there is commonly a complaint of bad taste, while inspection of the nose gives indications of the presence of pus. Frequently, too, these conditions are confined to one nostril. It must, however, be remembered that simple polypus may be unilateral, and also that bilateral disease of the antrum is by no means of very great rarity.

Again, in some cases the growths look like common mucus polypi, but they are associated with purulent discharge. It will, I think, often be found that in such cases there is a marked tendency to rapid recurrence, and it may be desirable to take away a portion of the middle turbinated from which they usually spring. It must, in such cases, be considered an open question whether the polypi result from suppuration in the ethmoidal cavities, or cause it.

A difficulty which sometimes confronts us is the association of large polypoid masses with empyema of the antrum where the former obviously depend upon the latter. It is then, I believe, better to remove the polypi and cauterise the base as well as drain the antrum, for I have noticed that even after free escape of pus has been duly provided for, they tend to recur.

The methods of treating empyema of the accessory cavities have already been briefly referred to, but suppuration of the antrum seems to deserve more than a passing notice, because of its very frequent occurrence.

Here, too, there can be no doubt that a great deal depends upon the duration of the affection. Some authors recommend washing out the antrum by the natural orifice, and no doubt in recent cases a cure may be attained in this way. Opinion is, however, generally in favour of making an artificial opening. This may be made— (1), into the nose; (2), through the alveolar process; (3), through the canine fossa; (4), by removing the whole anterior wall of the antrum, as recommended by Jansen; (5), by combining opening into the canine fossa with opening from the inferior meatus.

There can, I think, be no doubt that in recent cases the best treatment is to extract a carious tooth, if it exists, and open through its socket into the antrum. A plate with a solid plug is then made by a dentist, and the patient syringes the cavity two or three times daily with an antiseptic. In those cases where there is no dental disease or vacant space through which the cavity can be entered in the gum, the propriety of opening through the canine fossa must be considered. My own experience has been that an opening in this position is extremely difficult to keep patent, but in recent cases this can be got over. In chronic old-standing cases, where there is a prospect of requiring through drainage for months and even years, I much prefer to open through the alveolus, as here, at least, we can make sure of maintaining patency of the channel. It has been recommended in such cases to open in the canine fossa, and plug the cavity with iodoform gauze, while Chiari applies the same treatment through an alveolar opening. I cannot, however, say I have found this method generally successful in obstinate and old cases.

Again, it has been advised to make a very large opening in the same situation, so that the whole cavity can be explored by means of the index finger, and even by sight. The walls may then be scraped, and any existing granulation tissue removed. Insufflation of powders has been advocated by some, but it is extremely difficult to carry out unless through a large opening, as the moisture clogs the insufflator; again, Grünwald has advised a spray of an ethereal solution of iodoform as a substitute for insufflation.

Opening through the inferior meatus of the nose is an operation which is gradually being given up for old-standing cases, as the orifice is difficult to maintain. Caldwell and Scanes Spicer have, however, employed it in combination with an orifice in the canine fossa.

Jansen, recognising the tedious nature of chronic antral empyema, has suggested dissecting up the gum in flaps, and then removing the anterior wall, excepting the infra-orbital foramen. The flaps are then stuffed into the cavity so that a permanent opening is established, which is closed by an obturator attached to a tooth. There can be no doubt that we often meet with cases which resist all ordinary methods, and it becomes a question whether or not Jansen's operation should then be employed. An opening through the alveolus, closed by a solid plug attached to a plate, enables the patient to wash out the antrum as often as is required, and he is generally thus kept in perfect comfort. My own inclination is in such cases to give this method a very prolonged trial before resorting to more heroic means.

In view of the extreme obstinacy of these antral suppurations after they have been allowed to remain for years, we ought, I think, to operate early in every case, when the extraction of a tooth and the introduction of a vulcanite plug, with regular washing through, will usually effect a speedy cure. The parallel in this respect with middle-ear suppurations is complete.

––––––

Mr Bell having complimented Dr M'Bride on his paper, said that one very remarkable change had taken place with regard to the view they took of middle-ear suppuration. Twenty years ago they knew very little about it, and did less. Nowadays he thought perhaps they were rather far on, thinking they knew a great deal about it, more than was warranted. Especially in the case of children it was a regular operation to open the antrum, even without other symptoms. That was a part of their routine treatment. He quite agreed as to the importance of not doing that in too great a hurry in chronic cases. They should simply be kept clean, not having so much to promise them in the way of cure, for the hearing was nearly gone in most cases. With reference to the different methods, he thought the great thing was to get into the mastoid antrum first, and then gradually work one's way upwards and backwards, cutting away all the softened bone, and taking care not to remove any more of the healthy bone than was necessary. He quite agreed as to the utility of the dry method after washing out. Let the cavity be filled with powder, and kept dry as long as possible. With regard to empyema of the antrum, which was the real practical point for surgeons, he thought when one got a really bad chronic case, one never got on until a satisfactory opening was made into it through the socket of a tooth. If the teeth were good, then one must be sacrificed. In one or two of the very worst cases he had seen, they had also to make an accessory opening in front through the canine fossa. He had never removed the whole anterior wall, which was not only a serious operation, but, as Dr M'Bride said, left a permanent deformity which had to be managed afterwards.

Dr M'Kenzie Johnston said he had been, in common with, he was sure, all the members of the Society, extremely interested in this very able paper by Dr M'Bride. It contained a great deal, and more than one of the subjects dealt with might be taken up. He should like to refer chiefly to the principal point in the first part of the paper, viz., whether it was wise to open in chronic cases early, or earlier than they were in the habit of doing, under the influence, say, of a subacute attack. Personally he thought such cases, *i.e.*, cases of over a year's standing, would undoubtedly benefit by opening. Victor Horsley and others had committed themselves to this opinion. But there was a difficulty in proposing that. First of all, chronic suppurations of the ear (by chronic he meant at least twelve months' old) were extremely common, and he was quite satisfied that patients would not submit to operation until the surgeon was prepared to say that it was necessary. He was sure the patient would not, and he had very grave doubts as to whether the majority of the profession were prepared to propose operation at so early a stage. But it would be a benefit to those cases in which discharge continued and complications appeared. He had hopes, as time went on, that they might be able to differentiate in these cases,—to be able to say that this case should be opened earlier than another which had also discharge. But at present they were not in that position, viz., to say whether a case should or should not be operated on simply because the discharge did not stop in twelve months. But when a case lasted longer, were they to operate or await symptoms? He would rather open at the earlier stage, if one could get the sanction of the patient and practitioner. If that were refused, then they had to wait until active symptoms set in. With regard to continuance of discharge in middle-ear disease, there were certain things which in themselves might maintain discharge without a great amount of disease affecting the antrum, e.g., presence of adenoids and various nasopharyngeal conditions might keep up a slight discharge. He assumed that all such things were eliminated before the serious operation of opening the mastoid was proposed. With regard to the curability of chronic cases he had nothing to add, because he felt that Dr M'Bride was correct in saying that absolute cure was a rarity. With regard to the methods of various surgeons he was also in accord with him. Personally he preferred, if possible, Schäffer's operation in the first instance, and would rather delay the more extensive one, because there was less oozing, and one saw better into the cells. The question of operation in middle-ear disease was one of great difficulty, but he believed as time went on they would operate earlier. With regard to the nose, Dr M'Bride had opened up a very wide question, and he had only to express his own preference, with regard to disease of the antrum of Highmore, for opening through the socket of a tooth, making it very large so as to have free drainage, and keeping it open by obturator and plug until the discharge ceased, then allowing it gradually to heal. At the same time he was aware that a certain number of cases would go on a long time, and it was impossible absolutely to get a cure.

Mr Wallace said that Dr M'Bride had left them very much in the position from which he would have expected him to carry them on, because it was to specialists that they looked for information as to when they were to operate in long-standing cases of otorrhœa. Dr M'Bride had asked the wrong people to tell him when the operation should be done, seeing he had so many opportunities of treating cases of chronic otorrhœa. He (Mr Wallace) recollected that Victor Horsley suggested that if after a year otorrhœa had not been checked, an operation ought to be considered; but, as Dr M'Kenzie Johnston had said, it was very difficult to make up one's own mind that it would be right to step in in such circumstances, and still more difficult to get patients to consent to operation. The patient was practically quite well; only a slight discharge from the ear, associated with deafness. To suggest an operation would only be to meet with refusal. It was a question that came up before the general surgeon constantly,—e.g., in the case of a tubercular joint, were they to do a trivial operation or attempt a radical cure? Were they to incise, excise, or, if the disease were in the tarsus, amputate the foot? In such cases they usually found, what Dr M'Bride found in otorrhœa, that treatment failed, and sooner or later they had to perform the major operation. He thought some information might be got from the bacteriological side. From the examination of the discharges some statistics might be got as to which cases should be treated radically and which not. Another point was the difference between adults and children. He would like Dr M'Bride to tell them what he had found in the treatment of ordinary suppuration in children as compared with similar suppuration in adults. Personally he thought he had obtained better results in adults than in children; the very reverse of what, from one point of view, he would have expected. In adults the bony partitions were stronger and the sinuses more numerous. In the child the partitions were more easily broken down and not so extensive. On the other hand, there was the fact that it was always more difficult to carry out after-treatment in the child than in the adult. In an acute case he thought the indication was to gain free access to the antrum, and have free drainage. If all the disease were radically removed, the result in the acute case would be good. In chronic disease with the bone more sclerosed, and probably organisms more deeply seated, it was only reasonable to suppose that the result of treatment would not be so successful. With regard to the nasal cavities, Dr M'Bride had again carried them so far and then stopped. No doubt some surgeons preferred one method of operation to another. He thought it mattered very little in an acute case. In a chronic it was of more importance. When one had to deal with the posterior ethmoidal frontal and sphenoidal sinuses, both diagnosis and treatment were extremely difficult. From one or two cases he had observed, when disease had affected either ethmoidal sinus—it was difficult to differentiate posterior from anterior—the results of treatment were not at all good. The patient was often left in as bad a case after as before treatment. With regard to the frontal sinus, he admitted the difficulty in diagnosis, but he thought that now and then they got pretty distinct evidence of frontal sinus affection, *e.g.*, in deeper-seated pain and more frontal headache than in the case of antral disease. If there were no discharge of pus in the inferior meatus, no evidence of ordinary antral disease, and at the same time acute symptoms pointing to the frontal, there should be no difficulty. Where there was antral disease, and the nasal chamber more or less covered with pus, it was more difficult. With regard to the method of opening the antrum, he again agreed with Dr M'Bride and Dr Johnston. Both referred to the extraction of a tooth. But extraction might have been carried out before active suppuration appeared, and the socket of the tooth might have become filled with new bone which was very sclerosed and difficult to pierce. One might make a large opening and get free drainage; but, as he thought Dr John Smith once said in a discussion at this Society, the opening remained patent afterwards and was difficult to close. In such a condition, he (Mr Wallace) thought it was better to open through the canine fossa. With regard to the removal of practically the whole anterior wall of the antrum, he had never done

y

it; but after such an operation, in three cases which he had seen, in one there was a very satisfactory result, in another it was not satisfactory, and in the third it was fairly satisfactory. It could only be justified when one did not get a satisfactory result from an opening either through the canine fossa or alveolus. Here, again, a distinction had to be drawn between acute and chronic.

Dr M'Bride said he had escaped with so little criticism that there was very little to be said in reply. Victor Horsley's opinion was something like this:—If any case resisted treatment for a year, then one ought to drain through the antrum. Reading between the lines, one might infer that this was regarded as leading to a cure. If one were of that opinion, then one was justified in recommending the operation. In acute cases with small perforation, one sometimes went on treating it for weeks, perhaps months, and still found no improvement whatever,—perhaps a tendency for the opening to become smaller, with a little pain. In such a case, slitting the membrane had no effect. The wound was healed the next day. One could not excise the membrane, because one expected recovery with almost perfect hearing. In such a case, opening the mastoid usually led to an early cure. He (Dr M'Bride) had operated on post-influenzal cases and on scarlatinal cases, and found the same satisfactory result. Chronic cases, however, comparatively rarely got right even after operation. If he himself had an acute otitis media he would agree to the opening of his mastoid. He was doubtful as to the expediency of the operation in chronic cases, unless some definite indication over and above a small amount of discharge existed. With regard to children and adults, no doubt there was a certain form of suppuration in children, with much pus and a good deal of disease of bone, which, he suspected, was very much worse in prognosis than the suppuration usually found in adults. As to the ethmoidal sinus cases, they were not always so difficult of diagnosis as Mr Wallace seemed to indicate. One found pus flowing from several points in and about the middle turbinated, and the method of treating was at the same time the method of diagnosing them. Grünwald wrote an elaborate monograph which might be summed up in a few words:—Put in a sharp spoon and follow up the pus until you come to the end of it. He (Dr M'Bride) did not agree as to the ease of diagnosis of frontal sinus conditions. In the first place, Mr Wallace absolutely put on one side the fact that one constantly had mixed infections. It was comparatively uncommon in his experience to have uncomplicated empyema of the frontal sinus. The antrum was generally first affected, and perhaps also the anterior ethmoidal cells. That fact, combined with the often sufficient drainage in such conditions, made one hesitate to recommend an operation, especially as most of his cases had occurred in young women, to whom a scar in the frontal region was a somewhat serious matter. If one wished to operate, the difficulty was how? In one case he attempted to perforate the frontal sinus from the nose. The case did remarkably well, the patient being afterwards able to insert a tube and wash out the cavity. He had never, however, been certain whether he had perforated the frontal sinus or one of the large anterior ethmoid cells. The patient, however, had been cured by the use of the tube, which had been specially made, and measurements would seem to indicate that the frontal sinus had been actually reached.

Meeting IX.—May 1, 1895.

Dr CLOUSTON, *President, in the Chair.*

I. ELECTION OF MEMBERS.

The following gentlemen were admitted Ordinary Members of the Society :—James Gibson Cattanach, M.B. C.M., 3 Alvanley Terrace ; J. S. Fowler, M.B., 3 Henderson Row.

Prof. Kocher, Berne, and Dr J. S. Billings, Washington, were elected Honorary Members of the Society.

II. EXHIBITION OF PATIENTS.

1. *Dr R. F. C. Leith* showed a case of INCIPIENT CASEATING PULMONARY PHTHISIS of over four years' standing, without any physical signs.

2. *Mr A. G. Miller* showed a man whose LEFT ARM he had amputated, by DISARTICULATION at the ELBOW JOINT, for PARAFFINE CANCER OF HAND AND FOREARM. There was extensive ulceration on the dorsal and palmar aspects, especially the latter. He was admitted to hospital on account of hæmorrhage from the ulnar artery. He was recommended to Mr Duncan, but came under Mr Miller's care on account of Mr Duncan being away. There was very little skin to come and go upon, and therefore it was impossible to amputate in the forearm. The best operation available was disarticulation at the elbow. A modification of the circular method was used. The wound healed by first intention, and the resulting cicatrix was shown to be most satisfactory.

3. *Dr Lundie* showed a BOY who four and a half years ago had his night-dress set on fire. He and his brother were playing in bed with matches. Practically the whole of the skin was burnt on the front of the chest from umbilicus to neck, and there were also burns on both hands and arms. At the end of a month there was a very large ulcer on the front of the chest that looked as if it would never heal. Mr Miles helped him to transplant to the

ulcer a number of large skin-grafts from a black and white fox-
terrier puppy,—some dozen, each about 1 inch square. The wound
took long to heal—about six months from the date of accident.
After the grafts were put on most of them appeared to melt away,
so that no remains of them were visible except black pigmented
cells on the granulation tissue, where black skin had been put on.
Cicatrisation, when it did begin, proceeded very quickly. Considering the severity of the burn, the cicatrix was wonderfully pliant.
Both wrists were burned on front, but the left less severely, and a
month after the accident, when the grafts were applied, it had
almost healed. The right had still a considerable ulcer, on which
a graft was put; and although it took about three months to heal,
yet the resulting cicatrix was somewhat softer and more pliant
than that on the left wrist.

4. *Mr Alexander Miles* showed a BOY who had been shown
to the Society about five years ago. Skin had been destroyed
by a burn from knee to ankle, except a small island on front of
tibia, about 1 inch by ½ inch. There was now a pliant cicatrix,
the result of grafting from an animal.

5. *Dr Allan Jamieson* showed—(a.) A case of IMPETIGO VARIOLI-
FORMIS. The patient was a girl of 15, who had been sent to him
by Miss Catherine J. Urquhart. She was admitted into Ward 38,
Royal Infirmary, on the 15th April 1895. The eruption began
nearly three months previously, as a single pustule on the left side
of the trunk. This was poulticed for two or three nights, and then
a number of fresh spots appeared, though the poultices were discontinued. The eruption came first on the back, subsequently on
the abdomen. She had evidently been but poorly cared for at
home. From observation since her admission, it was seen that
the earliest symptom consisted in the appearance of a vesico-
pustule or pock, varying in size from a pin-head to a small pea,
surrounded by an areola, which becomes larger as the pustulation
is more defined, and is sometimes distinctly raised. The lesions
are mostly discrete, though some, in particular over the loins and
sacrum, are pretty closely aggregated. Few are now in the active
stage. The condition present is either a blackish crust, surrounded
by a collarette of whitish epidermis, the areola persisting, or little
more than stains, some with a scale attached. Though copious on
the back, on the abdomen it is less pronounced, and the lesions
are more recent. It is accompanied with some degree of itchiness,
but has not been scratched. The resemblance to variola, both on
casual inspection and on more minute examination of the elements
of the eruption, is sufficiently close to justify the name. Three
other cases had come under Dr Jamieson's notice; two had been
recorded in the *British Journal of Dermatology* of last October.
The fourth was in a man of 47, in whom the eruption had existed
for two months; the lesions occupied the chest and back, and were

somewhat larger than most of those in the present instance. The treatment had been the administration of warm boric acid baths, under which a steady improvement was visible, though a few fresh vesico-pustules were still appearing.

(*b.*) A case of ERYTHEMA PERSTANS. G. E., 31, a healthy labourer, with a somewhat sallow complexion, but who had never suffered from rheumatism. He was sent to the Infirmary by Dr J. Aitken Clark on the 28th April 1895. When the eruption first appeared he was working indoors, in the indiarubber works, hence cold could hardly be a cause in this case. The spots and patches of which the eruption consists occupy the backs of the hands, both surfaces of the forearms, and slightly the upper arm. There are also one or two small spots about the knee. The smallest spots are the size of a shot, pink in hue, a little elevated above the surface, flat, and with a smooth, polished summit. Some would appear to originate at a hair follicle, others apart from one. The hairs, however, are themselves unaffected. They seem to enlarge individually or by aggregation. Thus patches, of which there are half a dozen, are the size of a shilling, and round or oval. Such are slightly scaly, purplish-pink in colour, the centre being a rather deeper tint than the periphery, the margin fairly, not sharply defined. The aspect of these larger patches is not unlike an erythema iris. Under the dermoscope the smaller fade entirely, the larger almost wholly. The eruption itches at night considerably. The urine, on examination, was found normal. Though in some respects resembling lichen planus, it approximates much more to an erythema, and should be regarded as an erythema perstans. Such cases are often benefited by salicylate of soda; but, encouraged by the success which has attended the suggestion of Dr Payne, 5-grain doses of quinine have been prescribed three times a day. Locally a calamine lotion containing carbolic acid gives most relief.

(*c.*) A case of EXFOLIATIVE DERMATITIS, limited to the hands, and affecting to a slight degree the sides of the feet, in a man with general but mild ichthyosis and hyperidrosis pedum. J. S., 23, a railway signalman. He has had all his life some amount of ichthyosis, especially of the arms and legs. He used to perspire on face and chest in warm weather. He has had uniform good health; the only complaint he had till six months ago was excessive sweating of the soles, which began after he entered the signal cabin three years since. Six months ago a blister formed on the inner side of the palm of one hand. Then a dry and peeling condition established itself, first on one, latterly on both hands. He ascribes the extension of the complaint to the use of an ointment containing 20 grains of salicylic acid in an ounce of vaseline. At present the epidermis of the soles is soft, soddened, and white, in consequence of the hyperidrosis. Along the inner margin of each sole there is a hyperæmic, though not quite continuous line, half

an inch broad, extending from the ball of the great toe to the commencement of the heel. This is made up of purplish-red smooth
patches, which nearly disappear on pressure. There is a similar,
but less marked condition on the outer side of the foot. The palms
and backs of the hands, as far as the knuckles, are vivid red.
The skin is thickened, so that the margin, which extends a little
above the wrist, is elevated and sharply defined, dry, constantly
exfoliating thin filmy flakes. There are several spots on the backs
of the hands, quite the same, and by the coalescence of such the
present state has been brought about. Under the dermoscope only
a faint coloration remains. Cases of this kind are rare. In one
similar one the condition extended till it became all but universal,
in spite of all treatment, yet on one occasion it wholly disappeared,
only to recur as bad as ever after a time. A case is recorded by
Mr Hutchinson in the second volume of his *Archives of Surgery*,
in a woman of 61, in whom a complete cure resulted from the continuous administration of opium in moderate doses for three months,
after the failure of many other remedies. In his case other parts
of the body, as the scalp, were affected, and the nails were also
diseased, but, like this one, the affection began on the hands.
Psoriasis sometimes passes into a condition indistinguishable from
this, but for psoriasis to commence on the palms is one of the
rarest things in dermatology.

(*d.*) A case of SCORBUTUS. Scurvy is now comparatively rare,
even among seafaring people. It is, however, occasionally met
with in those who habitually avoid the use of fresh vegetables or
fruit. It is interesting to note that the scorbutic habit does not
immediately follow on this hygienic deficiency. An example of
this is afforded by the instance presented. C. M., 49, turner, has
throughout life had good health. When in India he suffered from
guinea-worm. Till the date of his wife's death, three years since,
he was well attended to, but after that occurred he has lived alone,
done his own cooking, and in consequence has been careless as to
diet. Though he has had an egg at breakfast, he indulged in a "tea
dinner," subsisting on tinned meats, bacon, and bread, never on
any occasion taking either fresh vegetables, fruit, or milk. Still
till two months past he did not complain. Then he noticed red
spots come out on his legs and thighs, which persist, though they
are now less vivid. Then he experienced rheumatic pains in his
back, hip joint, knees, and in the feet just above the toes. He now
felt very weary, a troublesome cough came on, he was constantly
sleepy, and felt short of breath on exertion. There are numerous
punctate, dark, purplish-red, hæmorrhagic spots, seated at the
hair-follicles, on the legs and thighs, a large blackish purple ecchymosis behind and to the side of the right knee, and another, though
fading into yellow, in the loose tissue under the right eye. The
gums are spongy, in places almost fungating. The urine has never
been bloody or smoky, nor has there been bleeding from the bowel.

The heart and lungs are healthy.   He has been admitted for treatment into Ward 37, Royal Infirmary.

III. Exhibition of Specimens.

Dr Leith showed the TEMPORAL BONE of a girl, æt. 15, who died from symptoms pointing to tubercular meningitis.   She was only fifteen hours in hospital.   The real cause of death, as ascertained post-mortem, was a large abscess immediately below the convolutions, just at the junction of the parietal and occipital lobes, 2 ins. in diameter, and with a well-formed capsule indicating a duration of at least three or four months, and probably much more. It was nearly as large as a duck's egg.   There was extensive encephalitis in the neighbourhood, extending especially downwards and inwards, the greatest prolongation being towards the internal capsule, into which it would probably soon have discharged.   He examined the right ear and found a striking condition of the tympanum.   The lining of the middle ear was caseous, evidently from caries, and soft enough to be cut away with a knife.   The tympanic membrane was seen to be completely ossified, and showed a large perforation of size of porcupine quill at the upper end.   The ossicles were perfect.   The tubercular process had just extended towards the inner ear.   It did not affect the mastoid cells.   He believed the bone on the other side was also affected, but could not be absolutely certain.   The first symptoms appeared three weeks before admission,—headache and vomiting, which persisted for two days and gradually disappeared, but the headache persisted, and the patient remained in bed and became drowsy, and finally comatose. The eyes were not examined until after admission.   The house-physician examined the left eye and found marked optic neuritis.

There was no ear discharge, but Dr Leith found a plug of wax about 1 in. long filling up the external meatus.   The two specimens and photos. were shown.

IV. Original Communications.

1. THE PALLIATIVE TREATMENT OF JAUNDICE FROM MALIGNANT OBSTRUCTION.

By WILLIAM RUSSELL, M.D., F.R.C.P. Edin., Assistant Physician to the Royal Infirmary, and Physician to Queensberry House ; Lecturer on Pathology, Edinburgh School of Medicine.

MRS L. was admitted to Queensberry House Hospital on 18th December 1893, as she had sustained an intracapsular fracture of the femur which rendered her incapable of attending to herself in her own house, as she had hitherto done.   Her age on admission was 85, and no measures by means of splints or extension were taken with a view to bring about union of the broken bone.   In the course of some weeks she was lifted out of bed to an easy chair for several hours almost daily, this being beneficial to the general health and a preventive of back irritation and bed-sores. Such was the life the patient was leading in the early part of 1894. She was rather a short, plump woman, with a very contented and well-balanced mind, not looking her age by fully fifteen years, and with all her faculties intact and, on the alert. Her arteries were little thickened ; in fact, they gave as little indication of her age as her general appearance and mental faculties did. In April she suffered from slight dyspeptic symptoms, which were not thought much of until she began to show a suspicion of jaundice, confirmed by finding bile in the urine. The most careful physical examination of the abdomen at this time revealed nothing abnormal, and I hoped the biliary obstruction was due to duodenal catarrh. This is the hope to which I usually give my adhesion in such cases, although, as a matter of experience, I have not found that jaundice from duodenal catarrh is usual in persons over middle life. My experience has rather been that the hope with which I first regard these cases has had to give way before the development of evidence which puts the diagnosis quite beyond the pale of doubt and of hope. In young persons, and in younger adult life, on the other hand, a diagnosis of catarrhal obstruction which has been carefully made is usually correct. It soon became apparent that the obstruction in this case was not to yield to the remedies which are early successful when the cause is a duodenal catarrh, and I watched very carefully for the first evidence that might present itself which would throw distinct light upon the cause of the obstruction. My attention was necessarily most closely directed to the region of the pancreas, from the presumption that the cause would probably turn out to be situated in it. From time to time I therefore carefully explored the abdomen in that region, and the signs noted were the following :—The pulsation of the abdominal aorta was of course evident and marked, but I early noted that the pulsation appeared to become more marked to palpation, as if the vessel had become larger at that part, or as if there were something between the hand and the vessel, and overlying it, and to which the pulsation was communicated. This after a time could be fairly satisfactorily resolved into an elongated structure with a somewhat firm or tough sense of resistance, which from its position and shape was believed to be the pancreas. The normal pancreas cannot, as a rule, be felt with any measure of certainty, but when its consistence becomes increased and its tissue hardened, it can be felt if the abdominal parietes are not too tense or the abdominal wall not too laden with fat. While the pancreas became thus palpable, the absence of any palpable thickening above or to its right made it improbable that either the pyloric outlet of the stomach or the duodenum was the seat of material lesion. That the pylorus was not affected was further rendered probable by the absence of any gastric dilatation, or evidence of marked derange-

ment of gastric function. As time passed, the right extremity of
what was believed to be the pancreas increased somewhat in size
and at the same time in hardness, forming quite a tumour-like
body, which rendered it extremely improbable that there was a
mistake as to the structure affected. As to the liver, there was no
greater enlargement of it than could be explained by the
obstruction to its biliary outflow. No nodules or inequalities
were felt on its surface. The distended gall-bladder was felt as a
pyriform elastic body, not in its usual anatomical position, but in
the axillary line immediately under the tenth rib at its most
dependent part.

The jaundice had not existed long when the patient began to
complain somewhat bitterly of a general sense of *malaise* and discomfort, and of aversion to food from a persistent nausea. From
the continuous discomfort, and from the belief that the case
was one of pure pancreatic malignant disease, I represented to
her the possibility of having her symptoms alleviated and the
jaundice removed by means of an operation, while not holding out
any expectation of complete and radical cure. She was hopeful
that the jaundice would pass off, and regarded her age—85 years—
as too advanced to entertain the suggestion of operation, and I
made no further reference to it. Things went on thus for some
three months, the discomfort becoming greater, the patient's
strength necessarily progressively diminishing, and emaciation
slowly but steadily advancing. In fact, so great was the general
sense of discomfort, due to the deepening cholæmia, that she
began to press me to have the operation undertaken. I was very
loath to entertain the idea at this stage, as her general condition
had so deteriorated that I doubted the possibility of the operation
being moderately or temporarily successful; however, she was so
anxious to have it done, and both she and her friends were so
willing to run the risk which I quite plainly and clearly put before
them, that I asked my surgical colleague Mr Cotterill if he would
be willing to give her what small chance there was.

Her admission to Mr Cotterill's ward, on 25th September 1894,
was necessarily followed by a reconsideration of the diagnosis, and
my position was that the case was one of primary cancer of the
head of the pancreas; that there was an entire absence of evidence
that the stomach or liver was the seat of further malignant disease; that the tumour in the axillary line was the gall-bladder, and
not any other organ; that the disease appeared so confined to the
head of the pancreas that I did not think it had extended along
the bile-duct, so as to occlude the cystic duct; that, therefore, to
tap the gall-bladder would effectively drain the retained bile; and
that, if the operation could be performed with any measure of
surgical propriety, it might be risked.

Unfortunately after admission to the Infirmary various untoward
symptoms developed, which made the prospect of success still more

doubtful; and it was only after very full deliberation, and with many misgivings, that the operation was performed.

I need not dwell upon the care and manipulative skill with which Mr Cotterill did the operation; and he, I hope, will tell you of the method by Murphy's buttons which he adopted. Unfortunately, although not unexpectedly, the patient only lived for thirty hours after the operation, and it was at least doubtful if she would have lived longer had she not been operated upon. At the post-mortem examination the diagnosis was confirmed in every detail, and the seat of operation showed that nothing untoward had occurred there to hasten death.

I would not have thought of bringing before the Society a solitary case of unsuccessful operation upon the gall-bladder, undertaken largely at my request, were it not that it raises the important question whether this is an operation which we are to regard as legitimate merely as a palliative measure. The question might be regarded as being answered in the negative, to judge from the meagreness of the literature dealing with it, at least so far as I have yet been able to find. Operations upon the gall-bladder for the removal of calculi as a cause of jaundice or of colic have, of course, been frequent in more recent years, and the successes have firmly established the procedure as warrantable, and even necessary. Exploratory operations have also been performed in cases which have been found to be malignant; but, as I have said, there is a dearth of records of operations deliberately undertaken for the relief of the jaundice caused by malignant obstruction. The point is one on which it is desirable to form an opinion which can be applied in suitable cases, if, indeed, we are to grant the operation to be at all a justifiable one. Personally, I am decidedly disposed to favour it. I think an operation for the relief of the misery and discomfort of a deepening cholæmia is as humane a procedure as tracheotomy in malignant laryngeal disease, as gastrostomy for malignant œsophageal stricture, or enterectomy or enterostomy for malignant intestinal obstruction; and I do not see why we should shrink more from the one than from the other. In Mrs L.'s case, had the operation been performed at the time I recommended it, the patient might have been alive still; but, even if it had not materially lengthened life, it would have made months of life more endurable, and have saved her much of that languor, weariness, and nausea which were a daily and hourly burden. The advisability of operation would, of course, depend partly upon the possibility of making a diagnosis which could reasonably be regarded as accurate and complete. If the obstruction to the bile-duct were above the cystic duct, operative interference would be ineffectual; but with obstruction below that point, draining the gall-bladder would remove the jaundice. Thus a distended gall-bladder would indicate and warrant operation.

Then there is the question as to the influence involvement of the stomach should have upon the question, and I should put it thus: If the gastric symptoms are not only prominent, but clearly attributable to gross involvement of that organ, the removal of the jaundice would not give sufficient relief to warrant the operation. If, on the other hand, as was the case in my patient, the gastric symptoms appeared to be due rather to the jaundice than to coarse lesion, the relief of the jaundice would be followed by gastric relief. The presence of duodenal lesion would not contra-indicate operation. Even clear involvement of the liver would not necessarily be a contra-indication so long as the distension of the gall-bladder showed that the hepatic duct was not blocked. The most perfect cases for the operation would, of course, be those in which, as in my case, the lesion was confined to the head of the pancreas, and these are by no means uncommon.

Mr Joseph Bell said he had not had time to think the matter over. Dr Russell's paper was a model of what such a paper should be,—short, accurate, made them see the case, and gave them food for thought. He thought Dr Russell had made his point. There was no reason why they should not attempt to relieve such cases. The difficulty was the diagnosis, and Dr Russell had made an accurate and well-reasoned out diagnosis. He was right, the speaker thought, in asking Mr Cotterill to give the patient a chance. It was a pity it had not been done sooner, but it showed a great deal of courage in the physician to make the diagnosis and advise operation, and the surgeon to perform it in a woman of that age and in that condition. The operation of draining the gall-bladder was not in itself a serious one even at that age. They still lacked an account of what was done at the operation. Murphy's button, he understood, had been used. He very much doubted whether they would succeed in doing a curative operation in very old people with long-standing jaundice; probably to simply drain the gall-bladder would be safer. His own experience of the condition, both during life and at post-mortem, was against it. But draining the gall-bladder was, he thought, quite within the realm of legitimate surgery.

Dr G. A. Gibson said he did not know much about the subject practically, but for several weeks had watched a case on which a colleague had operated. The benefit from operation was very great indeed. It removed the pathological influence of the various biliary substances circulating in the blood, and thus gave the greatest relief. It certainly could not do any harm. Dr Noël Paton and Dr John Balfour, in a case of Mr Duncan's, had shown that drainage of the entire bile from the patient for a long time had not done the least harm. The patient was in better health now, three years after operation, than before. It was not a malignant case, but one of ulceration and cicatrisation in the biliary canal, which completely occluded it and prevented exit of bile by natural channels. As regards the nature of the operation, it was more a case for the surgeons to make up their minds about than for physicians, since the former had more opportunities of watching such cases after operation.

Mr Hodsdon made some remarks on Dr Russell's paper, and raised the question whether in cases of malignant jaundice it was not safer to simply drain the gall-bladder than to perform chole-cystenterostomy.

Dr Leith said he had made the post-mortem, and found a scirrhus cancer of the head of the pancreas, not involving the neighbouring glands or cellular tissue. There was great cicatricial contraction, with small areas of cells. The pressure was only on the end of the common bile-duct, the interstitial part within the wall of the duodenum. Dr Russell had another extremely strong argument in favour of operation for relief of turgescence of biliary channels. So far as his pathological knowledge guided him, the simpler opera-tion appeared to him better than cholecystenterostomy. There was distinct danger in allowing the bile to stagnate in the biliary channels. He had seen two or three cases, but one was especially prominent in his mind. It was under the care of Drs Grainger Stewart and Gibson. The common bile-duct pre-sented a stricture ½ inch long, owing to new growth, the channel being reduced to size of No. 1 catheter. Biliary ducts, in-cluding cystic duct and gall-bladder, were greatly engorged. Complete dilatation throughout. The damming back of the bile in the interior of the liver caused a deleterious element to transude, which led to necrosis of areas of liver tissue, not true abscesses, although they had been described as such. They were sometimes extensive, and formed a suitable *nidus* for septic organisms, which could readily make their way up through the turgescent bile-ducts. Getting into the necrosed areas, they set up real abscesses. He had seen that sequence of events happen more than once. It was extremely common in horses; he did not know why. In them it did not pass on to abscess formation as in man. There was risk of the abscess formation becoming general. He had seen pericarditis result from it. The tapping relieved tendency towards early death by abscess formation or pyæmia.

Dr William Russell, in reply, said that, in the first place, he had to thank Mr Bell for the flattering words which he had applied to his short, unambitious paper. He must say he tended somewhat strongly to hold that it was the duty of the physician to settle matters of this sort with reference to the gall-bladder as with reference to the pleura; to make up his mind distinctly what the local condition was, and then to ask the surgeon to come in and give what addi-tional light he could on the matter, and between them to settle whether it was desirable to operate or not. In all the cases of jaundice which were obscure, he thought the physician should be made responsible for the diagnosis. He would be exceedingly surprised to get any great light from the surgeon in any of the more difficult cases, however willing he might be to accept it were it forthcoming. He would not, in Mr Cotterill's absence, attempt to vindicate the course which he had decided to adopt in this case, viz., the connecting of the gall-bladder with part of the intestine. He did not feel qualified to express an opinion on that point. He agreed with Mr Hodsdon in thinking the other would have been the simpler method, and with Mr Bell in thinking that logically there was no reason why they should not thus relieve such cases. In some cases it was comparatively easy to make a full and complete diagnosis. In other cases it was exceedingly difficult.

2. THE PROBABLE LESIONS IN A CASE OF INCIPIENT CASEOUS PULMONARY PHTHISIS OF OVER FOUR YEARS' DURATION, WITH NO PHYSICAL SIGNS, BUT ABUNDANT BACILLI IN SPUTUM, WITH SOME REMARKS UPON THEIR DIAGNOSTIC AND PROGNOSTIC VALUE.

By R. F. C. LEITH, F.R.C.P. Ed., Pathologist to the Royal Infirmary ; Lecturer on Pathology, Edinburgh School of Medicine.

TUBERCULAR processes naturally engage a great deal of our attention in this country. When we remember that phthisis alone is accountable for about one-seventh to one-tenth of the total number of deaths in Britain, we may well consider that we can hardly spend too much time upon its study. I am induced to bring the following case of incipient phthisis before your notice on account of its somewhat unusual features, and also on account of the interesting pathological and therapeutical considerations which it raises.

William N. M., aged 43, clerk, a well-developed, healthy-looking man, of a somewhat dark and sallow complexion, first consulted me on 19th February 1890, complaining of a swelling of his scrotum. This proved to be a left hydrocele. It returned, and was treated a second time on the 2nd June, and this time successfully. While attending him during this second attack I noticed that he had a slight cough and a scanty expectoration. On being questioned, he said that he had frequently had a similar cough, but had not paid much attention to it. He had been more or less subject to winter colds so long as he could remember, and latterly these had been more severe. They had never incapacitated him from his work, however, and he had not considered them of any importance. He had had a good deal of cough during the previous winter, and it had recurred several times during the spring. It was often dry, but sometimes accompanied by a viscid sputum tinged with carbon pigment. It was not irritating or painful. I examined his chest carefully, but could find no evidence of any mischief whatever. Its expansion was good, and equal on both sides, resonant all over, and the respiratory sounds perfectly normal. I was inclined to regard the cough as due to chronic pharyngitis, with some laryngitis. He had a slight huskiness of speech. This had developed gradually, and had been in existence for a good many months. He had been a regular member of his church choir until about a year ago, and he thinks it was not present then, as his singing voice had been in no way affected. His general condition was eminently satisfactory. He was apparently in excellent health. He had a capital appetite, took his food well, and enjoyed it. He slept well and had no sweating at nights. He was in vigorous muscular condition, and took plenty of regular exercise, being in particular an excellent walker. His height was 5 ft. 10 in., and his weight about 11 stone, and the latter had kept pretty constant for several years back at any rate. His chest measurement at the level of the nipples was $33\frac{1}{2}$ inches during expiration, expanding $\frac{3}{4}$ inches during inspiration. The expansion was everywhere equal.

His family history is not of the best, as one brother died of phthisis at 33 years of age. This was nearly thirty years ago. Two sisters died in infancy from water in the head, and a brother from some accident during childhood. He has three sisters still alive, one older than himself, and all are healthy. The father and mother both died at an advanced age, and never suffered from any tubercular disease; and so far as we can ascertain there was no other case of tubercular disease in any member of their family.

I saw him occasionally during the summer of that year, and finding that the cough did not entirely disappear, although he might be for days without it, I again examined his chest most carefully, with as negative a result as before. His cough was almost restricted to the morning, being then mostly accompanied by a little expectoration. This did not seem to me to be in the least suspicious; however, I asked him to send me the morning sputum each day for a week. This I found to average somewhere about a drachm, sometimes a little more, and to apparently consist entirely of semi-transparent sticky mucus. Beyond a few carbon particles, it contained no specks visible to the naked eye, even when spread out in a thin layer upon a black photographic tray; but on examination with a hand lens I thought I could detect one or two tiny slightly opaque points. Having prepared a cover-glass film with a portion of the sputum containing one of these, I stained it by the Ziehl-Neelsen method. I did not expect to find tubercular bacilli, for such a purely mucous sputum seldom shows them, and I made the examination more on the ground of routine practice than on account of any suspicions which I entertained. We soon learn in a pathological laboratory not to be easily surprised, but I confess that I was considerably astonished on this occasion. The specimen presented almost the appearance of a pure artificial culture of the tubercle bacillus. It simply teemed with them (shown under the first microscope). It was now perfectly clear that the case, notwithstanding its innocent and simple appearance, was really one of great gravity,—viz., tubercular disease of some part of the respiratory tract, either the larynx, the main air-passages, or the lungs. I felt inclined to exclude the lungs on account of the entire absence of any symptoms or signs, and the main air-passages on account of the extreme rarity of a primary tuberculosis of this nature, and thus for a time feared that the patient was the unfortunate victim of a primary acute laryngeal tuberculosis. His huskiness of voice and the great numbers of the bacilli seemed to support this view. Hunter Mackenzie[1] says :—" In the sputum of laryngeal phthisis, especially if at all acute, bacilli are frequently present in enormous numbers;" and although Percy Kidd and Taylor[2] say "we cannot confirm the statement of Dr Hunter Mackenzie that the bacilli are always numerous when the tubercular ulceration of the larynx is present," it certainly appears to have been true in one of his cases at any rate, as shown by the illustrative Plate. I therefore made several laryngoscopic examinations, and fairly satisfied myself that there was nothing wrong with his larynx. The patient showed a singular intolerance to the laryngoscopic mirror, which neither cocaine nor ice seemed in the least to relieve, and I never really got a thoroughly good examination of his cords at any one time; but from the results of several attempts I felt pretty sure that his larynx was healthy. Dr Hunter Mackenzie kindly examined him for me at a later date, and corroborated this opinion. I now fell back upon the lungs, and for reasons which I shall presently give, considered that the presence of a cavity or cavities somewhere therein was more than probable. A minute examination of his chest elicited nothing. He was apparently perfectly sound and apparently none the worse for being the rich breeding-ground for such vast numbers of bacilli. I hesitated for some time about informing him of their presence and significance, as patients are apt to brood too much over such a condition; and the consequent depression of spirits reacts injuriously upon their bodily health. He received the sad intelligence extremely well, and I duly emphasized the great hope we had of recovery in such cases.

It was impossible for him to leave Edinburgh for longer than a month or so, and I confined my treatment mainly to dietetic and hygienic lines, making the former as rich as his powers of digestion would allow. He went to the country shortly afterwards,

[1] Hunter Mackenzie, *A Practical Treatise on the Sputum*, p. 49.
[2] Percy Kidd and Taylor, *Med. Chir. Trans.*, vol. lxxi., 1888, p. 351.

in the month of August, for his summer holiday, and when he returned the cough and sputum had almost disappeared. His condition remained much the same during the next two years,— the morning cough, though occasionally absent, never quite left him, and it was attended as before by a slight and pretty constant expectoration. Once or twice in the following winter and spring time he developed a slight coincident bronchitis, and his cough and sputum accordingly partook during these times of the characters natural to that condition, remaining at other times much as they had always been. A slight admixture of pus gradually appeared in the sputum during 1892, becoming more pronounced towards the end of the year, when he caught another of his colds. I had examined it periodically for tubercle bacilli during these two years, and each specimen presented much the same appearance as the first had done. Shortly after the pus began to appear little tiny specks of opaque, or slightly yellow material, were also noticed, especially with a hand lens. These were found to be caseous centres teeming with bacilli. During all this time his health might be described as unimpaired. The winter cold attacks were slight, and confined mostly to the larynx and trachea, with perhaps a few of the larger bronchi, and while they caused him some discomfort, they were not sufficiently serious to keep him at home. He was always ready and fit for his daily work at the office, and would probably under ordinary circumstances have paid little attention to them. His general health, weight, and condition remained the same, and his lungs were as free as ever from any abnormal physical signs. If we exclude the occasional signs noticed during his catarrhal attacks, I only twice detected anything suspicious, once early and once late in the year 1892,—viz., a few fine moist crepitations in the second interspace on the right side, about 1 inch outside the margin of the sternum. They were present only towards the end of inspiration and the beginning of expiration, and were quite transient, but apparently spontaneous, being heard for about two to three days only. I believed also that the bacilli had increased during this year, as it was hardly necessary to select particular bits of the sputum. Any part, even the most transparent, contained them, though not nearly in such numbers as the little solid specks.

On February 22nd, 1893, I received a message to the effect that he had been taken suddenly ill. I had last seen him fully three weeks previously, and he was then doing as well as ever. On going to his rooms I found him sitting in an easy chair by the fire reading the newspapers. He complained of a pain in his side, which was pretty bad when he walked, but did not trouble him much so long as he kept quiet. He had first noticed it on the morning of the preceding day, the 21st, and took a tablespoonful of castor-oil, as he had missed stool on the previous day. This acted well and without pain, and he was able to go to his office and do his work all day, walking home in the evening. The pain had not disappeared. He was able, however, to enjoy his dinner, and slept well that night; but on wakening next morning he noticed the pain at once. It was more severe than it had yet been, and this was all the more marked when he got up. The bowels were moved slightly, and he thought that this diminished the pain a little. He now first noticed that it was more marked on the right than on the left side. He was able to take breakfast, and walked to the office at his usual time. He had to give in, however, in the course of the afternoon, and come home. There had been no nausea or vomiting or headache. On examination I found distinct tenderness on pressure, an ill-defined sense of resistance, and a slightly increased tympanitis in the right iliac region. The rest of the abdomen could be freely handled, and there was no appearance of any swelling. His pulse was 98, and his temperature 100°. I believed that I had to deal with an acute appendicitis. The patient had committed no dietetic or hygienic error so far as I could discover. I mentioned fresh fruit, apples, etc., but he had not indulged in anything of this kind for some weeks previous. His bowels had been quite regular, and he had thus particularly noticed the single omission on the morning above mentioned, and took castor-oil to remedy it. He had been doing his usual routine office work, and had not required to undergo any unusual strain of any kind. He had not got wet at any time, and had always been well and warmly clad. He had felt perfectly well before the attack. I could, in short, find nothing which might be regarded as accounting for the condition, a common enough experience in appendicitis, except the tubercular affection of the patient himself, and I felt inclined to ascribe the present attack to the same source.

I need only refer shortly to this part of the history of the case. It was a fairly typical acute appendicitis, which ran a regular course, and, though for a time it gave cause for considerable anxiety, it progressed favourably towards recovery. It lasted about sixteen days. It is especially interesting to note that the pulmonary mischief was checked during the period of activity of the appendicitis. He never coughed at all during the first six or seven days, and but very little during the second week. The cough and expectoration began gradually to return. I examined his chest several times during this period, and found nothing. There was no sputum at all for about a fortnight, but when it did appear it was as full of bacilli as ever. It increased rapidly in quantity and the cough in frequency, so that by the time he was first able to leave the house, viz., the 17th March, the pulmonary lesion had seemingly made a considerable advance. Not only had he pretty severe coughing in the morning, but it often returned during the day, and the sputum, besides increasing in quantity, had become markedly purulent. There were also numerous moist sounds and prolonged expiration in the second interspace on the right side

2 a

close to the sternum. It is pretty generally observed, I think, that cases of pulmonary phthisis do better, run a more chronic course, and live longer where there is at the same time some other existent tubercular lesion, such as a joint affection, the latter serving to act as a diverticulum to the central lesion. It is possible that the appendix had acted in this way in this case. He was considerably pulled down, and had lost over a stone in weight.

Fearing a rapid extension of the disease, I strongly advised his going abroad as soon as he was able. Through the kind consideration of his employers he got four months' leave of absence, and was able to leave Edinburgh a week or two afterwards and stay in Torquay for over three months. He commenced work again at his office towards the end of August. During the time he was away he sent me fortnightly reports of his progress and specimens of his sputum. He gained greatly in strength and weight. He was 10 stone 2 lbs. when he went, and 11 stone when he returned. The cough and sputum both diminished gradually, the latter from over 2 ozs. daily to about a drachm. The bacilli generally showed a similar diminution, and as great care as possible was taken to select similar parts for examination. With due regard to the difficulty of forming a decision in such a matter, I am decidedly of opinion that the bacilli steadily diminished greatly in numbers during this time. His lung sounds were perfectly clear, and breathing natural; the moist sounds having entirely disappeared. He continued well after his return, and while at home for a short holiday at Christmas time 1893, he was told, after having undergone a very careful medical examination, that his lungs were as sound as a bell.

He has continued in excellent health throughout the whole of the past year, and from his appearance, as you saw him to-night, you would not think there was much amiss with him. He has been constantly at his work, and fit for it. He is not afraid to undertake a twenty to thirty mile walk, and enjoys other amusements in moderation. He suffers in no sense from mental or bodily languor or muscular weakness. He is not more anæmic now than he was four years ago. He sleeps well, and does not sweat at night. He has never had any pyrexia, except, of course, during the attack of appendicitis. His cough and sputum have both gradually increased, however, during the year. He occasionally coughs a good deal during the day, especially in damp and foggy weather. The sputum averages about ½ to 1 oz. in amount.

The specimen now shown is yesterday's collection. It is viscid and purulent, and shows several minute caseous foci. I have placed a stained specimen of it under the second microscope in order that it may be compared with that under the first, which is a preparation of the first sputum examined in 1890.

To all intents and purposes he is as well now as he was over four years ago.

Treatment.—It will suffice to mention the line of treatment adopted throughout:—1st, *Dietetic.* His food has been as rich as possible, and has consisted of a generous supply of nitrogenous carbohydrates and fatty foods, port wine and Burgundy, and cod-liver oil and malt, and their various combinations and modifications. Unfortunately, he cannot take the oil for any length of time, but can generally manage cream instead. He has also used the oil as an inunction. 2nd, *Hygienic.* He sleeps in a large airy bedroom, takes a certain amount of exercise both out of doors and indoors, and is most careful as to his being always well and properly clothed. 3rd, *Medicinal.* Besides expectorants and tonics when necessary, he has taken hypophosphite of lime without any apparent benefit. Various antiseptic inhalations were also perseveringly tried, apparently with some benefit, and he has now been taking considerable doses of creosote for some time. I have fancied when I left off these for a little that the symptoms became somewhat aggravated. It may become advisable to try the injection of prepared animal serum, if reliable material can be obtained.

From the facts of this case, as they have all along been present to my mind, I have tried to construct a picture of the pathological condition of the lungs. It is now about $4\frac{1}{2}$ years since the presence of the disease was demonstrated, and it may well have been present even much longer than that. If we regard incipient phthisis as meaning the disease localised to one apex, with or without physical signs—and this is the sense in which I have used it—then this case provides us with a good example, characterised further by apparently remaining in this stage all the time. So far as we can tell from the symptoms, general condition, and physical signs such as they are, the case has remained very much in a stationary condition. I am well aware that many physicians have met with cases so far similar to this in that the presence of bacilli in the sputum has been the first indication of the disease. Such cases are to be found not infrequently scattered throughout the vast range of the literature of phthisis, but the great majority of them had but a short spell of existence. In some death followed within a few months of the outbreak of the disease, in others not for a year or two, but in nearly all where the duration has been of any extent there were obvious indications from the physical signs that tuberculisation was slowly spreading. In such chronic cases, where the physical signs tell us that there are well-marked lesions in the lungs, the duration of life is often greater than it has been so far in this case; for we find that Laennec Louis and Bayle assign two years as the mean duration of life in phthisis generally, while Pollock,[1] from a study of 3566 Brompton Hospital cases, found that the further expectation of life was fair even at the end of two and a half years. Fuller,[2] in 118 cases at St George's

[1] Pollock, *Elements of Prognosis.* [2] Fuller, *Diseases of the Chest.*

Hospital, found the average duration mostly under eighteen months, whereas in 46 private cases it ranged from one to four years. Still more striking results are given by Theodore Williams and C. B. Williams.[1] Their analysis in 1000 cases in the upper classes gave an average duration in 198 deaths of seven years 8·72 months, and in 802 living of eight years and two months. Many of these had lived twenty years since their first attack. Some of these were cases of fibroid phthisis, which have the longest expectation of life; others had, besides the affection of the lung, a similar process in a joint, which, acting as a diverticulum to the central disease, kept it in check, and thus considerably prolonged the duration of life. In the light of these figures we cannot consider the term of four and a quarter years, during which we know that the disease has been existent in this case, as greatly exceptional. We are naturally enough led to inquire more particularly into a case of this kind, and to ask if we have any evidence beyond their clinical history of such quiescent tubercular lesions. And the answer is easy, for every pathologist is familiar with them. The lungs of patients who have died of some independent disease are frequently seen to show tubercular foci of a dormant or obsolete character. They are most commonly situated at or near the apex, and may be present in one or both lungs. They vary in size from a small pea to that of a marble or larger, and may be single or two or three close together. They may be placed within the substance, not showing upon the surface; but more commonly their position is indicated by a more or less depressed, irregular cicatrix upon the pleural surface. We can arrange them practically in two great groups, according as they have undergone a fibrous or a caseous change. Both these groups include changes differing somewhat in appearance from one another,—e.g., in the first there may be simply an irregular scar of fibrous tissue, or such a scar containing few or many little fibroid tubercles, miliary or larger; or a number of these fibroid tubercles more or less closely grouped together, without the appearance of a branching and contracting scar; while in the second we have caseous or cretaceous foci grouped together more or less completely. The agglomerated tubercles may be encapsulated by one general fibrous capsule, or if more discrete each may have its own capsule. Encapsulated smaller foci may be seen around a larger mass in the centre. Still further changes may take place. The caseous centre may become calcified, or soften and break down, resulting in a cavity. The pleura over the surface may become greatly thickened and adherent, the interlobular septa in the neighbourhood thickened and contracted, the bronchi dilated, etc. All the fibrous tissue, whether it be the radiating scar, or the fibroid tubercle, or the capsule of a caseous mass, is generally deeply pigmented. Sometimes these foci show giant cells, and

---

[1] Williams, *Med. Chir. Soc. Trans.*, vol. liv. pp. 112 *et seq.*

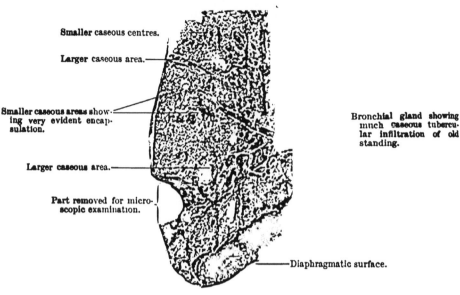

Healthy lung tissue.

Smaller caseous centres.

Larger caseous area.

Smaller caseous areas showing very evident encap-
sulation.

Larger caseous area.

Part removed for micro-
scopic examination.

Bronchial gland showing
much caseous tubercu-
lar infiltration of old
standing.

Diaphragmatic surface.

Fig. 1 shows a vertical section of the lung, made from apex to base. The bronchial gland is seen at the root
of the lung; its plentiful caseous infiltration is well encapsulated. A large branch of a bronchus is seen
just below it. Towards its termination a caseous focus is seen, entirely shut off by encapsulation
from it. Many caseous centres of various size are seen scattered through otherwise healthy lung tissue.
They are all completely surrounded by capsules, though this is best seen in the smaller ones in the
photograph.

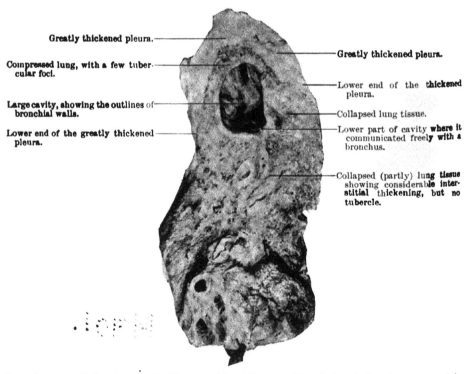

Greatly thickened pleura.

Compressed lung, with a few tubercular foci.

Large cavity, showing the outlines of
bronchial walls.

Lower end of the greatly thickened
pleura.

Greatly thickened pleura.

Lower end of the thickened
pleura.

Collapsed lung tissue.

Lower part of cavity where it
communicated freely with a
bronchus.

Collapsed (partly) lung tissue
showing considerable interstitial thickening, but no
tubercle.

Fig. 2 shows a vertical section of part of the upper lobe of the lung. The apical cavity is well seen surrounded
by compressed and collapsed lung tissue, with a few indefinite tubercles scattered in it. It was not
consolidated, and its relative size in relation to the dense white thickened pleura which surrounds it
like a cap is well seen.

sometimes not.   The fibroid forms, cicatrices and tubercles, do not show tubercle bacilli, while the caseous and even cretaceous foci generally do, although commonly in smaller numbers.   In all of them, however, the tubercular process is no longer active, but has retrogressed, and may be properly described as obsolete or dormant. I have seen a lung even riddled with cavities which could with justice be placed in the same category, as the walls were smooth and lined throughout by healthy fibrous membranes; and another extremely interesting, though unusual, which I have reproduced in the Photograph, Fig. 1.

Both lungs were affected.   They show numerous tubercular foci scattered throughout the pulmonary substance.   They are mostly about the size of peas, showing firm caseous centres encapsulated by firm and deeply pigmented fibrous walls of some thickness.   The surrounding lung tissue is quite normal.   Microscopic examination demonstrated plentiful bacilli within the caseous areas, but none outside the capsules.

It is quite probable, however, that all such lesions may not be tubercular, for some of them may have originated in dilated bronchi (isolated by an interstitial pneumonia), or in dried-up abscesses, or even in syphilitic growths; but the great majority are admitted on all hands to be tubercular.   In both of the above-mentioned cases the lesion was undoubtedly tubercular, and the patients died of independent diseases.   Out of a total of about 1400 necropsies observed by me in the Royal Infirmary of Edinburgh, such lesions have occurred about 165 times, or approximately in about 12 per cent.

Several writers have referred to them, and give interesting data regarding their frequency, relative to other diseases, age, sex, etc. Brouardel found them in the apex of the lungs of 60 per cent. of those over 30 years of age, whose bodies he examined on account of their having died a violent death.   Coats,[1] writing in 1891, gives the necropsies in the Glasgow Western Infirmary for the ten months immediately preceding as numbering 131; of these, 28 were cases of acute tuberculosis, and therefore unavailable; and of the remaining 103 there were evidences of healed tubercle in 24, but in only 20 of these was the lesion in the lungs.   This gives a proportion of 19½ per cent.   Harris[2] of Manchester had two years previously given a somewhat similar analysis of 54 cases in the Manchester Infirmary.   His term of involuted tubercle is, however, used in too wide a sense to be synonymous with obsolete.   He includes cases in which the tubercle was not dormant, and hence his proportion of 38 per cent. must be regarded as much too high. Kingston Fowler,[3] in a thoughtful paper written in 1891, gives the results at Middlesex Hospital from 1879 to 1886.   Out of 1943

[1] Coats, *Brit. Med. Journ.*, 1891, p. 935.
[2] Harris, *Brit. Med. Journ.*, 1889, p. 1385.
[3] Kingston Fowler, *Brit. Med. Journ.*, 1891, pp. 940 and 941.

necropsies, obsolete tubercle was found in 177, a proportion of 9 per cent. Sydney Martin[1] at the same time gave an analysis of 445 consecutive cases, also taken from the records of Middlesex Hospital, showing retrograde tubercle in 42 cases, or 9·4 per cent. Fowler also quoted Heitler's[2] statistics from the Institute of Pathological Anatomy at Vienna, based upon the records of ten years (1869 to 1879). Out of 16,562 necropsies obsolete tubercle was found in 789—i.e., only 4 per cent. It is a somewhat curious and instructive fact that while the cases of affection of one lung only were about equal, they were together far fewer than those in which both lungs were affected—e.g., in Fowler's own cases it was 71 to 106, in Heitler's, 134 to 655, although in Martin's it was 21 to 21. We are therefore amply justified in believing that such cases of local or apical tuberculosis, which, although ultimately obsolete, must at some time during the patient's life have been living and active processes, are not uncommon. Unfortunately, the clinical history of such cases is either unattainable or silent as to any symptoms or signs referable to the lungs. They may have been wholly latent during life, leaving only an indubitable anatomical record of their existence. In answer to the question, Are they clinically recognisable? Grancher[3] says :—" In almost all cases the tubercles are small and separate, incapable in the state in which they have been found, as well as in the course of their development, of modifying the respiratory sounds or vibrations. They are generally small masses of the size of a pea, at the extreme apex of the lung, and surrounded by healthy crepitant lung-tissue, or they are isolated fibrous tubercles scattered in small number in the centre of the lung." Now, as this condition can hardly be looked upon as quite the beginning of the lesion, it is hardly surprising that he holds, and many with him, that the " stage of germination " or " occult " stage of consumption, as it has been called, is quite beyond the recognition of the physician. He says, in fact, " In an individual suspected or not of tuberculosis, a few tubercles begin to develop slowly; embryonic cells and giant cells form and group themselves together, so as to constitute the follicular tubercle—that process lasts a long time, and is silent—and nothing appears changed in the health of the man doomed to phthisis; sometimes a little anæmia, a little debility, a slight cough, a little quickened respiration, nothing more." This is not much, certainly, and yet it is enough to make a watchful physician suspicious; and if he finds in addition, as he will often do, other abnormalities in the respiratory sounds, such as harsh, low-pitched, or jerky inspiration localised to and more or less constant in any particular area, I think he may venture upon a diagnosis of phthisis as at least probable. If this be so in the " stage of germination,"

[1] Sydney Martin, *Brit. Med. Journ.*, 1891, p. 944.
[2] Heitler, *Vienna Klinik*, 1879.
[3] Grancher, *Maladies de l'appareil Respiratoire*, p. 140.

it is equally or, indeed, more probably true in the somewhat more advanced stages which the obsolete tubercle just referred to represent. In some of these cases, at any rate, the skilled and careful clinician would be able to detect some sign of their presence, especially during the period of their activity, were his attention only sufficiently aroused to look for them. I am tempted, therefore, to give the following instance here:—Robert A., aged 54, was under the care of Drs James and Stockman, in the Royal Infirmary, for a combined heart and kidney lesion. Both of these physicians independently noticed a little dulness with some irregularity in the breath sounds at his right apex, and suspected an old apical lesion. His sputum was examined two or three times for tubercle bacilli, but none were found. He died on 13th January of the present year. The sectio showed, besides valvular heart lesions and chronic nephritis, a cavity about the size of a hazel nut at the right lung apex, containing a very small quantity of cheesy material, and communicating at its lower and outer margins by a small aperture with a small bronchus. Its wall was not thickened, hence, perhaps, the absence of the clinical signs of a cavity; and a few cheesy tubercular points lay around it. It was within ¼ of an inch of the pleura, which was much thickened by a simple chronic pleurisy in this region. I have reproduced the condition by means of the Photograph, Fig. 2.

Here, then, is an instance of one of these obsolete tubercular foci, perhaps a little more pronounced than usual, being in a sense diagnosable, and diagnosed during life. I made careful inquiries, with a view to ascertaining whether his clinical history revealed any symptoms referable to this lesion, and got nothing even so definite as in the well-known case of Sir Astley Cooper, whose body was opened after death in pursuance of his own wish, in order, if possible, to clear up certain phenomena which occurred during his lifetime. One of these was a hæmoptysis in his youth. He believed that he had suffered from an early phthisis. The result was that "at the superior and posterior part of the right lung was a depressed and somewhat contracted surface about the size of a sixpence; a section of which exposed a calcareous mass very uneven upon its surface, and about equal to the size of a small pea. It was placed about three lines distant from the pleura." (*St George's Hospital Reports*, vol. vi. p. 230.)

I have been led thus shortly to review these lesions, as the suggestion has occurred to my mind that the case under discussion at present may really be an instance. The physical signs are fleeting and of the slightest, but in their absence, from the characters of the sputum and abundance of the bacilli, we may make certain valuable deductions. The majority of clinicians are of opinion that the presence of a bacillary sputum signifies that destruction of lung tissue has taken place, and that the formation of a cavity has followed, communicating with a bronchus. Others, *e.g.*, Kidd and Taylor,[1] prefer to withhold their judgment. They say, "Whether it is necessary to assume the existence of a softening process in the lung in all cases where bacilli are expectorated we are not prepared to say." Theodore Williams,[2] on the other hand, holds that they may be found in connexion with tubercle formation and not only with softening and excavation,—for out of 106 cases of phthisis in which he found tubercle in the sputum, 9 were in the stage of early consolidation. This is further supported by the frequent occurrence of the bacillus in the sputum in cases of acute miliary tuberculosis. I have not yet personally found the bacillus in such a case where softening had not occurred, but numerous instances are on record, and I have, further, made post-mortem examinations upon several cases of this nature without visible signs of softening in which the physician under whose care the patient was has assured me that the bacillus was indubitably present in the sputum. I have looked for, but not found, the minute bacillary ulcers in the bronchioles found by Kidd and Taylor[3] in some of their cases of this kind. They suggested the probability of the discharge of the bacilli by these channels during life. The mere presence of the bacillus would not, therefore, entitle us to infer a cavity in our case, but when the great numbers are taken into account along with the amount of daily discharge, I think we may consider it certain that pulmonary excavation has taken place, and that at least a small cavity has been formed which is in free communication with a bronchus. The transient presence of moist sounds towards the apex of the right lung perhaps indicates that this cavity may be seated here. Experience teaches that such a cavity may exist and go on discharging for long periods of time without undergoing any material enlargement. The case of Robert A., of which the photograph has been given, may be taken fairly as an instance. It is practically a chronic abscess which secretes pus, but does not increase in size. The question of the possibilities of cure in phthisis is of the greatest importance. Many physicians at the present time hold that it is incurable after it has reached a certain stage, *i.e.* after it has become well established; and while this may not be the opinion of all, it is unfortunately too true that general clinical experience has not so far entitled us to take so favourable a view as is suggested by the observations of the post-mortem room. An undoubted disparity at present exists between clinical and pathological experience in this respect. Can any physician point to such a result as 19, 12, 9, or even 4 per cent. of cures in his cases of well-established phthisis. The very fact that Nature so frequently establishes such cures is most encouraging to us, and strongly suggests the advisability of doing

[1] Kidd and Taylor, *Med. Chir. Trans.*, vol. lxxi. 1888, p. 351.
[2] Theodore Williams, *Med. Chir. Proc.*, vol. vi., 1884, p. 371.
[3] Kidd and Taylor, *loc. cit.*, p. 352.

more than is at present done in dealing with the disease. Not only are separate hospitals necessary, but much good might be done by the establishment of bands or homes of nurses trained in the treatment of phthisical cases who could be sent to treat, or at any rate inspect, superintend, and guide the treatment of such cases among the poor in their own homes. I need not point out how little is done at present towards the treatment or amelioration of the immense numbers of cases of phthisis among the poor of our large towns. What an immense boon it would be to them and to mankind if a system were established by which they could all be controlled and supervised.

The great prominence which the bacilli took in the present case leads me to make a few observations upon their import- ance in the diagnosis and prognosis of phthisis. Their presence in the sputum at once indubitably stamps the case as one of tuberculosis of some part of the respiratory tract. Immediately after Koch's wonderfully clear and conclusive work became known abundant corroborative evidence quickly appeared. In 1882 Heron[1] examined 62 cases of phthisis and found them in all, Balmer and Fraentzel[2] 120 cases with a like result, and D'Espine of Geneva[3] gave a similar experience. A little later Fraentzel,[4] in a further examination of 380 cases, found them present in all but 5 cases, which were of the non-caseating variety, Theodore Williams[5] found them in 106 out of 109 phthisical cases and not in 21 cases of other lung affections, and Kidd and Taylor[6] in 91 phthisical cases and not in 9 others not phthisical. Gabbet, Dreschfield, and Hunter Mackenzie in this country, and on the Continent Ziehl, Zahn, Leyden, Ehrlich, Güttmann, Gaffky, B. Fraenkel, Heitler, May, and a host of others have all obtained similar results. Such evidence is practically overwhelming, and entirely overrules the few isolated cases in which the bacillus could never be detected in spite of repeated examinations, although the autopsy demon- strated that they were undoubtedly tubercular. Leyden has recorded two and Ziehl one such case, and once or twice such cases have come under my notice in the Royal Infirmary. It may be that in these cases the examination was not made frequently enough, or that the sputum was not sufficiently carefully sifted. All authorities are agreed that the early morning sputum is the best, as it is free from contamination with food and has little pharyngeal mucus, and represents the secretion of some hours of the air tubes, that it should be spread out in a thin layer

[1] Heron, *Lancet*, 1883, p. 189.
[2] Balmer and Fraentzel, *Berl. klin. Wochenschrift*, No. 45, 1882.
[3] *Rev médicale de la Suisse Romande*, Dec. 1882.
[4] *Deutsch. Med. Wochenschr.*, 1883, p. 245.
[5] Theodore Williams, *loc. cit.*
[6] Kidd and Taylor, *loc. cit.*

upon a flat glass dish with a black background (an ordinary black photograph dish does very well), and the small opaque specks or caseous pellets should be chosen, and that the examination should be repeated twelve or thirteen times if necessary. Wethered[1] says that he failed twenty times, and succeeded on the twenty-first in finding them in a case which the necropsy proved to be tubercular.

I have not personally found the bacillus in any case which a post-mortem examination showed was not tubercular, but I have once or twice been told they had been found by others in such cases where I could find no evidence of tubercle at the necropsy, and it may be useful to inquire how this may be explained. We may grant that the finder of the bacilli made no mistake about his methods, and that the bacilli were really there; nay, further, due precautions may have been taken to prevent any possibility of admixture from other sources than the patient himself, such as imperfectly cleansed spittoons, or even glasses or slides. Hadley[2] says he found bacilli perfectly stained in slides washed for some days in spirit and potash. Such sources of impurity must be carefully remembered in any large hospital; but, supposing that this has been done, and that there was no doubt about the bacilli being present in the patient's own sputum, it does not necessarily follow that the case is one of phthisis. The bacillus is ubiquitous, and therefore present in the wards of any general hospital where phthisical patients are admitted, and it is not surprising that a patient may inhale some of these germs, especially when the patient occupying the next bed happens to be a phthisical one. If long retained they are, of course, generally killed by the vital resistance of the tissues, but they may be coughed up soon after inhalation, and will then appear in the sputum. Zahn, Leyden, and Ziehl record cases of this nature; and recently Straus[3] has made some interesting observations of importance. He tested the dust, solid particles, and mucus of the outer nasal cavities of twenty-nine patients and ward tenders in two hospitals of Paris. The subjects of the test had all been resident in the hospitals for at least several months, but were not in any way tuberculous. The *modus operandi* was to remove the nasal contents by means of sterile cotton plugs, and transfer them to sterilised water or bouillon, which was injected into guinea-pigs. The animals thus inoculated from seven of these cases died rapidly of septicæmia or peritonitis, while those from nine others exhibited indubitable tuberculosis in from three to five weeks from the time of inoculation. The lesions were obvious, and showed the tubercle bacilli in every case. Thus nine out of the twenty-nine persons examined, nearly one-third, possessed active and virulent tubercle bacilli within their nasal cavities.

[1] Wethered, *Med. Soc. Trans.*, vol. xv. 1892, p. 302.   [2] Hadley, *ibid.*, p. 305.
[3] *Archiv de méd. expér. et d'anat. pathol.*, July 1894.

In unskilful hands the sources of error in the staining of tubercle bacilli are numerous.   None find out how numerous these may be, and sometimes how ingenious of discovery, better than the teacher of students.   It is not always in unpractised hands that these mistakes arise.   It is not a little startling to be told, as I have known happen in the case of perfectly sound men, that you had tubercle bacilli in your sputum.   Such mistakes may arise through a want of knowledge of the *why* of the process, though the *how* may be well enough known.   I can best illustrate this by a short summary of the steps to be followed in the process of staining. The Ziehl-Neelsen carbol fuchsin solution is the one I usually employ.   The fixed cover-glass film is held by a pair of bacteriological forceps, and a little carbol fuchsin filtered on to the film, enough to completely cover its surface.   It is then held over the flame of a bunsen till the steam rises.   This should be repeated two or three times during the space of two or three minutes. The cover-glass must not be allowed to get dry.   The carbolic acid combines with the aniline salt fuchsin (hydrochlorate of rosanilin) to form a bright red pigment, and also makes the capsule of the bacillus easily penetrated by the dye which becomes deposited in fine particles within its protoplasm. The stain is then poured off, and the cover-glass rinsed in water. A 25 per cent. solution of sulphuric acid is next added, and the red colour at once changes to a pale yellow.   It acts by converting the pigment in the cells or outside the bacilli into a colourless, readily soluble, triacid salt.   Hence everything but the bacilli (the sheaths of which it cannot penetrate) are decolorised.   This is by far the most important part of the process, and must be carried out carefully.   Imperfect decolorisation is the most fruitful source of error.   There is little fear of over-decolorisation, although it may occur, for after a time the acid seems to be able to penetrate the bacillary capsule, and then, of course, will act upon the pigment within the bacilli in the same way as it does upon that outside them.   We can easily ascertain if the decolorisation has been carried far enough by rinsing the cover-glass in water, when, if imperfectly accomplished, some red colour will return.   The water decomposes the colourless triacid salt into a non-acid red salt and free acid.   More acid may now be added, and the cover-glass again rinsed in water.   This should be repeated until no colour reappears on washing.   The danger of over-decolorisation is very slight, though it undoubtedly exists, and at times happens more quickly than at others.   If there is any reason to fear it, the last stages of decolorisation may be accomplished by washing with methylated spirit; but in all cases it must be complete.   It is better to run the risk of over than under decolorisation.   After complete decolorisation and subsequent thorough washing in fresh water to remove all trace of the acid, a solution of methylene blue is added for a few seconds.   The cover-glass is again rinsed in water, and placed at once upon a slide and examined; or if a permanent preparation be wished, it is allowed to dry in the air, and mounted with a drop of Canada balsam. The whole process is simple, and may easily be accomplished within three to four minutes. Having thus stained and found bacilli, can we venture upon any further opinion than that the case is one of tubercular disease of some part of the respiratory system? Does their number, arrangement, or special characters in any way guide us as to whether the seat of the disease is the larynx or the lung, or whether the case is acute, chronic, or stationary or advancing? As already mentioned, Hunter Mackenzie[1] says, "In the sputum of laryngeal phthisis, especially if at all acute, bacilli are frequently present in enormous numbers." Kidd and Taylor[2] deny this; but it is at once evident that, as pulmonary sputum also may contain enormous numbers, and as laryngoscopic examination is available, it is of little value, whether true or not, as a means of differential diagnosis. In the early part of our present case the mucous scanty sputum, with its very abundant bacilli, did suggest to me a laryngeal origin, but the laryngoscope negatived this. The bacilli were therefore of pulmonary origin (as I think we may exclude primary tubercular ulceration of the main air-passages, which is extremely rare), and their presence in such vast numbers was naturally suggestive of an acute process, and of a somewhat grave prognosis. The subsequent history of the case shows that this supposition would have been incorrect; but there are many other considerations which will guide us here, and prevent our attaching much importance to the numbers and characters of the bacilli in the sputum. Their multiplicity in the sputum may certainly point to their multiplicity in the lung, but the converse would be a dangerous doctrine to hold. A simple consideration of the relation of the bacilli to the various pulmonary tubercular lesions, as shown by sections, will at once demonstrate this.

In that most acute form, the acute miliary tubercle, and in early caseous tubercle, the lung lesions show immense numbers of bacilli, whereas the sputum may show none; while in fibroid tubercle, lung lesion and sputum alike show very few, or none. Again, in cases of rapid softening, both lung and sputum may show great numbers, or the reverse may be found, as in many cases of chronic cavities. Further, the lung may show many and the sputum few, and *vice versa*. Clinical observations on this subject are equally definite, for while in cases running an extremely rapid and acute course the sputum often shows abundant bacilli, it may show few; and further, while in chronic cases it frequently shows few, it may fairly teem with them.

Earlier observers, indeed, were led to different conclusions. Thus Heron,[3] from his 62 cases, concluded—(1), that if bacilli

[1] Hunter Mackenzie, *A Practical Treatise on the Sputum*, p. 49.
[2] Kidd and Taylor, *loc. cit.*   [3] Heron, *loc. cit.*

are persistent for some weeks in small numbers the case will probably run a long course; (2), that if they are present in large numbers in the early history of the case it will probably run a short course. He considered them to be few if only three or four were present in a microscopic field, numerous if thirty or forty were present. Balmer and Fraentzel,[1] from their 120 cases, concluded—(1), that when bacilli are numerous and well developed the prognosis is bad; (2), that they are exceedingly abundant in the most acute cases of phthisis; (3), that their number is greater when the destruction of the lung is rapidly progressing, and that the number is greatest toward the end of the disease. Further evidence was rapidly forthcoming, and on nearly all hands showed that such opinions were really untenable. The numbers and characters of the bacilli afford no valuable evidence of the severity or activity of the disease or of the gravity of the lesion. This is all the more obvious when we remember the varying relation shown by tubercular foci and cavities to bronchi, the unequal and varying powers of discharge shown by the same or different patients, the great possibility of variation of vital activity which the bacilli may possess in no way related to any physical differences they may show, and, lastly, the great difficulty of arriving at even an approximate estimate of the numbers present in any given quantity of sputum. While, however, we can place but little reliance upon the bacilli for the purposes of prognosis, we may make certain general inferences which may be of use to us. We cannot hold that there is any definite ratio between activity of disease and number of bacilli; but I think we may hold that, as a rule (which has many exceptions), they are numerous in acutely progressing cases, and scanty in chronic cases, that their steady diminution in number possibly means a tendency towards recovery, and that their complete disappearance is a good sign, indicating a retrogression of the disease, or at least a quiescent cavity. During the only period of their apparent steady diminution in the present case whilst the patient resided at Torquay, there was a marked improvement in his general condition. Diminution in amount of sputum and numbers of bacilli occurred at the same time as the general improvement in his bodily health; and I have more than once thought that a relapse in the latter has been accompanied by an increase in both of the former. I have also seen this in other cases.

I do not mean to overrate either the diagnostic or prognostic value of the presence of tubercle bacilli in the sputum. The general condition of the patient and the physical signs are far truer indications of the extent, rate, and progress of the disease. In the great majority of cases the physician will value, and rightly too, these signs and symptoms far more highly than a bacteriological examination of the sputum, though the latter may often enable him

[1] Balmer and Fraentzel, *loc. cit.*

to convert a mere suspicion into a certainty, or, as in the present case, where not even a suspicion existed, indicate at once the true nature of the case,—a discovery pregnant with importance alike to the expectancy of life and the prolongation thereof.

Dr Philip said he thought the Society was to be congratulated on Dr Leith's important contribution. He had, however, not limited himself to the elements in his case, but had introduced controversial subjects. It was impossible to discuss them all. In the clinical record there were three main points of interest. In the first place, the extreme abundance of the tubercle bacilli in the expectoration. Second, the relatively long duration of the case. Third, the comparative absence of physical signs. First, as regards the tubercle bacilli in expectoration, his experience differed much from Dr Leith's. Tubercle bacilli were frequently present in large numbers where the expectoration was not abundant. As regards statements resting on the numbers present at any given time, a great deal must be discounted in view of the fact that the discharge varied immensely from time to time in some cases. Sometimes they had for weeks or months discharges with all the appearance of pure cultures; at other times hardly any bacilli. There was now no reasonable doubt that the presence of tubercle bacilli in the expectoration—the fallacies suggested by Dr Leith having been eliminated—was proof positive of a lesion of the respiratory passages. As to long duration, they could enumerate a great many cases, lasting not only four and a half years, but ten or twelve years, where the course had been extremely chronic. Lastly, with regard to the question of physical signs, he was surprised at the title indicating complete absence of physical signs, but was gratified to learn that there were physical signs, and such physical signs as one might have expected with a course such as the case presented. Much depended on the determination and interpretation of physical signs, and this must differ in different hands. The principal interest in connexion with the case seemed to him to lie in the conjunction of these three points, each of which afforded very considerable scope for discussion ; and he thought the Society should be especially grateful, because too few cases of this class were brought before them, and the points were not yet thoroughly appreciated.

Dr James Ritchie said he had listened with interest to the paper, although he could have wished that Dr Leith had limited the field of discussion. Since Dr Philip spoke he doubted if he had appreciated Dr Leith's point, which seemed to him to be that there were no physical signs in the chest, although he had mentioned some signs. Dr Leith had asked for surmises as to the lesion in such cases. Possibly deep down in the lower lobes there might be foci such as Dr Leith had described. Cases did occur presenting indubitable signs in the bases after they had gone on for a considerable time.

Mr Joseph Bell asked the President if he recollected how often Dr Littlejohn used to say that phthisis was the most curable of all diseases ?

The Vice-President said that was also a saying of Hughes Bennett's.

Dr Clouston said that in connexion with this remark he well remembered the late Prof. Hughes Bennett forty years ago passing round the class just such specimens of cured tubercular foci, and asking triumphantly, in his vivid dramatic way, if phthisis were not a curable disease ?   His literary dramatic teaching power many in our own time would do well to cultivate.   In his opinion Prof. Hughes Bennett was the most vivid lecturer of the century in the Edinburgh Medical School.

Dr Leith, having thanked the Society, said he was interested in cases cited by Dr Philip as having lasted 5, 6, or 7 years without any physical signs referable to the chest.   It was not his experience that such clear sputum as his case had shown should contain tubercle bacilli unless it came from the larynx.   Having excluded the laryngeal cause he had ground for surprise.   With regard to the length of the paper, he wished to impress on those who were not pathologists true data upon which clinical aspirations might be based.   The specimens showed very rare forms of healed tubercle.

3. *Mr Miles's* paper, ON SKIN GRAFTING FROM THE LOWER ANIMALS, was postponed until next meeting.

Meeting X.—May 15, 1895.

Dr CLOUSTON, *President, in the Chair.*

I. EXHIBITION OF PATIENTS.

1. *Dr Clouston* showed a YOUNG WOMAN who had recovered from PROLONGED INSANITY under treatment with THYROID EXTRACT.   The thyroid was administered in the method recommended by Dr L. C. Bruce, in very large doses till a septic thyroid fever was produced. The temperature and pulse rose, and the appetite disappeared at first.   The thyroid after six days was withdrawn, and the patient nursed in bed for a short time.   The effect in successful cases was an extraordinary improvement in nutrition.   The extract seemed to have acted as a fillip to the trophic centres, and patients, after having lost 3,4, or 5 lbs., sometimes ¼ stone, during the administration, began to gain weight and put on up to 2 stones after the fever.   He had always thought that the induction of septic fever in insanity would produce a cure by giving a fillip to the trophic part of the brain. This girl was now aged 24.   There was a neurotic but not an insane heredity.   As she grew up she had a hysterical attack.

She had an illegitimate child in 1889, followed by an attack of mania, from which she recovered; became pregnant again in June 1892, and after her second illegitimate child, had another attack of mania. After the acute maniacal stage she settled into a secondary stupor, which began to be uncommonly like secondary terminal dementia. She was put under thyroid treatment, and almost at once began to brighten up and laid on flesh, and a complete mental change set in. After about fourteen days she began to pick up in a marvellous way, and within six weeks was perfectly well mentally, and had gained 2 stones in weight. She herself was quite clear that the medicine did something to her which wakened her up. Her constant statement was that she felt as if she had wakened out of a dream.

2. *Mr Cathcart* showed two YOUNG MEN with VENEREAL WARTS. These cases, he said, established an important point in the pathology of venereal warts which was somewhat obscure. It was generally supposed that they were due to irritation from gonorrhœal discharges, but he had had cases in the Lock Ward which made him doubt this. It was not always easy to get cases to demonstrate the point,—*i.e.*, cases of warts without gonorrhœa. One of the patients shown had had gonorrhœa before. At that time there were no warts. He had incurred risk of venereal disease from time to time; but latterly, about three weeks after getting rid of gonorrhœa, and after another connexion, began to feel discomfort in prepuce, which developed into a well-marked case of warts. The other patient had had connexion about New-Year time, had no gonorrhœa, but felt something uncomfortable, which developed into warts. Dr Cathcart himself believed that it was a specific contagion distinct from gonorrhœa, although he was not prepared to say whether it was an organism or an epithelial cell.

II. EXHIBITION OF SPECIMENS.

Dr Bruce showed specimens of the EMBRYO of FILARIA MEDINENSIS, and said that he had to thank Dr Argyll Robertson and Dr Patrick Manson for the opportunity of doing so. The parasite which acted as intermediate host was the minute freshwater cyclops, not quite so large as a pin-head. Under the microscope he showed two specimens of cyclops under low power, in the interior of one of which three embryos could be seen. The temperature was too low at present to see them moving, but if put in the sun or gently heated the embryos could be seen coiling and uncoiling inside the host. Under the third microscope the embryos were placed under low power. Specimens were extremely seldom seen in this country, and were therefore well worth examining.

III. EXHIBITION OF DRAWINGS AND PHOTOGRAPHS.

Dr G. A. Gibson showed—(*a*.) Three drawings of a BRAIN with right side diminutive, left side being well developed. There was a large cyst on the right side.   The patient, a girl æt. 20, had been sent by Dr Veitch to the Deaconess Hospital in a condition of status epilepticus.   She had alternately two right-sided fits of Jacksonian epilepsy, and one left-sided in succession.   He did not know the family history.   (b.) Two drawings were shown of a case of THROMBOSIS OF THE CEREBRAL SINUSES, spreading upwards in the choroid plexuses and veins of Galen,—in fact, into all the cerebral veins.   The patient, a woman æt. 25, died in the Infirmary.   Clinical features were stupor, severe occipital headache, then a rigid opisthotonic condition very like tetanus.   He had thought it might possibly be tubercular meningitis; but post-mortem examination revealed the thrombosis and red softening in internal capsule and optic thalamus of left side.   (c.) Photographs were shown of a man with DOUBLE FACIAL PARALYSIS,—one photograph showing patient with eyes open, the other showing him in the act of attempting to close them.   It showed the inability to shut the eyes.   (d.) There was also shown the photograph from a case of ALTERNATE PARALYSIS, total paralysis of 3rd nerve on left side, 7th nerve on right side, arm and leg on right side, ptosis, external strabismus, dilatation of pupil of left side, paralysis of right side of face, right arm, and right leg.   The lesion appeared to be of the crustal fibres of left crux cerebri, implicating the 3rd nerve there.   It appeared probable from the other clinical features that it was a case of hæmorrhage, but at the post-mortem examination they found thrombosis.

IV. ORIGINAL COMMUNICATIONS.

NOTES ON SKIN GRAFTING FROM THE LOWER ANIMALS.

By ALEXANDER MILES, M.D., F.R.C.S. Ed., Surgical Tutor, Royal Infirmary, Edinburgh.

MR MILES communicated the following short digest of his paper on Skin Grafting from the Lower Animals[1] :—

While fully appreciating the value of Thiersch's method of skin-grafting, he points out that it has the drawbacks common to all operations involving the use of a knife on the person of the patient, and the administration of an anæsthetic.   These can be overcome by employing the skin of young animals killed for the purpose.

After giving a short résumé of the work which has already been done on the subject, he described the method he employs.

He has used dogs, rabbits, kittens, and frogs as the donors of skin, the best results having been obtained from dogs, and the least satisfactory from frogs.   Young animals are always used.   The ulcer is prepared, as in other skin-grafting procedures, by being

---

[1] *Edinburgh Hospital Reports*, vol. iii. 1895.

made aseptic, and by being brought into a healthy state as regards its granulations, which must be neither redundant nor œdematous. The grafts are placed on the surface of the granulations without previous scraping.

The preparation of the grafts consists in killing the animal, and, after shaving its abdomen, dissecting up the whole skin, leaving behind the subcutaneous tissue. It is floated out in warm boracic lotion, and cut into pieces varying in size according to the raw surface to be covered in (from 1 in. by $\frac{1}{4}$ in. to 6 in. by 1 in.). These are firmly pressed into the granulating surface, close up to the margins, and edge to edge. A dressing of protective, gauze and wool, with a splint, is then applied.

The after-dressing is the most important part of the proceeding. It should be left undisturbed for at least forty-eight or seventy-two hours, and then the dressing should be changed with the utmost gentleness and caution. Subsequent dressings may be necessary every day, or every second day, according to circumstances.

Various complications were then referred to, and their treatment described. A graft which dies should be removed at once, to avoid septic changes taking place. Apparent sloughing of a graft is occasionally observed. It is due to the superficial layers of the skin being thrown off, the more vital deep layers living and growing. When pustules form on a recently grafted surface they should be punctured at once, and covered with an antiseptic dressing. Granulations sometimes grow up through grafts, destroying them. These are best removed with a sharp spoon. In all cases special precautions are necessary to prevent movement of parts until the grafts have fairly established themselves.

Details of ten cases treated by grafting from animals were given. The results of the grafting in four were perfectly satisfactory. Two patients recommended for amputation, and anxious to have it done, left hospital with useful limbs. In another an ulcer which had resisted ordinary treatment for eight months was healed in a week. In the fourth case an ulcer 16 in. by 12 in. was reduced to the size of a shilling piece, when it was attacked by erysipelas, to which the patient succumbed. Four other cases were only partially successful,—some of the grafts taking, others failing. Two cases derived no benefit whatever from the proceeding.

The resulting scars are stronger, and show less tendency to contract than those obtained by any other method of grafting. Pigment speedily disappears, and no hair, sweat or sebaceous matter appears on the new skin.

_____

The President complimented Mr Miles on his concise and practical paper, and said he would be interested to hear about the microscopic appearances.

Mr Joseph Bell said that Mr Miles had treated his subject with his accustomed ability and brevity. He would try to give an account of his own experience a good many years ago of the Reverdin method of grafting from animals. He did a great deal of it with good results. Since the Thiersch method came in, he had done none from animals; but in the old times he used sponges, and he wished to say a word with regard to how much of the skin remained in these cases. As regards the animals used, his were almost exclusively tame white rats. One or two of the house-surgeons had a fad for keeping them, and bred them on the premises. The bellies of the young of the white rat yielded an excellent plastic skin. Small pieces were used not larger than a threepenny or fourpenny bit. The hair was shaved off first, and it was of great importance not to take the subcutaneous fat. They put the grafts always on granulation tissue. He never scraped if he could help it. They could not put them close, but had to leave gaps. These being the days before antiseptics, they had every now and then secretion of pus. The grafts were placed on the granulations, and firmly compressed on the spot. With regard to dressing, Mr Miles had very rightly said, never dress before forty-eight hours. He quite agreed with him—forty-eight or even seventy-two hours. If one dressed before forty-eight hours, one was sure to come to grief. As to the method of dressing used by them, he thought it rather an ingenious one. It was very difficult to get grafts kept on a mobile part, especially thorax and abdomen. They used to provide pieces of gutta-percha tissue or protective tissue of about the size of ophthalmic lamellæ, or larger, $\frac{1}{4}$ inch in each direction, kept in boracic solution, and put on in large numbers one above another, like the scales of an armadillo. The upper layers slipped over the lower, and the graft was not moved. If they were put on five or six ply the grafts were enabled to stick. Mr Miles spoke of the upper part of the graft dying, the epithelial layer being cast off. It apparently entirely died, but it was only that the upper layer came away, leaving a transparent layer through which the granulations rose. It seemed to form a sort of basis for them. The grafts became "ghosts," but in a few days they found them turning up again. The President would remember the gentleman in whom twenty out of twenty-two grafts succeeded. They were Reverdin grafts, not animal grafts. But animal grafts also became ghostly, then formed a centre of "skinification," and met. Of course, he did not think this so good a plan as the aseptic method of Thiersch grafting. David Hamilton put it into their heads to use sponge grafting. The results were most extraordinary. When they put a thin layer of sponge over the part the granulations came through. They did not scrape away the granulations. The sponge seemed to act as a matrix or support for the granulations, which seemed to heal up over it. There was a wonderful case near Kinross, still alive so far as he knew. After five operations on breast and glands, there was a hole in the axilla, larger than he could cover with his hand, which nothing would cover in. A sponge was put into this, and eventually it healed, sponge and all. For a good many years she went about with this bit of sponge embedded in granulations. It acted as a graft. He thought the case was recorded in one of Prof. Hamilton's papers. The important point that he thought Mr Miles might get a hint from was the method of dressing grafts on chest and abdomen with small pieces of protective in great numbers, which might slip upon each other. That was really a "tip," so to speak. He was very sorry for taking up so much of the Society's time.

Mr Miller said he was sorry he did not hear the commencement of the paper, but what he did hear gave him great pleasure, all the more that he knew several of the cases, more especially the first. The boy had been admitted to his wards for amputation, but puppy-grafting saved him the necessity of amputating the leg. Besides expressing his satisfaction in hearing Mr Miles's paper, he wished to make one or two remarks on the subject generally. First, it was a curious fact, but a fact all the same, that whatever resulted in skin grafting, it was not true skin. He supposed Mr Miles had shown that in the earlier part of his paper. It was cicatrix. Put on what they liked, the result was cicatrix, let it be bits of skin, shavings, sponge, or whatever it was. No sweat glands, sebaceous glands, nor hairs appeared, simply a layer of fibrous tissue with epithelium on it. The other remarkable point—and one not, he thought, explained to them yet—was that whatever they put on did good, more or less. Of course some things did more good than others. Skin, of course, was the best thing, but sponge also did good, and, more than that, a graft put on, even although it died, did good, and the good was very easily demonstrable. Let a granulating surface—let them say 5 in. by 2½ in.—be covered by any substance of the kind referred to—skin or epithelium—epithelium sowing (Mr Lister's method) also had a practical result; or let it be sponge, the immediate result was—by immediate he meant in the course of a day or two—that they saw the granulating surface become smaller. The final diminution in size, he took it, was largely due to contraction, but it was also due considerably to commencing cicatrisation. Then supposing that the ulcer had ceased contracting and cicatrising for some considerable time, let skin or sponge, or whatever it was, be put on, cicatrisation would immediately commence. That fact, he thought, stood in need of explanation. He had never failed to find diminution in size of the ulcer for the time being. Of course he assumed that the granulating surface was healthy. With regard to sponge-grafting, to which Mr Bell had referred, he thought it mainly useful for production of granulations. It also helped cicatrisation, but not so well as skin-grafting did. It was, however, he thought, the best thing for producing granulation on a non-granulating surface,—glazed, bare, raw, unhealthy surface. Therefore it made a good commencement for skin-grafting. With regard to the use of lower animals, he thought the puppy had been the most useful animal. A great many of Mr Miles's experiments were conducted in his wards when he was his house-surgeon. Frog's skin hardly did any good at all, and kitten's, curiously enough, had not proved so successful as puppy's.

Mr Cathcart said he would like to emphasize what he thought was the special point of Mr Miles's paper. He did not think the results would probably be better than those of the Thiersch method, but he thought the simplification of the plan—as Mr Miles said, the removal of the necessity for giving chloroform—was a great advantage. They were also indebted to him for having drawn attention to the plan of leaving the granulation tissue unscraped. They could certainly thus cover over a larger surface without inconvenience. The results were quite as good as those of Thiersch. Pigs, he thought, might be useful, but they were expensive. He had tried kittens, and found more difficulty in shaving them than in the rest of the operation.

Dr James asked if there were any microscopic sections of skin resulting from grafting? A good many years ago when sponge-grafting came in vogue he could not help thinking that in skin grafting it was not so much that the skin grafts took root, as that they afforded something to the granulating surface which supported and in some way or other allowed the granulation to become developed, as it were. He remembered Dr Hamilton's simile in connexion with his sponge-grafting. Fine pieces of sponge on granulating surface acted exactly like a pea-trainer. The peas, if left to themselves, rapidly went to the bad. He should like to know if there had been any observations as to how long bits of the skin remained grafted. He thought that they became gradually absorbed and their place taken by fibrous tissue with epithelium over it.

The President said that it would certainly, he thought, be extremely interesting to hear if any of the three professional pathologists present had had any experience as to what constituted the outer surface of the grafts when they had healed.

Mr Miller claimed that the case of the boy shown at last meeting was proof of what he had said.

Dr James suggested that the resulting tissue might be called skin.

Mr Miller replied, if that were to be the definition he gave up his point, but in that case how were they to define a cicatrix?

Mr Wallace said it was quite reasonable to suppose that no hair or sweat glands should be present, because in making the Thiersch graft they did not cut deep enough to take glands, but only took the tips of the papilla, just enough to draw blood. In the case of the Thiersch graft it was interesting to note how, as

Mr Miles had said, the superficial layers came off and the graft became transparent—as Mr Bell had said, ghost-like. If they used small pieces they very often disappeared, but in a few days they came up once more. If closely examined they could be seen to dip into the granulation tissue, producing an umbilicated appearance, and from the margins the epithelium gradually spread. He agreed with Mr Miller in this, that when they used grafts they had an increased growth of epithelium at margins even at some distance from the grafts. Mr Bell had mentioned the method of putting on protective in an imbricated fashion. That was the method Thiersch recommended, and which he (Mr Wallace) always used. It had the marked advantage of allowing the discharge to escape. If the discharge were pent up it kept the grafts sodden, and tended to delay growth. Several interesting questions had been raised with regard to the method of grafting used. One he thought of importance was this:—What was the relative merit of skin taken from a puppy as compared with Thiersch grafting? Bier, he thought it was, had stated that although at first the Thiersch graft was red and adherent, it gradually took on more the appearance of skin, became movable, and, indeed, sooner or later it was impossible to tell where the graft had been applied. Would that be so also in skin taken from a puppy dog? With regard to relative advantages, he thought it depended on one's facilities for getting material. They could, as a rule, without difficulty get the patient to consent to the administration of an anæsthetic, and could take large portions from the front of the thigh. If they took only the superficial layer no cicatrix formed. Personally he rather leant to Thiersh's method than to grafting from lower animals.

Mr Miles, in reply, said that with regard to the question of histology he had searched carefully and had found no record of any microscopic examination. One was too anxious to get healing to be willing to disturb the cicatrix afterwards. In one case which proved fatal erysipelas had destroyed the graft before death. He was very much interested in Mr Bell's method of protecting grafts by layers of protective. He had read Thiersch's description, and he did not recall that he dressed in that particular way, but he might be mistaken.

(*Mr Bell*, interrupting, said his method was at least twenty years old, and preceded that of Thiersch.)

He had never used young pigs; the cost would often preclude their use. The scar in grafts from animals was, he thought, better than that resulting from Reverdin or Thiersch grafts. One could not distinguish grafted skin from healthy skin after a time. He had had no difficulty in getting animals. There were always plenty of kittens and pups about.

Meeting XI.—June 5, 1895.

Dr CLOUSTON, *President, in the Chair.*

I. EXHIBITION OF SPECIMENS.

1. *Mr Shaw M'Laren* showed a RIGHT KIDNEY removed for malignant disease, the aorta and vena cava split open, with malignant glands around them. Three years ago the patient began to suffer from a slight intermittent hæmaturia. This continued with more or less fluctuation until lately, when the bleeding became much more profuse and constant. A swelling appeared on the right lumbar region, causing the belly to protrude, and yet was not noticed until pointed out by the doctor who attended him, a week before his admission to the Infirmary here. The diagnosis was a malignant condition of the kidney, in absence of symptoms pointing to the bladder. He (Mr M'Laren) removed the kidney by an anterior abdominal incision, it being far too large to be removed between the ilium and the ribs. The incision was between 7 and 8 inches long, and extended almost from ribs to groin. He found it necessary to make another incision straight back into the posterior lumbar region. After that the operation was easy enough, except for pretty smart venous hæmorrhage. However, these malignant adenomas shelled out pretty easily as compared with tubercular kidneys, in which there were troublesome adhesions. Salt and water were twice transfused. There was extraordinary absence of shock afterwards. The patient only survived three days, but did not die of shock. He could move in bed, and change from one side to the other. He did not die of suppression of urine, because he made water plentifully within a few hours of death. He did not die of peritonitis. As a friend of his (Mr M'Laren's) remarked, he missed his kidney somehow. At the post-mortem there was little to note except that the ligatures held firmly. The only other point of interest was perhaps the position of the colon, which never came into the field of operation at all. As for microscopic appearances, the disease seemed to have spread to the glands, and had almost eaten its way into the inferior vena cava. It turned out to be a malignant adenoma, and Dr Leith stained some of the urinary deposit and almost certainly diagnosed it to be a malignant adenoma.

Mr M'Laren also showed a photograph of a MALIGNANT ADENOMA OF THE SCALP. It looked like an epithelioma, but was really not so. A glandular cancer of the skin was a comparatively rare form of tumour. It was removed a month ago. It was sent to the College of Surgeons' Museum, and Mr Cathcart had prepared the section on view that evening. The little bunches of epithelioid cells of which it was composed bore a remarkable resemblance to the cells of sebaceous glands.

2. *Dr Leith* said he had several specimens to show of surgical and pathological interest:—(*a.*) SKELETON OF VERTEBRAL COLUMN, PELVIS, AND LEGS, WITH LIGAMENTS, from a case of double dislocation of the hip. They. rarely had an opportunity of dissecting such cases, although they were common enough. The patient was a girl of 8, who walked well enough, but with the peculiar waddling gait. Muscles of calf and thigh were very much wasted. Dupuytren mentions 26 cases, of which 22 were double, and in females. Four only occurred in males; while Brodhurst gave 36 cases—28 in females and 8 in males. Seven were single and the rest double. There was no true pathological explanation of the frequency in the female sex. The only explanation that had been brought forward had been found to be false. Other interesting points were the position of the head of the bone, the condition of the different parts of the pelvis, and the prominence of the great trochanter. The transverse diameter was increased, and the antero-posterior diameter diminished. The sacrum was stunted, and there was compensatory anterior lordosis in the lower lumbar region anterior. There was also in this case slight lateral curvature of the legs, and lateral curvature of the spine, probably due to rickets. With regard to the causation of this condition, there were three suggestions:—1. Violence *in utero* or during birth. 2. Some disease like morbus coxæ during fœtal life, or distension of capsular ligament. In this case the capsule was hourglass-shaped, dilated at attachments, but diminished midway. There was no ligamentum teres on one side, and a little window he (Dr Leith) had made in the capsule also showed its probable absence on the other side. The head of the femur was much smaller on the one side than on the other, and this was suggestive of a former hip-joint disease. The acetabulum was generally said to be absent, but it was not so in this case. So far as the acetabulum was concerned, there was no reason why the surgeon should not attempt reduction. The capsule, however, being hourglass-shaped, prevented that. The dislocation was either upwards and a little outwards, as in this case, or simply upwards, or upwards and inwards. The only other cause suggested was some error in development, and this was nothing more than a suggestion.

(*b.*) The next three cases were conditions of HYDRONEPHROSIS of some interest. The first showed three preparations from the case of a man, æt. 36, who died with all the symptoms of urethral fever. Urethral fever was stated by Ferguson to be common in cases not previously catheterized, and uncommon where instruments had been freely used. The fulminating type of fever which was present in this case is mostly seen in cases of stricture whose average age is less than eighteen months. The case presents an exception to both these general rules, the stricture having been in existence for about 20 years and catheterization having been fairly frequent. He attended the Old Infirmary twenty years ago complaining of difficulty of micturition. He had an instrument passed with difficulty, and was well for two years thereafter. Three years ago a catheter was passed in the New Infirmary. He was lost sight of for some time, and returned last year in June with a history of cystitis which had lasted for about a month. He was then apparently free from cystitis. He was catheterized and dismissed. He returned to the Infirmary on January 17 of the present year, and became a patient of Dr P. H. Maclaren, who found a fine stricture of a corkscrew character just behind the bulbous portion of the urethra. No fever followed upon catheterization until the 20th, when he had a severe attack, the temperature rising in a few hours to 105° F. and remaining up all night. At 5.30 A.M. next day it was 105·°8 F., but gradually fell upon the administration of quinine and antipyrin. He was all right next day, and was dismissed a few days afterwards. He returned to hospital on the 6th of March and had his stricture dilated. The surgeon started with 2-5 and went up to 5-8 Lister's bougies. There was no constitutional disturbance. He got on pretty well, but returned on 23rd May to Mr Duncan's ward, again complaining of difficulty of micturition. A No. 5 catheter was passed without difficulty. Temperature rose almost immediately, and in a few hours reached 103°. It remained up in spite of treatment, and next morning was 104°. In the afternoon, about 3 o'clock, the patient complained of distension of his bladder, which was up almost to the umbilicus. At 4 o'clock the temperature was 107°·8 in spite of quinine. The catheter was again used, and quinine, antipyrin, and a sponge bath were administered. An ice-pack afterwards brought it down to 104°, but for a little only, as it quickly rose again to 107°, and kept up until his death at 10.30 on that evening. This was thirty-six hours after admission. At post-mortem, the obstruction, a stricture about ⅝ inch long, was found behind the bulb. The bladder was permanently hypertrophied and dilated, and a considerable amount of hydronephrosis was seen on the left side. There was an obvious bend where the pelvis joined the ureter. The first portion of the ureter was tacked on by old adhesions to pelvis of kidney, so that he had no hesitation in deciding that the condition must have existed a long time. Indeed, he believed it was one of those congenital bends that predisposed to hydronephrosis on one side, denied by so many authorities. Another interesting point in the case was the existence of minute abscesses in two wedge-shaped areas shown in the photograph. They had disappeared now from the specimens. They were related to the general condition : how ? was the problem. A catheter had been passed less than thirty-six hours before death. The abscesses must have existed before that. There were indications of a possible cystitis of a latent, dormant character, which might make the case really independent of urethral fever.

2 d

The man was of low vitality. It may be a case of urethral fever superimposed upon a pyæmia lit up shortly before it.

The next case was an example of an advanced left hydronephrosis, either congenital, or started by a calculus long since passed down the ureter. There was a mere rim of kidney substance left. The pelvis was dilated, and at its junction with the ureter the lumen was not sufficient to admit a fine bristle, while a minute quantity of urine passed down. To compensate, the other kidney was markedly hypertrophied. The patient had been sent in by Dr Miles for a hugely dilated bladder. The first night he drank his urine, and this made the nurse suspect that he had diabetes mellitus. This was afterwards found to be the case. There was no hypertrophy of the prostate. The patient's low mental condition, and his inattention to the calls of Nature, were elements in the case. There was no other explanation of the greatly dilated bladder, which had reached to the ensiform cartilage. It measured over 10 inches long.

The other case showed kidneys, ureters, and uterus with a three months' fœtus *in situ* from a woman æt. 30, who was three months pregnant. She died of embolism in the brain, due to mitral endocarditis. Here was a condition of double hydronephrosis, both pelves being dilated. Both ureters were markedly dilated, so much so that he thought at first one was a coil of bowel. There was no pressure from the pregnant uterus, as had been suggested in these cases; and there was actual narrowing of the ureter in both cases at the position of reflexion of the peritoneum. He had really come to the conclusion that this was also a congenital condition. It happened to be double. Unless the impaction of the pregnant uterus in the pelvis was able to cause the condition, he had no other explanation than that it was congenital. The absence of all urinary trouble pretty clearly indicated that the condition of the uterus had nothing to do with it. The case was further illustrated by photographs.

The last specimen was that of a cystic kidney from a man æt. 63. It was a good example, and suggested clearly two points with regard to that disease. Almost every portion of the pelvis was filled with urinary calculi. Whether these were antecedent or subsequent it was difficult to say, but interesting in relation to the suggestion that these cysts were related to obstructive conditions. The other kidney was affected but slightly. If they were congenital it was difficult to see how they could have developed so slowly. He had seen them at 65 or 66, but never so slight as in this case at such advanced ages.

3. *Dr Elder* showed a BRAIN with hæmorrhage into Broca's convolution and the part between Broca and the internal capsule. The peculiar interest of this specimen was that the part of Broca involved was the posterior part; and he had found on looking up

the record that there were very few cases where such a specimen had been produced,—very few cases where the posterior part of Broca alone was involved in hæmorrhage or obstructive lesion. He was able to observe the case from the beginning, and could ascertain exactly the symptoms. The symptoms were almost those of bulbar paralysis. The paralysis was on the right side of the face, and almost entirely limited to the lower part, the part around the eye not being involved. There was paresis or paralysis of the muscles of the lips or the angle of the mouth, also paresis of the muscles of the tongue and throat, and those involved in swallowing. There was no paralysis of the leg or arm. The only other symptom was dilatation of the right pupil, and this came on towards the end of the case; it was not seen at the beginning. The anterior part of Broca's convolution was not involved—*i.e.*, the posterior part of the third frontal convolution and the adjacent part of the ascending frontal convolution had also escaped,—the part which Horsley and Ferrier had pointed out in the anthropoid apes as connected with the vocal cords. The vocal cords in this case were not involved. The patient had difficulty in speaking, but no real motor aphasia. It was easy to understand what ·he wanted to say. He had difficulty in moving the muscles of articulation, but he succeeded always in saying what he wanted to say. The hæmorrhage looked extensive in the specimen, but that extension was a small wedge-shaped process into the interior of the brain, which did not involve the internal capsule, and was anterior to the motor fibres from the leg areas. Two drawings of the lesion were handed round.

II. EXHIBITION OF PATIENTS.

1. *Dr Allan Jamieson* showed a case of PSORIASIS with a peculiar CRATERIFORM arrangement of scales. The patient was a healthy man, aged 36, with a doubtful history of having had a chancre sixteen years before. For the last three years his diet had consisted of dry food,—sometimes fish, more often tinned meat, or ham, with an egg in the morning, but very rarely indeed any fresh green vegetables. The present affection was noticed in February as a small patch on one leg. Since then it has extended widely and symmetrically. On the forehead and sides of the cheeks are numerous isolated yellowish-red blotches, elevated a little above the surface, varying in size from a pin-head to a pea, and bearing scanty greasy scales. On the chest and back are oval or circular reddened patches, some of which have coalesced into wide areas. These are distinctly raised above the surface. On these, chiefly arranged close to the margin, are fairly thick yellowish-white scales. The appearances on the face correspond rather to a seborrhœic dermatitis, the type of scaly spot described by Unna; but those on the trunk differ in no respect from an ordinary psoriasis. On

the outer aspect of the forearms, however, the condition as regards the arrangement of the scales is peculiar. (It is not now quite so marked as when he was admitted to Ward 37 in the Royal Infirmary a week since. It is better seen in the drawing handed round.) There the general colour of the affected part is a pinkish-red, the scales are heaped up, thick, and very adherent. In numerous places they are piled up so as to form a truncated cone, with a crater-like depression, which seems black or dark. The elbow is affected, as well as the patellar region, where, indeed, the scales were very thickly massed. On the legs and thighs the appearances are like those on the chest; on the upper arm the patches are small and scattered. Dr Robert Robertson kindly afforded him the opportunity of studying this remarkable case. Already, under prolonged alkaline baths and inunction with salicylic vaseline, much improvement has taken place in the parts subjected to their action—all the body, except the right forearm.

2. *Dr Norman Walker* showed a case of ECZEMA and a case of LUPUS ERYTHEMATOSUS in an early stage.

3. *Professor Fraser* showed a RABBIT immunized against cobra poison. He said he must first express his indebtedness to the Society for the privilege they had accorded him of thus interposing in the proceedings. The opportunity of seeing one of these animals, which he proposed immediately to lay before the Society, might, however, never again occur, and the condition that the animal was in had never previously been produced. Before he showed it he should like to make a few remarks, in the way of historical statement. What had induced him to make these experiments, on which he had been engaged for some time, were, in the first place, statements of travellers describing the remarkable performances of snake-charmers, and also of the descendants, in Africa especially, of some ancient sects who, since the time of Pliny, were famed for the impunity with which they manipulated the most venomous serpents, which were actually seen to bite some of the exhibitors. Onlookers who expressed ridicule or doubt regarding the performances, or hinted that fraud or imposture was employed, were invited to handle the animals, and in several cases they were bitten, and died a few minutes afterwards. The performers also were seen to be bitten by the serpents, and it appeared that some of them actually, as a usual part of the performance, ate the venomous serpents. Further, there had been long an idea that venomous serpents were immune against their own venom, and that of other venomous serpents. It was almost impossible to conceive of their existence if that were not so. The mere conditions of their social intercourse, not always very friendly, would otherwise have led to the extermination of the race long ago. They had, moreover, experimental evidence that serpents were apparently immune. In almost all

the work done with serpent's venom there had, however, been a lack of exactitude. The quantity necessary to kill any animal had not been clearly defined; but still that work seemed to show that serpents were immune not only against their own venom, but also against the venoms of other serpents. These had been the starting ideas in his own mind, and he thought since 1879 he had been collecting venom in order to obtain a sufficient quantity to put these ideas to experimental proof; for it occurred to him that if that experimental proof led to the result that the statements were correct, then it was clear that the first and most important and vital step had been taken in finding a means for treating poisoning by these animals, because there must be something in the serpent itself which rendered it able to counteract the effect of the venom, and it would be for experiment to determine where that substance in the body was to be found—in the blood, liver, or any other part. Having been found, it was clear that it could be applied for the purpose of antagonising the venom in the human being. The progress of the investigation had been slow, but he had now collected venoms from India and from many other parts of the world: rattlesnake poison from Weir Mitchell of America; venoms from Australia and Africa; and cobra venom from Dr Cunningham, a graduate of this University, and now occupying an important post in the Indian Sanitary Department. It had been demonstrated in this country by Sewall of Oxford, and also by Kanthack of King's College, that a faint degree of immunity could be produced in animals, but all the experiments terminated fatally in a short time. Even in the absence of a definition of the minimum lethal dose, these experiments appeared to show that a certain amount of immunity could be produced. Only recently, several observers in France, working with the venom of the viper, had obtained similar results. It was strange that this had not attracted more attention, seeing that so much interest was being taken in the subject of immunization. These experimenters appear to have obtained slight indications that the blood-serum of the viper could act therapeutically. This had since been more definitely proved by Calmette of the Pasteur Institute. As to his own experiments,—in the first place, in regard to immunization, he found it difficult to immunize animals, more difficult than with diphtheria toxine, for this reason, that the death-producing quality of serpents' venom was much greater than that of the diphtheria toxine. The minimum quantity killed within a few hours; while in the case of diphtheria it was a matter of several days, and so also with the other toxines of disease. The result of that was that one found it extremely difficult to produce immunity. His first experiments, like those of Calmette and others, generally resulted in a fatal termination before reaching a high degree of immunity; but after many efforts, it was found how fairly well success could be secured; and he would refer to

the diagrams which represented the immunization history of two
animals. They illustrate two of the methods on which he proceeded.
The dark line at the bottom represented the minimum lethal dose;
everything above that was greater than this dose, in proportion to
its distance from the line. Distance from left to right represented
time in days. In the first place, the dose was only $\frac{1}{10}$ of the
minimum lethal, which was repeated at intervals of two or three
days. In about three weeks one gave about half the minimum
lethal dose, and then one came up to the minimum lethal; and then
at longer intervals $1\frac{1}{2}$ min. lethal dose; and then one got to two,
and then gradually after five months one got up to the top of the
diagram, where one gave fifty times the minimum lethal dose to
one animal. As for the other diagram, in this instance he started
with half the minimum lethal, repeated fourteen days after, and
then after seven days increasing as before. He found it necessary by-and-by to make the intervals longer. In this case the
experiment was also carried on to fifty times the minimum lethal
dose, and the animal was still alive. He would show it to the
Society. The rabbit ate well, was in good health, and was perfectly
strong. Another curve showed the weight, which had increased
during the immunization. There were no bad effects, except a
little rise of temperature after each dose for about twelve hours.
This rabbit got its last dose on 29th May, and it had a perfectly
normal temperature now. Its virile powers were unaffected,—
were, indeed, increased and energetic. That represented the
highest point to which he had reached. The animal had had
enough venom to kill two horses or 320 rabbits of its own weight.
The last dose it had received was enough to kill fifty animals of
the same weight and the same species in about three hours. He
had not yet made any observation with the blood-serum of animals
which had been immunized to this high degree. Observations on
the blood-serum had been made on animals immunized to thirty
times the minimum lethal dose. When a minimum lethal dose of
the venom was added to the serum of an immunized animal, and
injected immediately after mixing, perhaps only a few seconds
after the two had been put together, he found that $\frac{1}{250}$ cub. cm.
of serum would then prevent death. That was with the serum
of an animal immunized against thirty times the minimum
lethal dose. But that did not represent the antidotal power; for
when put into separate parts of the body, the venom in one part
and the antidote in another, the quantity required to be very much
greater, which indicated, in his view, that it was not a physiological
but a chemical antagonism between the two substances. The
serum was, however, much superior to any other substance that
had been used as a chemical antidote. He showed another rabbit,
also in good health, which was illustrative of the therapeutic
power of the serum, derived from an animal immunized thirty
times, to prevent death. This animal received twice the minimum

lethal dose, a quantity which would kill in little more than an hour after having been injected subcutaneously; then the serum was injected thirty minutes afterwards, when already toxic symptoms had occurred in the animal. After the serum or antivenin was injected the animal almost at once began to recover, and it finally altogether recovered. He had been working on the line of definition, and trying to define the smallest quantity of the antidote that would prevent death after different lethal doses and conditions of administration of venom. As to the treatment of poisoning in man, it appeared from the statistics of various men, especially Sir Joseph Fayrer of India, that in a large number of the cases that had been recorded of death from serpents' venom, 75 per cent. of the deaths occurred at a period greater than three hours after the infliction of the bite. Twice the minimum lethal dose would probably kill in about two hours; therefore it seemed that in the majority of cases the victims had not received much more than the minimum lethal dose, and that was always very favourable for success of any antidote. The result of the experiment in the animal which he had placed before the Society probably, therefore, represented a condition of difficulty in the treatment which was greater than the condition of difficulty in the majority of cases which would require to be treated in man. Transcending, however, their practical importance in the treatment of snake bite, the facts were of much value from the standpoint of general therapeutics, and from their obvious bearing on the brilliant new field of therapeutics, that of serum therapeutics, which had been inaugurated within the last few years.

The President said he was sure the Society were exceedingly obliged to Professor Fraser for the account he had given them of his brilliant researches, and congratulated him heartily on his results. It was the third time he had appeared before the Society this session, and he earnestly hoped that in future sessions they might see him as frequently.

IV. ORIGINAL COMMUNICATIONS.

1. CHRONIC AND TUBERCULAR PLEURISY.

By ALEXANDER JAMES, M.D., F.R.C.P. Ed., Physician to the Royal Infirmary ;
Lecturer on Practice of Medicine, Edinburgh.

THE connexion between pleurisy and tubercular processes is one which has made itself apparent to almost every investigator. Every one knows that in tubercular disease of the apices, apical pleurisies terminating in adhesions are almost invariably present; and every one, too, has met with cases in which, with tubercular apical disease, pleurisy of the lower parts of the lung, followed by effusion, sero-fibrinous, but very commonly hæmorrhagic or purulent, has occurred. Again, in the experience of most of us, instances have been met with of individuals, apparently healthy, becoming affected with pleurisy with effusion, and in whom the disappearance, usually rather tardy, of the fluid has revealed the fact that there is disease of the corresponding lung. In such cases the continuance and increase of the fever and sweating, the loss of flesh, the cough and spit, and the physical signs, soon make it manifest that this lung disease is tubercular in nature. More careful enquiry, then, makes it equally evident that this tubercular lung disease has existed, though all unknown to the patient, previously to the attack of pleurisy, and that thus the attack of pleurisy has been, again, simply a complication of tubercular lung disease.

In all these instances the pathological explanation of the occurrence of the pleurisy is the same, viz., that it has been set up by the transmission through the interfascicular lymphatic spaces of tubercular or other morbid products from tubercular foci in the substance of the lung to its surface.

But there is another connexion between pleurisy and tubercular mischief which I wish now to refer to more particularly. It is that pleurisy may be the precedent, instead of the succedent, to tubercular disease. Thus, how often do we find that an individual who, at the age of 30 or 40 or 50 succumbs to tubercular phthisis, has informed us that five or ten, or a greater number of years before, he has suffered from one, or several, attacks of pleurisy. It is difficult to get precise data on this point; because, in the first place, it is difficult to follow up individual cases for the number of years required; and, secondly, because it is impossible in such individuals to be certain that the attacks of pleurisy were not in reality secondary to tubercular lung disease which had either healed or remained latent for all those years.

Whilst admitting that in many of these instances the pleurisy has been secondary, I cannot but hold the opinion that in certain of them it has been the primary condition. Believing, as I do, that in tubercular disease the soil is more important than the germ, I would interpret the occurrence of a pleurisy in such cases as indicating a lowered nutritive power in the respiratory and other tissues, which renders them specially vulnerable to the tubercle organism. But I think that in certain cases of chronic pleurisy occurring in older people who have never ailed previously, we have specially valuable evidence on this point, and to these cases I wish now to direct attention.

R. M., aged 50 years, a blacksmith, was admitted to Ward 30 November 24, 1894. He stated that he was suffering from pleurisy, and had been ill two months and a half. His family history showed no tendency to tubercular disease, and was indeed particularly good. His habits and general surroundings were unexceptionable; and although at his work as a blacksmith he had been exposed to the usual risks of strain and changes of temperature, he had never been conscious of having received harm thereby. He had had no previous illnesses, and gave no history whatever of accidents.

His present illness had begun on the 5th of September previously, with shivering, headache, and general feeling of unwellness. On the day following, however, he had gone to his work; but he states that, on sneezing, he suffered from such a severe pain in his right side, that he went home and took to his bed. He lay in bed evidently feverish and ill, and on the 19th September the doctor attending him ascertained the presence of pleuritic effusion on his right side. During all this time he states that he had little or no cough, and only pain in the side when he took a long breath. Lying in his bed, he did not complain of any shortness of breath; but he states that he was sleepless at night, and troubled then with sweatings. After about three weeks in bed, he improved so much that he was able to go about. He seems to have been taking his food well, and gaining strength; but he states that whenever he attempted to climb stairs, or move about more actively, the shortness of breath showed itself. He came through to Edinburgh about four weeks ago for a change; but still feeling the shortness of breath, he called upon and was examined by Dr Stockman, who finding the right pleural cavity almost filled with fluid, recommended him to Ward 30 of the Royal Infirmary.

State on Admission.—Height, 5 ft. 8 in.; weight, 10 st. 4 lbs.,—used to weigh about 12 st. His development is good, but his muscularity has fallen away very much since his illness began. His temperature varies between $97°·5$ and $100°$; his pulse between 100 and 108. On physical examination of the chest, we find the condition as represented in the diagrams A and B. There is dul-

A

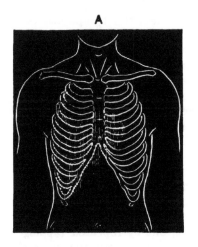

B

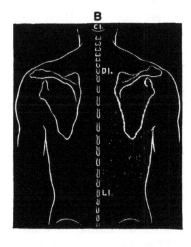

ness, more or less complete, with absent fremitus and absent breath sounds over the whole of the right chest, except at its upper part

2 e

anteriorly. Here there is an area where, with a tympanitic percussion note, the vocal fremitus is markedly increased, the breath sounds are harsh, vesicular, with prolonged expiration, and the vocal resonance, like the fremitus, is markedly increased. Over this area also crepitations are occasionally heard with inspiration. Over the left side of the chest, with the exception of somewhat exaggerated breathing, nothing abnormal can be made out. Examination of the heart shows the impulse beat in the fourth interspace about ½ an inch external to the left nipple line.` On auscultation of the heart nothing abnormal can be heard. The second pulmonary sound, however, is slightly accentuated. The liver is displaced downwards, about 2 in. below the costal margin. Examination of the digestive, urinary, nervous, and other systems reveals nothing abnormal.

And now a little more as regards the physical signs in this case. We recognise that the percussion dulness and the absence of fremitus, vocal resonance, and heart sounds over the greater part of the right side, indicate pleuritic effusion, and that this effusion causes the displacement of the heart to the left side, and of the liver downwards. The tympanitic percussion note over the upper part of the right chest is explained on the ground that here there is relaxed lung tissue, and to this also the increase of the vocal fremitus and resonance, the loud and somewhat hollow character of the heart sounds, and the occasional crepitations, are to be ascribed.

In this, as in all similar cases of chronic pleural effusion, one has a great difficulty in being sure as to whether or not the lung apex is free from phthisical disease. The marked increase in the fremitus and resonance, the loud, hollow, and almost bronchial character of the breath sounds, and, above all, the crepitations, all suggest this. But these signs, and with them the tympanitic percussion note, can all be brought about by the pleuritic effusion; and in this case they were so, for, as will be seen by-and-by, the post-mortem revealed that the lung itself was absolutely free from phthisical disease. At the time, however, we contemplated the possibility of there being some tubercular apical disease.

We prescribed for this patient rest in bed, nourishing diet, counter-irritation in the form of blisters to the side, and a mixture of potassium iodide and syrup of the iodide of iron. With a temperature varying between 97° and 100°·5, a pulse of about 104, and respirations about 20, we found at the end of three weeks that the condition of his chest was practically unchanged. We determined, therefore, to draw off the fluid, and bearing in mind the possibility of the existence of lung disease, we did this, not by taking off a large quantity of fluid all at once, but by repeated tappings every seven days or thereabouts, and taking away quantities of from 10 to 35 ozs. at a time. The first tapping was performed on December 19, and the tappings were continued till February 9, the total number of tappings being ten, and the total quantity of fluid removed being 130 ozs. During all this period, however, no improvement occurred. The temperature kept oscillating between 98° and 101°, the pulse about 104 or 108; the patient's weight kept very much the same, and examinations of the chest indicated that there was only a very slight diminution in the quantity of the fluid. About February 15 he made complaint for the first time of some pain on the left side posteriorly, and his temperature began to rise, oscillating between 99° and 102°. What appeared to be fine crepitations, with some impairment of the percussion note, was made out to be present at the left base, but in a few days effusion there was manifest, and he complained of dyspnœa. Although, after a few days more, the temperature fell to what it had been before, he was never so well as he had been. He suffered from attacks of dyspnœa, and quantities of fluid, varying from 20 to 60 ozs., were removed, at one time from the right pleural cavity, at another time from the left. In this state, gradually though surely losing ground, he continued till about the 15th of April, when his temperature was noticed to be rising again. On the 23rd of April, with a temperature varying from 99° to 101°, an examination of his chest showed the greater amount of fluid to be in the left pleura. I then determined to have his left chest incised and drained, and this was done on the 24th of April, a piece of rib being resected and about 15 ozs. of sero-fibrinous fluid removed. Considering his weak state, he bore the operation wonderfully well, but he never gained strength, and his temperature falling to normal, he died on April 27th.

The following was the result of the post-mortem examination :— Left pleural sac obliterated by adhesions of some standing. The lung weighed 2 lbs. 4 ozs., and showed a chronic subacute pleurisy. There was a small amount of fluid at that part of the pleural cavity corresponding to the lower lobe, which was collapsed. Miliary tubercles in great numbers were found in the thickened pleural membranes and adhesions. The upper lobe was œdematous, and the lower collapsed, both showing miliary tubercles in great numbers. The right lung weighed 1 lb. 12 ozs. The pleural surface was thickened like that of the left lung, but it was more collapsed, a large quantity of fluid being present. The pleuritic membranes and adhesions, and the lung itself, were studded with miliary tubercles. The peritoneum, liver, spleen, and kidneys all showed miliary tubercles.

In this case, the sequence I believe to have been, a left-sided pleurisy with effusion and formation of false membrane, little or no absorption of the fluid, and great increase correspondingly in the thickness of the false membrane. After some months, pleurisy and effusion of the other lung, with similar want of absorption power as regards the effusion, and thickening of the false membrane. Eventually acute miliary tuberculosis, due to the weakened tissue nutritive power allowing the tubercle bacillus to take root, this miliary tuberculosis beginning first in the lowly vitalized tissue of the pleuritic membrane, and spreading thence to the lung and to the serous coverings of the liver, spleen, and kidneys.

I may state here that I am well aware that it might be argued that in this case the pleurisy had been tubercular from the commencement, and that its course and unfavourable termination had been due to its tubercular nature.   But I would point out that this patient's family history and personal history were absolutely favourable.   He gave absolutely no history of cough previous to his illness, and he had no cough when admitted, nor for several weeks afterwards.   In time a cough developed, with muco-purulent expectoration, but this was simply bronchitic.   The spit, examined repeatedly, never showed the tubercle bacillus, and it is interesting to notice that even a few days before his death, when we may be certain that miliary nodules were present in pleuritic adhesions and in lung, the most careful search failed to discover bacilli.   The fluid removed from his chest at the repeated tappings, carefully examined, showed neither tubercle bacilli, pneumococci, nor, indeed, any organisms whatever.   Further, the post-mortem examination revealed no evidence of old-standing tubercular disease.   I am, therefore, of opinion that the sequence of events was as has been stated.

But a further piece of evidence in favour of this view is that cases of pleurisy presenting symptoms similar to the one just given, and running a similar course, may be met with in which the post-mortem examination reveals no tubercle whatever, neither recent nor old.

Of this the following is a very fair example :—J. H., æt. 47, worker in a brewery, was admitted January 16, complaining of pleurisy.

His family history was particularly good, his parents having died at the ages of 85 and 83.   He had always been able to take care of himself, and had had no previous illnesses.

His present illness had begun on the 1st December previously with a chill and cough, and pain in the right side.   He had kept in bed for about three weeks, and then got up, but as he felt that he was troubled with breathlessness, and was not improving, he sought admission to the Infirmary.

On admission he was found to be somewhat reduced in weight ; his temperature varied between 98° F. and 101° F.; his pulse was usually about 104; his appetite was poor, he had thirst and occasional sweatings.

As it is mainly the course of the case and the pathological appearances which are of interest, I shall now summarize these.

State of chest on admission, January 16, after six weeks' illness : Marked dulness on the right side, extending as high as the third rib in front and as high as the spine of the scapula behind, with absent fremitus, resonance, and breath sounds.   A tympanitic note above the dull area in front.   Liver not apparently displaced. Heart slightly displaced to the left.

On January 19 right chest tapped, and 30 ozs. of sero-fibrinous fluid withdrawn.

On January 30 no improvement in the state of his chest or in his general condition.

On February 1 it was noted that he had had a slight shivering on the previous day, and that there was some pain and a pleuritic friction murmur at his *left* base.

On February 27, with a very slight diminution in the quantity of fluid in the right chest, it was noted that fluid had accumulated in the left chest, the dulness reaching as high as the seventh rib in the scapular line.   As he was suffering from dyspnœa the right chest was again tapped, and 25 ozs. of sero-fibrinous fluid withdrawn.

On May 9 examination revealed some diminution in the quantity of fluid in the right chest, with increase of that in the left, so that percussion of the chest posteriorly showed areas of dulness very much alike in extent on either side, the upper limits reaching as high as the sixth ribs in the scapular lines.   As his dyspnœa was distressing, an effort to relieve it was made by tapping both sides of the chest, 16 ozs. being thus removed from the right side and 23 ozs. from the left.

On May 23 he had a severe shivering, and his pulse and temperature rose rapidly.   His cough became aggravated, and was accompanied by a viscid and rusty pneumonic spit.   Becoming rapidly weaker and weaker, he died on June 2.

On post-mortem examination the pleuræ of both lungs were found to be greatly thickened, the lungs were adherent to the chest wall above, and collapsed below, owing to the pleuritic fluid. In both of them the greater part of the upper and middle lobes were found to be the seat of catarrhal pneumonic consolidation. There was no appearance of miliary or old tubercles in the lungs or elsewhere.

These two cases seem to me illustrative of a type of cases of chronic pleurisy which is not uncommon.   It occurs in men about the age of 50.   It is apt to run an unsatisfactory and unfavourable course, and usually terminates by miliary tuberculosis or catarrhal pneumonia after five or six months of illness.   Such cases are seen from start to finish more in outside practice than in hospital. They not infrequently come into hospital, but they much less frequently die there; for, feeling as weeks or months go by that they are making no progress, they desire to go home, and they are for long not so utterly feeble as absolutely to be precluded from taking the journey thither.

As already stated, much can be said as to whether or not these cases are tubercular from the beginning.   As I have previously stated, I am inclined to think that many of them are not; and I base my opinion on my interpretation of the clinical and pathological features which they present, and also upon the general principle that the powers for harm of the tubercle organism can only be exercised on tissue the nutrition of which is below par. Be the explanation, however, what it may, the treatment in all these cases is alike, and to this I wish now to direct attention.

With such patients the ordinary treatment of pleurisy—rest, dry-dieting, counter-irritation by blisters or tincture of iodine, mercurial inunctions, cardiac tonics, diuretics, laxatives, etc.—is found to be of very little use. The pleuritic membrane seems to be so thick, and the chest so immobile, that reabsorption by bloodvessels and lymphatics cannot take place. One feels with such cases that if one could favour the performance of respiratory movements, as by allowing the patients to move about, to ascend stairs, or to take light dumbbell exercise, one could do good. But this plan of treatment, so useful when the quantity of fluid in the chest is small, is not only not beneficial, but positively injurious in those patients where the quantity of fluid is large, and in which feebleness and dyspnœa come to be prominent symptoms. The plans of treatment which may be tried therefore are—

(1.) Repeated tappings,—that is to say, the removal of small quantities of fluid (10 to 30 ozs.) at intervals of four to seven days.

(2.) Diluting the effusion. This may be done by withdrawing a certain quantity of fluid and allowing to flow into the pleural cavity a less quantity of warmed saline solution.

(3.) Free drainage, as is practised in purulent effusions.

Let us now say a little about those plans in detail.

(1.) *Repeated Tappings.*—This is the plan of which I have had most experience, as it is the one to which I always give the first trial. It imitates Nature as well as she can be imitated in the circumstances, for, the quantity of fluid removed at each tapping being small, there is no undue stretching or tearing of false membranes, and the tappings being at short intervals, the lung expansion obtained by one operation is retained and added to by the subsequent one. The quantity of fluid removed at each tapping should not be large,—not above 25 or 30 ozs: I think that with larger quantities loculi are more apt to be formed. Further, if a small aspirating needle be used, the patient does not much dread the repetition of the operation.

This plan is often wonderfully successful. I have seen it act sufficiently in cases where I hardly expected it. Thus in the following case, where from the commencement I thought that free drainage would be required, it was markedly efficient.

J. B., aged 55, a labourer, was admitted to Ward 30, April 30, 1895, suffering from pleurisy with effusion.

Family History indicates a slight tendency to heart disease and phthisis.

Social History is always good. He has always been temperate, and his home has been comfortable.

Previous Illnesses.—Had influenza in Melbourne five years ago. Was ill about a fortnight, but completely recovered. Four years ago he fell about twenty feet, landing on his chest. He states that his chest was badly bruised, and he was laid up for two months, but did not then see a doctor.

Present Illness.—This seems to have begun in the beginning of March last, with severe pain in the left side of the chest, aggravated by breathing and coughing. He states also that at the beginning he had severe headache, and was feverish. He was treated by rest in bed, and by poultices and mustard plasters applied to the chest. He states, however, that he has been feeling no improvement, the pain is as bad as ever, and he has shortness of breath. He therefore sought admission to the Infirmary.

On admission his face was noticed to bear an anxious expression; his lips are dry and rather cracked, the alæ nasi move freely in respiration.   His temperature was—morning 97°·5, evening 100°. Pulse varied between 80 and 90; respirations about 30 per minute. There was loss of appetite, thirst, slight coughs, and night sweats. The small amount of opaque mucous spit showed no tubercle bacilli.

On examination of the chest the right side was seen to move freely, the left hardly at all, and the condition on percussion was as shown in the diagrams C and D.   Over the whole of the dull area

C

D

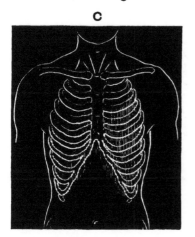
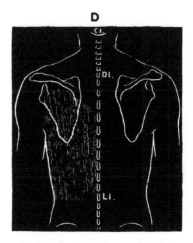

there was absent fremitus, resonance, and breath sounds; and below, the dulness could be made out to extend distinctly below the lower margin of the ribs.   Above the dull area, especially in front, the vocal fremitus and resonance were increased. The cardiac impulse could be felt in the fourth right interspace, and cardiac dulness could be made out to extend 1½ inch to the right of the right border of the sternum. The heart sounds were normal. The liver was in its normal position, except that its left lobe was distinctly depressed.

Examination of the chest posteriorly revealed dulness on percussion on the left side, extending as high as the spine of the scapula in the scapular line.   Nearer the vertebral column the dulness was not so high, so that, as was remarked, the "curved line" was just beginning to show itself. The other organs and systems were normal. He was treated by rest in bed, and a mixture of potassium iodide, syrup of the iodide of iron, and tincture of digitalis, with half an ounce of brandy every four hours. As the dyspnœa was troubling him, as he was very feeble, and as counter-irritants had been employed before his admission without effect, it was determined to withdraw some of the fluid. The chest was accordingly aspirated on May 31,—19 ozs. of distinctly hæmorrhagic fluid being drawn off.

The blood-stained character of the effusion corroborated what we had been suspecting, viz., that this, if not a tubercular pleurisy, was very likely to become one in time, and so we determined to treat it by tapping at short intervals.   This was accordingly done on June 2 and June 7,—10 ozs. being removed on the first, and 25 ozs. on the second occasion.   On both of those occasions more could have been drawn off, but the occurrence of pain warned us that it was better to desist.   After the tapping on June 7, distinct improvement showed itself, and on June 11 the condition of the chest was as shown in the diagrams E and F, a distinct improvement

E

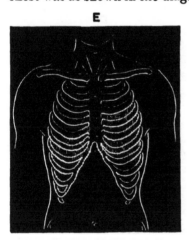

F

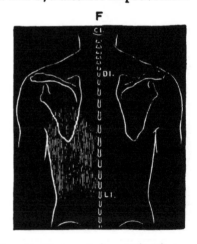

also showing itself in the pulse, temperature, and respirations. Still there was fluid in his chest, and on June 14 I aspirated again, drawing off 22 ozs. It was noted that the fluid on this occasion, though still blood-stained, was lighter-coloured than it had been on the previous occasions.   On June 18 the improvement in the condition of the chest was very marked ; the tympanitic stomach note was no higher than before, but the heart had returned to its normal position, and the curve of the curved line was flattening out (Diagrams G and H). He was allowed to get up, and en-

G

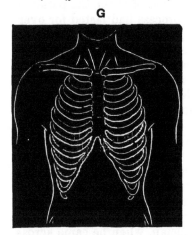

H

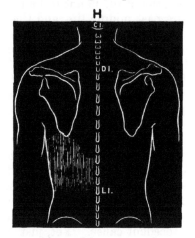

couraged to move about. His progress after this was uninterrupted, and he was discharged practically well on July 8.

(2.) *Diluting the Effusion.*—This may be done by drawing off a quantity of fluid, say 10 or 15 ozs., and allowing then to pass in a smaller quantity of saline solution, warmed to a temperature of about 100°, and of course rendered carefully aseptic; repeating the operation every five or six days. It is conceivable that, in cases of delayed absorption, should the delay be due to the constitution of the fluid itself, this operation, repeated two or three times, would tend to be beneficial. Concerning it, all I can say is, that in my experience no harm has resulted from its employment; but whether any subsequent improvement in the course of the malady was to be ascribed to the withdrawal of the pleuritic fluid or to the introduction of the saline solution, I do not at present know.

(3.) *Free Drainage.*[1]—This may be accomplished either by free incision, resecting a piece of rib or not, as may be deemed necessary, and the insertion of a tube, or else by puncturing the chest with a trocar or cannula, and inserting a piece of rubber drainage-tube through the cannula, then withdrawing the latter, leaving the drainage-tube in the opening. In either case the utmost care must be taken as regards antiseptics, cases of sero-fibrinous effusions being much more likely to go wrong than are empyemas. The patients for which this mode of treatment may be tried should only be those which have not been benefited by repeated tappings, in which it is certain that there are firm pleuritic adhesions, and in which the amount of fluid is not too great—not more than 40 or 50 ozs.

I have seen several cases treated by drainage, but if I am unable

[1] For cases of sero-fibrinous effusion treated by free incision and drainage see West, *Brit. Med. Journal*, April 27, 1895, and Rutherford Morison, *Brit. Med. Journal*, July 13, 1895.

to chronicle instances in which the results were so satisfactory as
to make me recommend the procedure, I feel that for this the
operation itself is not to be blamed. In most of them, the patients
were past middle life, and the pleuritic process had lasted for over
two months. In two of them, at least, there was already existent
tubercular disease. When one reflects on the great probability
that had these been cases of purulent instead of sero-fibrinous
effusion, operative treatment would not have yielded any less
unsatisfactory results, one feels entitled to anticipate from this
operation distinctly better results in time.

Dr Affleck said he had very little to remark. Most physicians
would agree with the position that Dr James had taken up.
Anything he had to say would be entirely from the clinical standpoint. From abundant experience in tackling cases of pleurisy he
found himself more and more regarding it in the light of a
symptom,—not but that pleurisies might occur alone without any
antecedent cause. Yet, just as a physician, when he came across
a case of peritonitis, tried to get behind it and ascertain the cause,
so in pleurisy, he thought clinical observation justified the statement that in a large number of instances there was something
underlying the case, either in the lung or in the constitution at
large. The pleura was very responsive to irritations of the lung,
and he thought Dr Leith and all pathologists would bear him out,
that when they had trouble in the lung they were very apt to have
trouble in the pleura. Therefore when he came across a case of
pleurisy he was very anxious to find out the cause. That a great
many pleurisies were tubercular he thought there could be very
little doubt, and the position taken up by Dr James was, he thought,
thoroughly sound. Pleurisy might be tubercular in its origin, or,
he thought, there was clinical and pathological evidence that
pleurisy from being apparently simple might become tubercular.
That pleurisy might be tubercular in its origin they knew from
the fact that it was often the starting-point of a general tuberculosis. The pleurisy might be an incident in an antecedent
tuberculous process in the lung. All pleurisies occurring in young
people, particularly in delicate young people, had to be viewed
with great suspicion, for many of them were, he believed, tubercular,—probably primarily tubercular in the pleura. There was a
considerable analogy, he thought, between the peritoneum and the
pleura in relation to tubercle. They found, for instance, cases of
tubercular peritonitis where the peritoneum alone was affected,
where they had considerable effusion, where sometimes without
treatment, but where, he thought, more decidedly with treatment,
the cases could be entirely cured. There were other cases where
the peritoneal inflammation was part of a more widely-spread
tuberculosis. These cases were very much less favourable.
Surgery had, however, done a great deal for the peritoneum, and

he was able to speak of no fewer than ten cases of tubercular peritonitis occurring in his own wards in the hospital, where the abdomen had been opened and drained, and where the patients had all recovered. The cases most favourable for it, of which there were a good many, were those in which you would think the peritoneum alone was affected, cases occurring with ascites or peritoneal effusion; if they were simply opened and drained, without being washed out, they got perfectly well. They might get well if left alone, but probably not. They sometimes became putrid, and infective processes got added and the intestine became affected. The cases complicated with diarrhœa were not so good, but simple cases of peritonitis were very suitable for operation. He had seen the intestines studded over with tubercle when the incision was made, and yet the children got quite well. He did not say that the analogy between the conditions was absolutely close clinically, but there was an analogy. They had cases of tuberculous pleurisy where the tubercle was primarily in the pleura. There were cases of that kind that, in the opinion of all authorities, did sometimes get well without any treatment at all. There was every reason to believe that a tuberculous pleurisy, so long as it was confined to the pleura and not in the lung, might get well. He might mention instances. A boy was brought in with bad tubercular peritonitis, abdomen swollen, and temperature high. He was just going to have him operated on when he noticed that the abdominal swelling was diminishing very much, and he therefore thought it would be better, as the swelling was going down, not to interfere. The swelling almost entirely disappeared in the abdomen, but pleurisy was set up on the left side. There was distinct evidence of it,—pain, and all the phenomena of pleurisy with effusion. He was tapped twice, and a large quantity of fluid was drawn off. Symptoms disappeared, and the pleurisy greatly improved. The boy got better and was sent home. He was sent back again, and this time he had diarrhœa very badly. It was quite clear that nothing could be done. He sank and died. Post-mortem there was abundant evidence of tuberculous peritonitis, also of tubercular meningitis, but no evidence of the pleurisy which had been there before. It was a question whether the method of treatment by free drainage was not better than aspiration for those cases where pleurisy was tubercular and the lung not involved. Tubercle, he thought, had a slenderer hold of serous membranes than of pulmonary parenchyma. As long as it was in the serous membrane alone, it might be got rid of. They knew it was got rid of from the abdominal serous membrane. He spoke from a clinical and not from a pathological point of view. As a matter of fact, they found that repeated tappings often did no good. Cases went on from bad to worse, and culminated either in free infection of the lung or in general tuberculosis. He agreed with Dr James that such cases occurring in middle life began as pleurisies—whether purely tubercular or not he did not know—but developed into phthisis. He repeated that it was a reasonable consideration whether it would not be well in such cases to open the chest and drain freely rather than resort to mere temporising methods of aspiration.

Dr Philip said he had listened with great interest to Dr James's paper. He (Dr James) had advanced two theses, one pathological and one therapeutic. With regard to the pathological thesis, he confessed that he was not altogether able to follow Dr James. He was aware of the difference of opinion that existed, and had for long been forming his own conception from pretty close observation on the point. Clinically he had found it difficult to get hold of a case of pleurisy with effusion, about which he had seriously to swither. He had seen a large number of post-mortems in this connexion, and he had not yet found a case such as Dr James described without evidence of tubercular infection. Excluding kidney and malignant disease and other such ascertainable causes, he had not yet found a case of chronic pleurisy without trace of tubercle present. He should like to ask on what other hypothesis than a specific one they could explain a pleurisy with effusion that became so intractable. The onus of proof lay with those who maintained that the tubercle, admittedly present even in Dr James's case, was a subsequent rather than a causal factor. With regard to the second thesis—the therapeutic one—it seemed to him very largely a question of the stage at which they had to deal with pleurisy with effusion. There could be no doubt that there was a great difference between a recent pleurisy with effusion and chronic conditions. If they had a comparatively healthy serous cavity, the sooner they exhausted the fluid the better, with suitable precautions as to the quantity taken away. But if they were dealing with a pleurisy with effusion which had lasted, it might be two, three, four, or five weeks or more, it seemed to him distinctly wise to consider such a major operation as Dr James had suggested, and if he limited his interference by free incision to these latter cases, he (Dr Philip) for one would certainly incline, from his own present knowledge, to agree with him.

Dr Leith said he had pleasure in listening to Dr James's paper, especially as this was a region he (Dr James) had made his own. He confessed to a disappointment from the pathological point of view. The light which he expected to obtain he had not obtained. Dr James would forgive him if he (Dr Leith) differed from him. He spoke from the pathologist's point of view, and would indicate some things he wished the physicians to do for them. Dr James spoke of pleurisy during the course of phthisis. He did not apprehend from Dr James whether he regarded pleurisy occurring during the course of phthisis to be tubercular or not. If he meant that it was tubercular pleurisy, then he (Dr Leith) found no pathological evidence that it was so. The pleurisies that occurred subsequently to a phthisis were not tubercular, but purely a tissue reaction of an inflammatory kind, which must be regarded as of a curative nature.   There were two kinds.   He might represent on the board the two pleural surfaces, here a necrotic area of caseous phthisis.   If it reached the pleura quickly it would cause a necrosis which was acute, and, like any other foreign body, set up an acute pleurisy which spread from that area.   That was very dangerous, because it was almost invariably followed by pneumothorax.   The other form, which was a little more common, was that this cavity as it reached the surface, as it always tended to do, exuded an irritative toxine, which was rarely a tubercular toxine, and thus set up a chronic pleurisy which covered the surface and prevented pyopneumothorax.   He thought chronic pleurisies during the course of phthisis were always of that nature.   Let them take the other condition, pleurisy preceding phthisis.   He took it that Dr James gave them two classes of cases.   He (Dr Leith) preferred to recognise three classes,—viz., those occurring in young people in good health where pleurisy was the first clinical symptom passing on without interruption to an undoubted phthisis.   To say whether or not that pleurisy was tubercular was practically very difficult, if not impossible.   Another class of case was where the patient had a basal pleurisy and got better, then a few weeks or months afterwards he had apical disease.   Whether that pleurisy was tubercular was also extremely difficult to say.   Dr Philip spoke of such cases, but he had left it doubtful.   Those patients were usually weakly, of sedentary habit, and they overworked themselves.   They had very little information as to that class of case.   He came now to the last class of case, which was the main feature of this paper,—viz., pleurisies occurring in old people.   They were undoubtedly the chief lesion that such patients suffered from.   They suffered from it for months, and Dr James's patient had been suffering from it for two and a half months before admission.   Dr James, in giving his able criticism of that case, said he believed the tuberculosis was a condition of a few days, that it occurred in the wards of the Royal Infirmary.   He (Dr Leith) made the post-mortem, and he entirely differed.   The tubercles were primary tubercles, and of many weeks' duration.   They were primary tubercles in the pleura, and the condition that carried off the patient was an acute tuberculosis starting from this primary focus.   That condition was undoubtedly blood-poisoning, and to say that they had no evidence of primary tubercle existing in the pleura for many weeks, even for months, in this case, he ventured to say as a pathologist, was not quite correct.   He agreed with Dr Affleck that they had primary tubercular pleurisies in these patients which might go on for months.   He did not see why they should not go on for years.   General tuberculosis, however, might carry the patient off at any time.   In the first place, they could tell the physicians how the tubercular pleurisy started.   It might reach the pleura primarily by the blood.   It might be from the peritoneum, as Dr Affleck had instanced.   Next, and this was very frequent, it started from tuberculous bronchial glands, which might have existed for many years.   It might start from the vertebral column, and in certain cases, he granted Dr James, there might be pleurisy precedent.   That tubercular pleurisy reached the pleura from the lungs, he ventured, as a pathologist, to doubt.   It might perhaps do so, but although there might be many foci throughout the lungs, he had never seen tubercular pleurisy developed from them.   Anatomists informed them that the lymphatics of the lung communicated freely with the subpleural lymphatics, and these by stomata with the pleural cavity ; and yet it was curious how in anthracosis, for example, the pigment readily reached the deeper layer of the pleura, but never the pleural cavity ; while, on the other hand, some affections of the pleural surfaces—*e.g.*, tubercular pleurisy—did pass for a slight distance into the lymphatics of the lung.   Perhaps the direction of the lymph currents might account for this. Physicians, he thought, ought to investigate the question whether pleurisy with effusion rendered the ground favourable for the growth of tubercle or the opposite.   Pathological evidence was a little doubtful.   He had cases where the tubercles were mainly related to the other lung, which was not compressed.   In other cases they were more numerous in the compressed lung than in the other.   They ought not to take it for granted that compression of the lung favoured tubercle.   With regard to treatment, he spoke from the physiological and pathological standpoint.   Why should not the physician inject tuberculin in doubtful cases to find out whether the reaction occurred.   The tubercle bacillus is rarely found in the products of the pleural paracentesis, but the absence of all organisms is in itself suggestive.   There was one other point.   As Dr James had said, the fluid always quickly increased if drawn off.   But if the depressed lung favours tubercle, the quicker it was drawn off the better.   It should be done, if necessary, every second day or every fourth day.   But Dr James mentioned the introduction of serous fluid to replace that drawn off, and a very wise and reasonable thing it was to try anything new which gave prospect of success.   What he (Dr Leith) wanted to ask him was —Whether the defective powers of absorption of the pleura had not been suggested as one reason for the persistence of the pleurisy ?   They had caseous pleura covered with lymph that entirely choked the lymphatics, and such a condition as that would render absorption difficult.   Moreover, in old people the pliability of the chest was greatly diminished, the costal cartilages calcareous, and it was said that the inflammatory condition favoured the calcification.   On these grounds he doubted the wisdom of putting in fluids.   It was, however, a point for experiment. As to free incision, if sufficient antisepsis were employed he did not see why it should not be done. He would go even further, for why should not the surgeon strip off a little of that lymph, which with its tubercles covered the free surface of the pleura, if he could get at it?. A free incision under antiseptic precautions in these cases could, he thought, do no harm. The danger was the absorption of the tubercle bacillus from its local seat into the blood, and thus a fatal result from general tuberculosis. Free incision, drainage, and scraping might even help to prevent this.

Dr Affleck said—Might he remind the Society of what Hippocrates did? He sometimes bored a hole in a rib, sometimes incised in an intercostal space, and poured in wine and oil. A piece of rag with a thread was stuck into the hole. He took it out each day and poured in wine and oil until the temperature fell and absorption took place.

Dr Stiles said there were other serous membranes besides the peritoneum and pleura. They had tubercular joints. The question was whether in chronic cases a simple pleurisy became tubercular, or was the condition tubercular from the first? He thought they would gain some light from what happened in the case of the synovial membrane of joints. Dr James had said his cases were chiefly in middle-aged or elderly people. A form of tubercle of the synovial membrane, to which Volkmann gave the name "tubercular empyema," occurred in the joints, especially of elderly people. It began with a little thickening of the serous membrane, effusion, first serous, then sero - fibrinous, ultimately sero-purulent. The disease lasted many years, was intractable, and ended in distinct tubercular disease of the synovial membrane. These cases have been shown to be tubercular from the first, and he was inclined to believe with Dr Leith that the cases referred to by Dr James were probably tubercular from the first; first very chronic, and then from some cause or other becoming more acute. Then as regards Dr Leith's view that pleurisy following tuberculosis of the lung was not tubercular, but was simply a reaction due to irritation, that, he must confess, he could not understand from what they met with in tubercular disease of joints, because when the disease began in bone and then actually made its way towards the surface either through synovial membrane, capsule, or the articular cartilage, the moment the tubercular focus burst into the joint, when it penetrated the cartilage the caseous material was set free, and they had very rapidly developed general tubercular disease of the synovial membrane, beginning at the surface and passing inwards. If they made a section they found the same structure as in a tubercular abscess,—a caseous layer internally, then tubercles, then a fibrous layer.

(Dr Leith, on being appealed to, insisted that a mixed affection did not occur in the pleura, although mixed contents might escape from a pulmonary cavity into it, the resulting pleurisy being simple or purulent, but not tubercular.)

When the tubercular focus reached the synovial membrane, and did not penetrate, what they met with was local tuberculosis in the synovial membrane, but the rest of the membrane became pulpy and thickened without any tubercle in it. The views he had given were based on Prof. Watson Cheyne's work on Tubercular Disease of Joints.

Dr James Ritchie said he viewed with increased suspicion all cases of pleurisy, especially with regard to life insurance, if there was a history of tubercle in the family; but he did not agree with those who held that nearly all cases of pleurisy with chronic effusion were tubercular, because there was a very large number of cases occurring in rheumatic individuals and along with Bright's disease; and, again, in old people with chronic bronchitis with considerable thickening of bronchial tubes, pleurisy occurred as a secondary lesion.

Dr Philip explained that he excepted cases of malignant disease, or with other ascertainable cause.

Dr Cathcart said that in reference to the interesting remarks of Dr Stiles, it seemed to him not quite fair to argue from synovial membrane to serous pleura. They had in the lung an element not present in joints, namely, risk of organismal infection through air passages. The synovial membrane secreted a fluid which was probably very much increased when the part was inflamed, whereas in the pleura the effect was rather to produce adhesive lymph, which might close up the aperture. He could not quite see that Dr Leith could actually state that tubercular pleurisy could never occur secondarily, but he thought that Dr Stiles' analogy would not hold so strongly as at first sight it seemed to do.

Dr James, in reply, said that he had to thank members of the Society for the way in which they had received his paper, and for the interesting discussion it had brought about. He would first express satisfaction at the general opinion expressed being in favour of incising and draining in these cases of sero-fibrinous pleurisy. One formed one's own opinion, and tended to stick to it if one thought it right, but he would feel greatly supported in his future work by what he had heard that night. His experience hitherto had been in favour of operation. As regards pathology, the point was—Was the tubercle first, or was the inflammation first and the tubercle afterwards? He preferred to take the big broad view, and held that unless they had the tissue below par as regards nutrition, the tubercle could not step in. The cholera bacillus could do no harm unless the intestine were below par. It was not our swallowing or inhaling bacilli that did the damage, but that some tissue in the body was below par. With the pleuritic process the tubercle bacillus got a nidus which it would not otherwise obtain. As regards this individual case, he had been looking up his notes again, and it was difficult to say when the miliary tubercular process supervened. One could say four or five weeks, at any rate.

2. The following is an Abstract of

SOME NOTES ON THE SURGERY OF THE BLADDER.

By DAVID WALLACE, M.B., F.R.C.S. Ed.

MR PRESIDENT AND GENTLEMEN,—I have on two or three occasions within the last five years brought under the notice of the members of this Society some points regarding the value of Cystoscopy, and to-night I propose once more to draw your attention to the usefulness of Cystoscopic examination as an aid to diagnosis in obscure genito-urinary affections, but more particularly to those in which hæmaturia is the chief or only symptom.

In a short paper, in Vol. I. of the *Hospital Reports*, on " Hæmaturia as a Symptom," I pointed out that the old dicta regarding the time of occurrence and the appearances of the blood as guides to diagnosis are very frequently fallacious, and I related cases illustrative of the mistakes into which we might be led. It is now very generally recognised that the appearances, etc., of the blood are unsafe guides ; but it was only the other day that I examined a patient who had been treated for three years for a supposed kidney affection, whereas the disease from which he suffered was a tumour of the bladder.

Mr T., æt. 55 years, had been a singularly robust man until December 1891, when, without any known cause, he passed blood in the urine. In the course of a day or two the urine was quite free from blood, and he had no recurrence of bleeding for nearly a year ; then again, without any apparent cause, blood appeared, and at intervals of some months during 1893 and 1894 he noticed blood in the urine. I cannot say what examination of the water showed during that period, but the hæmaturia was the only symptom from which he suffered. In the last months of 1894 and the beginning of this year the urine was very frequently examined. It contained no crystals, no tube-casts, but red blood corpuscles and a few pus cells or leucocytes, and also a few small-tailed cells in clusters of four or five. These cells were such as might come from the bladder. He had no pain at any time, but complained of some weakness in the small of the back. There was no frequency of micturition except when there was blood in the urine. When I saw him, just after a railway journey, the urine, which for some days had been clear, was brown, but contained no blood-clots. There was no red blood at the end of micturition, and he said there never had been.

Cystoscopic examination was made under chloroform, when the upper part of the bladder was found healthy, and not rugose. At the right inferior part of the wall, just above the right ureter, a tuberculated ulcerated growth was seen projecting into the bladder, while just below it there was a smooth mass irregularly raised from

2 *g*

the bladder wall. A suprapubic cystotomy was performed, and the tumour as far as possible removed. Microscopically it was proved to be an epithelioma.

On 5th April of this year I examined a patient in Sir Thomas Grainger Stewart's Ward. Arthur, æt. 49. In November 1894, for the first time, without any cause, he noticed blood in the urine. This was not increased by movement, and there was no frequency or pain. In April 1895 he complained of pain in the right side, and palpation of the right lumbar region caused pain, although no abnormal swelling was detected. The pain did not pass into the groin. The urine contained blood, but no pus, nor tube-casts, nor special cells.

Cystoscopically.—The bladder was healthy, slightly rugose anteriorly and laterally. Right ureter raised on a conical projection, and from this, at irregular intervals, dark brown urine (? blood) was emitted.

Diagnosis.—Bladder healthy ; probably stone in right kidney.

In these cases, it may be asked, could the diagnosis not have been made from the symptoms apart from cystoscopic examination ? Thus, in the first, where there was no kidney pain nor tube-casts, was the condition not most likely to be a bladder affection ? I reply that there were no definite bladder symptoms, and he was treated for three years for kidney disease. In the second, there was no bladder pain, while pain was felt in the loin : this pain, however, was not at all characteristic of kidney affection, and it is not at all uncommon to have pain referred to distant parts from the disease. The following case exemplifies this :—

Miss G., æt. 43, had suffered from frequency of micturition and pain at the neck of the bladder for nearly four years. At intervals of some months' duration she was better, but until six months ago (that is, after three and a half years) she complained of no pain in the kidney. She was treated during three years for cystitis, but derived no benefit. I examined the bladder cystoscopically, and found the bladder to be apparently quite healthy ; no areas of congestion, and no ulceration. Not even the hyperæmia that is frequently seen in cases where pus passing from the kidney has given rise to irritation at the neck of the bladder. From this examination, and from the symptoms which had more recently developed, the condition seemed to be renal. Tubercle bacilli were found in the deposit in the urine, and an exploratory incision of the left kidney was recommended.

In another patient, Miss D., æt. 25, whom I saw two years ago, the symptoms were precisely similar to those of Miss G. Examination of the bladder cystoscopically discovered no disease. Three months later, the symptoms having continued, but pain having developed in the loin, I cut down on and excised the kidney, which was riddled with abscesses.

In another patient, a girl of 10, the symptoms were frequency and pus in the urine, but no kidney pain at first. In that case also the bladder was healthy, but the kidney, when excised, contained numerous abscess cavities.

Then if we' take the appearance of the blood as a guide, bright red blood is thought to come from the bladder. The phrase goes, " The redder the blood the nearer the urethra the origin." I could quote various cases illustrative of the fallaciousness of this dictum, but the following may suffice:—Mr L. was recommended to me by Dr Edward Carmichael. In February 1894, without any cause, there was blood in the urine. No clots; the blood was all through the urine, and was bright red,—there was rather more at the end of the act of micturition. No other symptoms. The bleeding continued for twelve hours, and then the urine was perfectly clear. Six days later he travelled by rail to Dundee, and again there was bleeding; on this occasion, however, preceded by acute pain in the right iliac region, and while this lasted there was frequency of micturition. Fourteen days later he had another severe attack of pain, but no bleeding. On the 23rd of March this patient passed a small portion of oxalic acid calculus, and has never had another symptom.

These cases go to prove, I think, that too much stress should not be placed upon the appearance of the blood in cases of hæmaturia, and further, that such appearances, even when taken along with other symptoms, may be fallacious.

There is one feature in the bleeding which does, however, point more directly to the bladder, and that is, if at the end of micturition some pure blood comes away—but even this may occur in cases where the bleeding from the kidney is very severe, while in bladder cases it may be absent. With regard to the disease present in such a case, even when the bladder is the seat, we cannot definitely say what it is—it may be a tumour, prostatic congestion, or a calculus.

Before I pass from the subject of cystoscopy in such cases as I have referred to, I desire to advert to one other point regarding it. I wish to refute as strongly as possible the view held by some that the cystoscope causes intractable cystitis,—a condition which is fraught with extreme danger, and may hasten a fatal result. I assert that the cystoscope *per se* does not give rise to cystitis if it be used in suitable cases and with proper precautions (I have in a previous paper stated what these precautionary measures are), but I freely admit that if during the preliminary measures needful for the examination, or if during the examination itself any septic matter be introduced into the bladder, there is a great risk of septic cystitis being set up, just as there is in any examination of the bladder or in catheterisation. Every one is familiar with the tremendous risk of sepsis in cases where there is enlarged prostate with residual urine. Keyes, in a paper in the *American Manual of the Medical Sciences*, shows how great the difficulty is to avoid the introduction of septic organisms. Even with the most careful antiseptic precautions, the lotions may be sterile and the instruments aseptic; the orifice of the meatus may have been carefully washed with an antiseptic, but we cannot ensure that the urethra is free from organisms, and they may be pushed in front of the instrument into the bladder. How often after the introduction of a sound or catheter does sepsis result, although, as far as possible, every precaution be taken to avoid it. I have seen many such cases, and I always feel that there is no class of case where a surgeon's anxiety is greater than in one of enlarged prostate with residual urine, more particularly if complicated by hæmaturia.

Tumours of the Bladder.—In the initial stages of tumour of the bladder, hæmaturia is a symptom of the first importance. In a paper which I read two years ago before this Society upon " Cystoscopy in Tumours of the Bladder," I drew special attention to the features of the bleeding, which seem to be of great value as an aid to diagnosis. Since then numerous other cases of that disease have been under my care,—in all 33 cases, and consideration of these strengthen my belief that—

1. Bleeding is, in the majority of cases, the first symptom observed.

2. That it is usually intermittent in character.

3. That the amount of the blood, its colour (red or dark-brown), and duration are not pathognomonic; and

4. That the quantity of blood may be wholly out of proportion to the size of the tumour.

There are various difficulties which prevent accurate statistics being formed in relation to tumours, but from the cases which I have been able to thoroughly follow out I am led to draw the following conclusions:—

1. That the majority of bladder tumours are malignant.

2. That pedunculated tumours, which microscopically have all the characters of benign growths, may be recurrent and prove rapidly fatal. I have published, in the paper to which I have already referred, two such cases in which ultimately the death of the patient ensued after local recurrence. In one of these the patient, aged 55, was operated on by Prof. Chiene in July 1892. The tumour had a pedicle about the thickness of an ordinary lead pencil, and was, as far as one could judge, thoroughly removed. Six months later a large mass was found in the lower part of the abdomen, and the patient died in less than a year after the operation. In the second case there were multiple growths, but pedunculated. This patient was operated on on five occasions, and eventually died with all the symptoms of recurrence locally, and with, further, an enormous new growth in the region of the suprapubic wound. His first bleeding was in 1889, and he died in 1893.

3. That although the tumour is probably malignant, and complete removal impossible, suprapubic cystotomy is in some cases

most beneficial, and should be had recourse to in cases where bleeding alone, or bleeding and pain, are reducing the strength of the patient. In one stage or in two stages an endeavour should be made to remove the tumour as thoroughly as possible. The rest thus given to the bladder causes the hæmorrhage to cease, and diminishes or wholly alleviates the pain. Cicatrization of the wound takes place, and the tumour grows much less rapidly. I know that this is an opinion contrary to that of some surgeons, but I have observed marked benefit accrue in several cases. To one of them, already reported, I may allude, viz.,—a gentleman, 43 years of age, on whom I operated suprapubically, and removed an epithelioma which infiltrated the muscle tissue of the bladder wall. He made a good recovery, gained weight, had a complete cessation of bleeding and other symptoms, lived for eighteen months after the operation, and for sixteen of these did not have a bad symptom. He died suddenly, after a three days' illness, from probably blockage of a ureter and renal implication.

One has only to operate on an enlarged prostate by the method of two stages to be struck by the rapid decrease in size of the growth and the general improvement of the patient, after the preliminary cystotomy.

4. As a corollary to the second point, I may say that I believe malign growths may have originated from benign tumours. In the discussion which followed a paper I read at this Society, Mr Duncan took exception to this view; but I think the following case is one which goes to prove that it is at any rate in some instances correct:—

W. D. suffered from extroversion of the bladder. In 1889 Mr Chiene removed a polypoid mass, which microscopically was shown to be a simple adenoma. There seemed to be no infiltration of the bladder wall. A year later a new tumour on the original site was present, tuberculated in character, and quite analogous to an implanted papilloma. This was removed, but recurrence took place within a year. Again it was removed, but two years later a new growth was present with all the characters of an epithelioma. It was indurated, and infiltrated the bladder wall, and was accompanied by enlarged glands in the right iliac region. Removal was not attempted, and the patient died apparently from exhaustion four months after he last came under observation.

Enlarged Prostate.—The following seem to be the operative procedures usually adopted:—

I. Cystotomy—(a) Perineal, (b) Suprapubic.
II. Cystotomy, with removal of a portion of the prostate.
III. Forcible dilatation of the prostatic urethra.
IV. Castration.

In certain cases any one of these may be followed by alleviation or temporary cessation of the dangerous symptoms, but I believe, leaving castration out of account for the moment, that suprapubic cystotomy is the method most likely to be followed by permanent success.

I advise that, depending on the condition of the patient and the state of the urine, septic or aseptic, the operation be simply cystotomy, or cystotomy *plus* prostatectomy, always having in mind that the complete operation may be done in two stages.

Allow me to quote a case in which I assisted Prof. Chiene.

A patient, 71 years of age, suffered from an over-distended bladder, hæmaturia, great frequency, and pain. Want of rest was gradually wearing down his strength, and the loss of blood had rendered him markedly anæmic. The urine was septic, and for several years he had used a catheter.

Suprapubic cystotomy was performed. A large prostate was present, with a well-marked middle lobe projecting into the bladder.

The operation from time of anæsthetic to returning to bed was about twenty minutes. The patient rallied, and immediate benefit from the operation was obtained. 1. The bleeding stopped. 2. Frequency and pain disappeared. 3. Appetite, etc., improved. Ten days later the middle lobe was excised.

In this case temporary benefit was certainly obtained—What of permanent recovery? In what does permanent recovery consist? I take it that especially two things are desired.

1st, That atony of the bladder be recovered from; and

2nd, That no further prostatic enlargement takes place.

In September 1893, Mr M., æt. 71 years, was sent to me by Dr Paxton of Norham. For two and a half years he had used the catheter thrice daily or oftener, and during all that time had been quite unable to pass any urine naturally. He complained of pain, frequency every half-hour night and day. Prostate per rectum size of a cricket ball, hard, but tender. Urine alkaline, with deposit of pus. He was rapidly losing weight, and life was very miserable.

Milk diet, rest, washing out of bladder, etc., did no good, and in the beginning of October I performed suprapubic cystotomy, and at the same time removed a large mass of the prostate.

In seven weeks this patient returned home, and since the date of operation has never required a catheter. He passes his water with ease and with force, and has no frequency and no pain.

This is not an isolated case. The old view that if atony of the bladder exists along with enlarged prostate it cannot be recovered from is quite erroneous. When suprapubic cystotomy is performed and free drainage permitted, the bladder contracts, the muscle fibres regain their power, and atony is recovered from, at any rate in some cases.

The points in favour of the operation are these:—

1st, Rapidity.—The bladder can be opened into in three or four minutes. No preliminary distension is required, although it is advantageous. No Peterson's bag is needed.

2nd, It relieves retention instantly, and gives the bladder complete rest.

3rd, We can immediately gauge the size, etc., of the prostate.

4th, In cases of atony it gives the bladder the best chance to recover its muscular tone.

5th, If sepsis be present, it renders washing out easy, and topical applications may be adopted.

6th, The prostate immediately commences to contract, but in case of need at a second stage the prostate may be excised.

7th, Hæmorrhage ceases. Frequency is rendered *nil,* and pain disappears.

It may be argued that in old people it is dangerous to keep them in the recumbent posture for any length of time, but there is no objection to the patient sitting up in bed before the wound has healed.

With regard to the risk of the prostate again growing, it is said that it does not do so; and certainly in the case I have quoted two years have nearly elapsed without any recurrence of the symptoms of prostate enlargement.

Recently, the operation of castration has been recommended, but although the results gained by various surgeons seem most encouraging, we must recollect,—*1st,* That sufficient time to judge of the permanent effect of the operation has not elapsed. *2nd,* That now the operation has been performed on numerous cases, bad results have been frequently reported. *3rd,* The operation cannot overcome certain of the indications so rapidly as suprapubic cystotomy, *e.g.* retention, sepsis, hæmaturia.

Meeting XII.—July 3, 1895.

Dr CLOUSTON, *President, in the Chair.*

I. ELECTION OF MEMBER.

Ernest George Salt, L.R.C.P. & S.E., 50 George Square, was elected an Ordinary Member of the Society.

II. EXHIBITION OF PATIENTS.

1. *Dr Allan Jamieson* showed two cases of skin disease :—(1.) A case of HYDROA VACCINIFORME, or Hutchinson's Summer Eruption. A well-grown girl of 7, from the neighbourhood of Edinburgh. There is no history of a similar, or, indeed, of any skin disease in the family or relatives. Limited to the exposed parts—the face, hands, and wrists—it began two years ago, and though worst in the warm months, and subject to exacerbations and remissions, it has

never wholly disappeared. She was brought to the Royal Infirmary, and admitted into Ward 38 on the 27th of May 1895. The affected parts were then pretty thickly covered with crusts and scabs, the general aspect closely resembling what is seen in impetigo contagiosa. After being poulticed with boric starch poultices for a few days, the surface, though rough and eczematous looking, was clean, and on the backs of the hands, and to a lesser extent on the margins of the auricle, there were seen flat scars, the result of previous attacks. Her mother stated that fresh outbursts occurred at intervals of about three weeks, preceded and accompanied by great itchiness. In accordance with the views of Dr Bowles as to the effect of brown and yellow in preserving the skin from the action of the irritating elements of the sun's rays, a paste containing salicylic acid and resorcin, but coloured a deep brown by the incorporation of some umber, was thinly applied to the face and the hands. So long as this was used no amount of exposure to the tropical heat which has lately prevailed caused any uneasiness, or developed any eruption. The paste was then discontinued, and in a day or two the face became swollen to a slight extent, covered with red itchy papules, and eventually with small vesicles. The backs of the hands were similarly affected. The use of the paste was resumed, applying it solely to the left side of the face and back of the left hand. It will be seen that the skin on these is smooth and soft, but on the unprotected parts, on the right side, the skin is red, irritable, and eczematous. There is some unavoidable transference to this side also, hence the skin even there is to a certain degree protected, and thus the disease is not at its worst.

(2.) A case of ICHTHYOSIS, illustrating the effect of purely local treatment. J. T., 34, Co. Durham. Is an only child, with a marked tubercular history on her mother's side, but none of any skin affection in parents or collaterals. She has herself been delicate, and subject to asthma and bronchitic attacks on exposure. Has had measles, but without any effect on the condition of the skin. The ichthyosis is stated to have commenced when she was three months old, and to have first shown itself on the head, but as she has been liable to eczema on face and arms, there is some doubt as to the accuracy of this. There is also some difficulty in ascertaining positively whether the ichthyosis is worst in warm or cold weather, since the eczema which accompanies it is most troublesome in warm weather, when one would expect the ichthyosis to be at its best. She suffers from indigestion and constipation. She perspires very little, chiefly in axillæ. When admitted to Ward 38 on the 12th June 1895, her state was as follows:—The skin of the face, arms, and hands exhibited a leathery thickening, could be with difficulty pinched up, and was in places cracked and oozing. The shoulders and upper part of the back were dry and rough; the lower part, the flanks, round the umbilicus, on the nates, the skin felt harsh and dry, and seemed as if it had been dusted over with flour, which adhered firmly. The thighs and legs appeared as if painted over with a thick coating of lime. On the outer aspect of the thighs this was broken up into bands, a third of an inch broad, separated by narrow furrows, which ran diagonally upwards and outwards. On the front of the legs the epidermal accumulations were extensive, forming large, rough, almost warty areas, only here and there broken up into the usual quadrangular patches, but this pattern of arrangement was more evident on the patellar region. The hair was plentiful, the nails unaffected. The treatment ordered consisted of a daily warm bath, in which a resorcin salicylic soap made by Messrs Duncan, Flockhart, & Co. was employed to remove the epidermic masses. After the bath a strong resorcin ointment, 10 per cent., was well rubbed in. As the result of three weeks' such treatment, the skin of the trunk is now soft and smooth, little if at all different from the normal integument. That of the arms and hands is now dry and free from fissures, but is still leathery and shagreen-like. The subcutaneous fat is deficient, and the muscles atrophic. Improvement here must be a slow process. The warty plaster-like plates on the lower limbs have disappeared, and the skin is everywhere nearly as smooth as normal. The furrows between the plates are now felt to be slightly raised, the skin between them being flat and polished. These are atrophic lines where the skin had been unduly stretched in consequence of the unyielding nature of the ichthyotic areas. The skin can now be kept in good condition by the occasional use of the same medicated soap, followed by inunction with glycerine of starch, to which a little resorcin may, if necessary, be added. She states that she has only once been as well before, and that was after nine months' consecutive treatment in a hospital by lotions and ointments.

2. *Dr Norman Walker* showed a little boy with SKIN AFFECTION OF THE BACK. On his admission the diagnosis was doubtful. Some held that it was lichen, others that it was lupus erythematosus. Dr Jamieson's diagnosis of lichen turned out to be the correct one.

3. *Dr James* showed a BOY, æt. 15, at present in his ward. Two years ago he got a severe injury to the front of his head—fractured several of the bones. He was brought to the Infirmary, and Mr Caird enlarged the external wound and removed several pieces of bone. There was hernia cerebri, but it was got back; the wound healed, and he was discharged fairly well after eight months. He remained fairly well until last Christmas, when he took an epileptic fit. The pulsation of brain was visible in the soft area. In inspiration it seemed to fall, and in expiration to rise. He would show the pulsation by means of a water manometer communicating with a tambour bandaged to the pulsating area on the

2 *h*

head.   The column of water rose and fell with the pulse, and also
with respiration.   When he made any muscular effort the water
rose markedly, also when he held his breath.   They had also
taken tracings showing pulse, respiration, and time in seconds.
Very slight mental effort meant extra bulging and extra pulsation
of the brain, such as repeating the alphabet, adding up a column
of figures, reading.   The effect of merely attracting his attention
was remarkable.   What had struck him (Dr James) most was the
extreme slightness of the stimuli that caused the changes.   He
thought at first that the apparatus had gone wrong, but found that
it was not so.   They intended also trying the effect of difference
of temperature.

The President complimented Dr James on his interesting case.

III. Exhibition of Specimens.

1. *Dr Leith* showed a number of RUPTURES OF ABDOMINAL
VISCERA which might be of interest from a surgical and medico-
legal aspect.   First, a RUPTURE OF THE PANCREAS, in a boy aged
4, caused by the kick of a horse.   The rupture was partial, affecting especially the anterior part of the gland, and to an even
greater extent the peritoneum covering it.   It is to be carefully
remembered that the ascending layer of the transverse meso-colon,
which covers the pancreas anteriorly, does so most intimately,
without the intervention, even in fat persons, of any appreciable
fatty or fibrous tissues.   Hence hæmorrhage from the gland substance would most likely flow into the lesser omental sac.   In
this case it was not so, but into the retroperitoneal tissue above
the gland.   The case is referred to more fully in his paper on
" Ruptures of the Pancreas, etc." [1]   Such ruptures are rare, only
seven being, so far as he can find, previously recorded.

Second, a RUPTURE OF THE DUODENUM, almost at its junction
with the jejunum where it crossed the vertebral column.   This
was present in the same case, and the condition of the bowel
showed that it had been fairly full at the time of the accident.
It was to be especially noted that there was no bruising of the
external abdominal wall.

He also showed a case of RUPTURE OF THE LIVER; that of a van-
man who had been struck by the pole of a tramway car in the
epigastric region.   There was no external wound or bruise.   The
left lobe of the liver was almost entirely separated from the right.
He found two tears in the left main branch of the portal vein.
The man had been brought into hospital suffering from collapse
and signs of internal hæmorrhage.   Mr Annandale and Mr
Thomson performed laparotomy at once, but it was of no avail.
Ruptures of the liver were rarely met with in Edinburgh, though
by no means uncommon in some other places.   They might be

[1] This paper appears at page 250.

roughly subdivided into subcapsular and complete. The former might be successfully treated by rest and ice, but the latter were much better grappled with by laparotomy. Surgeons did not now fear to cut freely into the liver if necessary, and could control even severe hæmorrhage from its substance.

The next case was one of pretty severe RUPTURE OF THE KIDNEY in a man of about middle age. A tree fell upon him across the loins, and caused other severe injuries besides this. The rupture involved the capsule, but chiefly affected the posterior surface. This was a point of much importance, as when the anterior surface was involved, the peritoneum was likely to suffer, and blood and urine escape freely into the abdominal cavity, thereby greatly increasing the gravity of the case. Lesser ruptures might arise from comparatively slight injuries, but such severe ruptures as the present were only caused by some very severe injury.

He also showed a CEREBELLUM WITH MULTIPLE TUBERCULAR TUMOURS, well seen on both superficial and sectional view Tubercle is probably the most common form of brain tumour, and oftener single than multiple. They tended to be round and near the surface, but in the present case they were very irregular indeed, and deep in the substance as well as near the surface. They rarely softened in the centre, and were mostly firm and of a pale yellow colour, as in the present case. Symptoms and results were various. In this case the symptoms had given rise to doubts between bulbar paralysis and general paralysis of the insane, but in no way suggested a tumour of the cerebellum.

The BRAIN from the same case showed chronic hydrocephalus from pressure on the veins of Galen.

He also showed Specimens and Photographs from a case of PER-FORATIVE APPENDICITIS. The patient, a woman aged about 50, had been ill for about a fortnight, being attended by a dispensary student, before being seen by Dr Thin. From the history and the physical signs he suspected an appendicitis, and recommended her admission to the Royal Infirmary. Notwithstanding her great obesity, he was able to make out a swelling in the right iliac region. On her admission to Dr Wyllie's wards, she had an extensive gangrene of the right side of the vulva, from which an erysipelas spread over the upper part of the right thigh. A gangrenous patch also appeared in the middle line of the abdomen, in the position of a deep cutaneous fold a few inches above the pubis, caused by the great obesity. There was a marked protuberance in the umbilical region, suggesting an omental hernia or a large lipoma. The case terminated fatally. At the post-mortem a large omental hernia (now shown) was found. The gangrene of the vulva was traced upwards in the deep tissues of the anterior abdominal wall to a large gangrenous abscess in the substance of the abdominal wall in the right side. This passed upwards as far as the lower margin of the ribs, and was found to directly communicate with a large retro-cæcal abscess.

From this abscess another perforation passed through the iliacus fascia into the substance of the iliacus muscle, whence a large gangrenous tract passed beneath Poupart's ligament into a large gangrenous abscess among the muscles of the upper part of the thigh. The vermiform appendix was seen to stretch almost directly inwards at the upper internal part of the retro-cæcal abscess. It was adherent by its apex to the under part of the ileum, and showed, about 1 inch therefrom, two distinct perforations with tumefied margins. No concretion, kink, twist, or other abnormality in the vermiform could be detected. The whole case was a most interesting and peculiar one. Similar erratic outlets of retro-cæcal abscesses were not unknown, though rare. In a case of Dr Philip's, the abscess ran upwards in the lateral abdominal wall outside the peritoneum, and discharged itself into the right pleural cavity; and in another recorded by Dr Coats, it crossed the middle line above the pubis, and having ascended to the diaphragm, discharged itself into the left pleural cavity. The course and sequel of the lesions in the present case are well seen both in the specimens and photographs; first the appendicitis, then the perforation, then the retro-cæcal abscess, then the gangrenous abscess of the lateral abdominal wall travelling down to the vulva and the thigh, and, lastly, the erysipelas.

2. *Mr A. G. Miller* showed the BRAIN from a case of ABSCESS in TEMPORO-SPHENOIDAL LOBE arising from SEPTIC MIDDLE-EAR DISEASE. —P. W., æt. 15, plumber; admitted to Ward 31, 10th May 1895; admitted to Ward 12, 27th May 1895.

Complaint.—Vomiting; pain in belly; headache; discharge from left ear.

History.—Pain in belly and vomiting came on suddenly about a fortnight before admission to Ward 31. Checked by medicine and diet. Was able to be up and going about ward. Discharge from left ear for ten years; at times offensive. Patient is completely deaf on left side. Memory affected for about a year; speech slightly affected; very drowsy; answers quite intelligently. Was giddy and fell off chair about two months ago; headache since then. Gait peculiar; staggers to left; would fall if not assisted; before coming in had difficulty in turning street corners. Double optic neuritis—diminishing; has existed for some time. Paralysis of VI. on left side. Pupils do not respond to light, but to accommodation. Slight paralysis of tongue. Blue line on gums (?) Temperature 97° to 98°·4; always subnormal. Family history tubercular; a brother had glands; father and mother died of colds.

29th May 1895.—Ear reflected forwards; posterior wall of meatus chipped away; bone very thin; cranial cavity opened into almost at once; tympanum scraped out. Nothing found; no improvement.

6th June.—Slight weakness and congestion of right hand; no reflexes; water dribbles constantly.

7th June.—Suddenly became unconscious. Temperature rose from 97° to 103°. Trephined above left ear; trocar passed into brain; several ounces of very fœtid pus evacuated. Abscess syringed out and drainage-tube inserted. Patient never recovered consciousness.

Died next day (8th June) from septicæmia; temperature 105°; body greatly emaciated.

Remarks by Mr A. G. Miller.—Case remarkable as example of large cerebral abscess with very few and not very marked symptoms. Optic neuritis, headache, giddiness, paralysis of sixth, slight paralysis of ninth, and Argyll Robertson pupils. To these may be added the subnormal temperature and the history of chronic discharge (septic) from the ear. The diagnosis was in favour of intra-cranial abscess, but whether in temporo-sphenoidal lobe or cerebellum was not apparent. The first symptom that indicated distinctly implication of the temporo-sphenoidal lobe was the slight paresis of the right hand, followed next day by unconsciousness. Trephining was at once resorted to, but too late. Patient never recovered consciousness, but died next day. This case has impressed me with the opinion that in cases in which we suspect a cerebral abscess, if we would give the patient the benefit of the doubt, we should trephine and explore—first in the temporo-sphenoidal region, and then, if necessary, in the cerebellum. If we do not operate, the patient is certain to die. Operation gives a chance, and the patient should get the benefit of that.

3. *Dr Edward Carmichael* showed a specimen of SARCOMA OF THE SKULL which had been taken from a woman who died in Craiglockhart Poorhouse. The convolutions of the brain were depressed, but there were no symptoms until within the last few weeks. A Photograph and Drawing were also shown.

IV.—ORIGINAL COMMUNICATIONS.

1. ON THE TREATMENT OF FRACTURES NEAR A JOINT BY REST, AIDED BY MASSAGE AND PASSIVE MOVEMENT.

By A. G. MILLER, M.D., F.R.C.S. Ed., Lecturer on Clinical Surgery ; Surgeon to the Royal Infirmary, Edinburgh.

Mr Arbuthnot Lane[1] and Mr Marmaduke Shield[2] have recently drawn attention to a question which must have suggested itself often to surgeons—Is the result of treatment in cases of fracture near a joint usually satisfactory? Mr Lane uses very strong language in saying that it is not, and Mr Shield partly agrees with

---

[1] *Clinical Journal,* 17th April 1895.   [2] *Ibid.,* 15th May 1895.

him. The former attributes unsatisfactory results to malposition and effused blood, the latter to thrombosis of the deep veins.

Without going any further into the arguments of these gentlemen, I venture to say that I consider the present methods of treating fractures near a joint unsatisfactory, because I find not unfrequently that the injured limbs are stiff and comparatively useless even after a long period of treatment. As examples, I take fractures near the elbow, wrist, and ankle. And if any one doubts that the results of these injuries are often unsatisfactory, I would ask him to visit the out-patient department and convalescent home of any large hospital.

Taking as granted that the result is often unsatisfactory, I ask, What is the cause? There is no doubt that different causes may operate in different cases, and probably more than one in each; but the main cause I believe to be *the long period of rest maintained for the treatment of the fracture.* Mr Lane, in the lecture already referred to, says that unsatisfactory results arise "chiefly in consequence of rigid cases." Mr Shield speaks of "abominable and rigid apparatus," and long-continued rest, as leading to adhesions, etc. Let us see how the long continuance of rest leads to stiffness and uselessness.

In the case of a fracture near a joint, there is generally a double injury. The joint is damaged, more or less, by the same force that fractures the bone. We have then not a simple fracture, but a fracture plus a sprain. If the limb be put in a rigid apparatus, and kept there for some weeks, the fracture is being treated properly enough, but the sprain is ignored. Now this practice[1] has arisen, I believe, from the fear, hitherto uppermost in the surgeon's mind, of non-union of the fracture. In my experience, however, ununited fractures are very rare, while stiff limbs are very common.

Rest alone does not cause anchylosis. A healthy limb may be put up in a rigid apparatus for weeks, and yet quickly recover its mobility when the apparatus is taken off. On the other hand, let a damaged joint, say a sprain, be put up in plaster for some weeks, and it will take as many weeks of massage to make it useful.

Let us see, then, how this occurs, and let us take a case of Pott's fracture as an example. Besides the fracture of the fibula there is tearing of ligaments, damage to the synovial membrane and to the tendons and their sheaths. There is effusion of blood and serum into and around the joint. Now if this state of matters be left to itself, it is quite evident that adhesions and contractions may form which will materially interfere with the subsequent usefulness of the foot and ankle.

How is this difficulty to be met? Are we to treat the sprain, therefore, and ignore the fracture? By no means. No more than

---

[1] Of treating the fracture and ignoring the damaged joint.

we are to treat the fracture and ignore the condition of the joint. We have to treat the two injuries simultaneously. Rest for the fracture, and massage and movement for the joint, effusion, etc.

Let me take as an example the patient which I have the honour of showing to the Society this evening. The case was one of fracture of both bones of the leg in the lower third, slightly compound, and accompanied by much bruising and effusion of blood into the cellular tissue. The limb was put up in a box splint made by two pieces of wood rolled up in a sheet and well padded. This splint was opened down twice a week, and the leg carefully and gently massaged, and the ankle moved with every precaution to prevent movement of the fractured surfaces. The result in five weeks has been, I think, most satisfactory.

If any one should be nervous about the taking down of a fracture twice a week, let me remind him that the proper treatment of a fracture often obliges the surgeon to take off the splints several times during the course of treatment. The swelling that results almost immediately after a fracture subsides considerably in a few days, and any apparatus that has been applied becomes loose, and has to be readjusted. The padding used to prevent undue pressure becomes felted and hard in some places, or the limb from some other cause may become uncomfortable, and the splints have again to be removed and replaced. In this way, or from other causes, fractures have generally to be "taken down" and looked at several times during their treatment. If this has to be done once or twice for the benefit of the fracture, why not five or six times? And if the fracture has to be taken down for the purpose of readjustment, why not apply a little massage and careful movement at the same time?

The advantages of this combination of rest with massage and passive movement are:—1. Complete rest is provided for the union of the fractured bone, except for a few minutes once or twice a week. 2. Swelling and effusion are got rid of more quickly by the massage. 3. Adhesions are prevented by passive movements.[1] 4. Union of the fractured surfaces is probably facilitated by the massage. 5. Time is saved. _____

Mr Joseph Bell said he had not the slightest doubt that the case had been a bad fracture well mended. It had been oblique, as one could still feel, and it reflected great credit on Mr Miller. He was very glad indeed that Mr Miller did not give in to the very latest fancy of the present day, the ambulatory treatment of fracture. He (Mr Bell) was reading a long paper about it last night. That was the new fad. The patient was to walk about in ambulatory splints. Before he said anything he would direct the attention of the Society, and especially of his younger friends, to one point

[1] Voluntary movement I consider most dangerous, and believe that it may be a likely cause of ununited fracture.

which struck him very forcibly. He had been reading several of the papers of the present day. He thought the younger surgeons were laying on themselves a burden of responsibility which they had no right to do. They implied that fracture should be treated with absolute success. There were certain fractures in the vicinity of joints from which, do as they liked, they would have bad results. Many of them knew that for many years he had taught as Mr Miller had been telling them to-night. Fractures near the elbow generally occurred in young people, and he had taught that they should be kept quiet for a period corresponding to the age of the child, a day for each year,—*e.g.*, a child of five years for five days, of ten years for ten days. He never had the least anxiety as to ununited fracture in the vicinity of the elbow. He could not say that he ever had an ununited fracture of the shaft of the humerus or femur in his practice. For Colles' fracture he had given up splints. He thought them quite unnecessary. No man in his senses thought of tying up the fingers. He did not think they needed splints. A turn or two of plaster or a bandage would suffice. It was more for the sake of the public than for the sake of the parts that they used splints. He saw a very bad case of Pott six days ago, a few hours after it happened. His only treatment was to give it free and full massage. The patient had been tossing about with high temperature and swollen limb before the massage. After massage she expressed herself as very much better. She would require to be kept quiet, but not much splinting would be needed. With reference to the question of sprain, he was glad to see Dr Laing there, who knew more about it than most of them put together. He had never seen a sprain that one needed to wait very long in. He had a pretty bad one himself, but got it well rubbed and an elastic bandage put on. He was not confined for half a day. Probably most of them had read an interesting paper by Mansel Moullin, in which those views that Mr Miller had expressed were strongly emphasized, and especially the point that Mr Miller had referred to, that there was not merely fracture, but also an injury to the joint, and that probably the joint injury was the more important of the two.

Dr Laing said he could only speak from the massage point of view. As Mr Bell had said, as soon as effusion was over there was no reason why the sprain should not be treated by massage, and on the second or third day by movement also. A patient with average bad sprain should be able to walk in a week, as a rule, and it was important that it should be a free, good, and correct style of walking. Before trying to walk, the movement should be both passive and active against resistance, so as to cultivate the power. The fracture itself, with careful massage, was apt to be much sooner mended and better mended than if left in a stiff splint the whole time. He had seen ununited fracture treated by massage success-fully. By encouraging the circulation and nourishment of the bone the fracture would certainly unite better.   Careful massage should not in any way require any movement of fractured bone. There was no necessity whatever in massaging the leg to have any risk of moving the bone, and he would go further than Mr Miller, and have the fractured limb treated oftener and treated longer, as Mr Bell had pointed out.   The more gentle the massage the longer it would take, and, as Mr Miller had said, they became much more free in their treatment after the first few days.

Mr Alexis Thomson said he thought he might say for the younger members present that they were much indebted to Mr Miller for impressing on them the improved methods of treating fractures, more especially the fracture shown them to-night.   He did not imagine Mr Miller would have them believe that by this means they could get rid of the stiffness that followed in all fractures of joints,—*e.g.*, in the elbow joint they might have absolute stiffness amounting to anchylosis. He referred to those cases of comminuted fracture in which they had displacement of fragments.   No splints that they could apply would command the fragments, and no massage would keep them in their place afterwards.   As Mr Watson Cheyne had written, the best method was to cut down and fix the fragments either by wire or pegs made of ivory or steel. In private practice it was very much easier to carry out massage than in hospital practice.

Mr H. J. Stiles said he would like to make one remark.   Dr Laing and Mr Bell said that the best time to begin massage in severe sprain was after twenty-four or forty-eight hours.   He would like to know what was the best treatment during these twenty-four or forty-eight hours.   It was during that time that they had extensive hæmorrhage, more especially round the ligaments, tendinous sheaths, and so on, about the joint.   The blood, when organised, would favour the production of adhesions, and he thought, there-fore, that the best treatment during the first twenty-four hours was to put on cotton wool and a domett bandage.   This should not be confined to the region of the joint, but should be begun on the distal side, and the cotton wool should be carried right up,—*e.g.*, in the case of the ankle joint, as far as the knee.   In twenty-four or forty-eight hours they got ecchymoses extending up beyond the knee, even in an ordinary sprain of the ankle.   The blood having been distributed in this way in a thin layer over a large area could be more easily acted upon by the subsequent massage.

Mr Miller, in reply, said that he might mention that the man en-joyed the massage immensely.   Mr Bell had very properly drawn attention to a point which he did not think it necessary to refer to, that there were certain fractures which nobody could turn out satisfactorily; but with many fractures this method that he had referred to had very satisfactory results.   Indeed, he had no hesitation in seconding what Dr Laing had said as to the absence of risk in moving fragments.   With regard to the treatment of sprain, of course the application of cotton wadding and bandages was very good ; but even if they did not employ these, they spread the ecchymosis up to the knee and above it. In this case he had spread the ecchymosis away above the knee. Massage itself would spread the ecchymosis very well if they started early.

2. RUPTURES OF THE PANCREAS : THEIR RELATIONS TO PANCREATIC CYSTS, WITH SOME REMARKS UPON TREATMENT.

By R. F. C. LEITH, M.B., M.A., B.Sc., F.R.C.P. Ed. etc., Lecturer on Pathology, Edinburgh Medical School ; Pathologist to the Edinburgh Royal Infirmary, etc.

INJURIES of the pancreas are rare. The size, shape, and anatomical position of this organ are in the main responsible for the comparative immunity which it enjoys. Being about 8 to 9 inches long, 1 inch broad, and somewhat strap-shaped, it lies transversely across the posterior abdominal wall at the level of the first lumbar vertebra, the tail being a little higher than the head. This corresponds pretty nearly to a transverse line drawn across the anterior abdominal wall, about 3 inches above the umbilicus.

It will thus be obvious that blows or injuries received in front must be directed over a very limited area indeed in order to reach it ; and not only so, but their force must be expended more or less directly backwards and not obliquely upwards or downwards, and that, too, about the middle line, so as to crush the organ against the unyielding vertebral column. Not even all such blows will succeed in injuring the organ, for it is deeply placed, being protected in front not only by the anterior abdominal walls, but by the stomach, lesser omental sac, and the ascending layer of the transverse mesocolon. Posteriorly it is also, though less effectually, protected by certain soft structures, which to a certain extent act as buffers between it and the inner rigid bony framework. These are from right to left, the portal vein and the inferior vena cava, the two crura of the diaphragm on either side of the aorta, with the root of the superior mesenteric artery, and the left suprarenal capsule and kidney. The bony framework of the chest completely protects it from violence directed from behind, and hence we find only instances of injury resulting from violence received in front. There is some reason to believe that it may be slightly injured in cases where the force has not been expended directly over it in the middle line, but towards the left side, or even with a direction from below upwards ; but in order to effect any serious laceration of the gland substance the violence must be inflicted not only in the middle line and directed backwards, but be of very considerable severity. As the neighbouring organs, the liver, spleen, stomach, especially if full, and kidneys are all more exposed, and thus more liable to suffer, it follows that such a rupture of the pancreas, uncomplicated with rupture in any other organ, is not likely to be met with. This is amply demonstrated by our experience of the cases which have unfortunately proved fatal. In these the injury to the gland substance has generally been great. Of the more fortunate cases we cannot speak so positively, as in the absence of an exploratory laparotomy we must remain more or less in the dark as to the precise nature of the lesions.

I propose to consider the cases under two divisions,—1st, Those in which a fatal issue followed early upon the injury; 2nd, The milder ones, in which the immediate results of the injury were apparently temporary or slight, and quickly recovered from, and in which the main evidence of pancreatic involvement rests on the subsequent formation of a pancreatic cyst.

FIRST GROUP.—*Cases in which a fatal issue followed early upon the injury.*—I know of only nine cases altogether, of which seven have been previously recorded. Of the other two, one was received into the Royal Infirmary, Edinburgh, and the other, particulars of which have been kindly sent me by Dr Goldmann, into the Surgical Hospital at Freiburg, in Baden. In only two of these nine cases is it expressly mentioned that no other organ than the pancreas was injured. In the remaining seven other serious injuries were present, viz., rupture of the lung in one, of the spleen in another, of the duodenum in another, and fracture of ribs along with other internal injuries, such as rupture of the liver, kidney, or spleen, in the other four.

CASE 1.—A child, Adam W., aged 4 years, was playing one forenoon with some companions near his father's horse and cart in the Infirmary grounds. In the temporary absence of the father they had been teasing the horse, when it suddenly kicked out, striking the lad, evidently in the pit of the stomach, with its off hind foot. He fell forcibly against the wheel of the cart, but picked himself up apparently more frightened than hurt, and with the help of his companions climbed up into the cart. His father returning shortly after, and learning what had happened, did not think seriously of it, but kept the child with him until he went home for his dinner. Shortly afterwards the mother noticed that the child was not looking well. He complained of a numbness in his left arm, which he was unable to move. His father, fearing that the arm was broken, carried him to the Royal Infirmary, and he was admitted to Ward 9 under the care of Professor Annandale, to whose kindness I am indebted for permission to refer to the case. The left humerus was found to be fractured transversely in its lower third, but there were no signs of any other injury. His head, chest, and abdomen showed no bruises, and pressure elicited no pain. Later in the afternoon he did not look so well. He was evidently suffering from shock and pain, and obscure symptoms of some abdominal mischief began to appear. His condition became more grave as the evening wore on. The shock deepened towards collapse, and although it was fairly certain that there was a serious abdominal lesion, the symptoms and signs were too indefinite and diffuse, and the general condition too serious to render an exploratory laparotomy advisable. He gradually sank and died about ten hours from the time of receiving the blow. The necropsy was made by me about fourteen hours after death. The usual rigidity and lividity were observed. There was a bruised appearance around the lower part of the left upper arm, which showed the usual displacements of a fracture of the lower third of the humerus. There were no other marks of violence and no bruising or discoloration anywhere upon the body. On opening the abdomen a quantity of fluid (about 1 pint) was seen lying freely in the peritoneal cavity among the intestinal coils. It was clear and dark brown in colour, and had a peculiarly pungent but not fetid odour. The general peritoneal surface showed a certain amount of injection and slight loss of gloss, but no hæmorrhage.

On raising up the great omentum with the transverse colon, nothing further was observed except the appearance of a very slight amount of yellowish fluid between the intestinal coils just below the transverse mesocolon. On gently displacing the more superficial coils, it became more plentiful, and was evidently specially located posteriorly in this position. It was of a yellowish colour, with slight granular, cheesy-looking material in it, closely resembling the contents usually found in a stomach containing partially digested milk. It suggested a rupture of the duodenum in this position, and I presently found one close to the termination of the third part. The amount of the escaped contents showed that this part of the gut had been fairly full at the time of the injury. This would favour its rupture. Indeed, I think we may safely say that subcutaneous rupture of the collapsed bowel really never occurs. I have seen it follow a perforating wound but not a contusion. It will be remembered that this is one of the commonest sites of intestinal rupture, for here the gut is more or less fixed and rests upon the vertebral column. The tear in the present case was through the whole wall for about ⅔ of its circumference, the peritoneal coat still being intact in the other third. The Photograph (Fig. 1) shows the rupture and the natural undisturbed relationships after raising the omentum with the transverse colon and removing the superficial intestinal coils. There was another small tear about ¾ inch long in the mesentery of the jejunum a short distance lower down. There was very little hæmorrhage. The margins of the peritoneum in the neighbourhood of the tears showed a little infiltration with blood-clot, and there were a few petechiæ in the transverse mesocolon, but nothing further. The transverse colon was then displaced downwards and the pancreas exposed. The ascending layer of the transverse mesocolon and the underlying pancreas were both found to be torn. The rupture in the gland was a little less extensive than that in the mesentery. It ran vertically from above down-

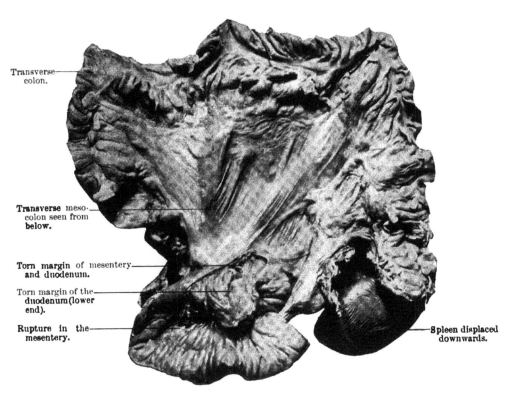

Transverse colon.

Transverse meso-colon seen from below.

Torn margin of mesentery and duodenum.

Torn margin of the duodenum (lower end).

Rupture in the mesentery.

Spleen displaced downwards.

FIG. 1 shows the rupture in the duodenum. The ends have been filled with cotton wool and separated from one another for the purposes of demonstration.

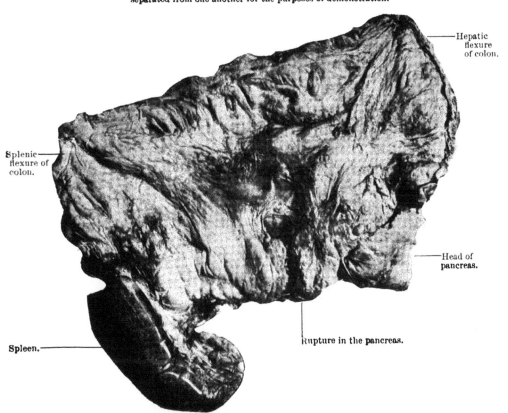

Hepatic flexure of colon.

Splenic flexure of colon.

Head of pancreas.

Rupture in the pancreas.

Spleen.

wards with a slight obliquity to the right, passing through its whole thickness at its upper border, but through a part only towards the lower border. The main duct and splenic vessels were uninjured. The line of rupture was almost directly over the aorta, and on being continued through the transverse mesocolon became continuous with that in the duodenum. This was probably the line of chief impact of the horse's hoof; the organs having been crushed between it and the vertebral column. Its position in the pancreas about the junction of the right with the middle third is well seen in the Photograph (Fig 2.) The ruptured ends had separated a little from one another, and were infiltrated to a slight degree only with blood. There was practically no blood in the lesser omental sac, which, except for the tear already mentioned in its posterior wall, presented a perfectly normal appearance. Blood had effused from the rupture as the retroperitoneal cellular tissues contained a certain quantity of diffusely spread blood-clot. It might amount altogether to about 3 ozs. It passed mainly to the left above the pancreas towards the spleen, reaching its hilum and infiltrating also a little downwards. It did not pass behind the pancreas except just at the tail, where it spread itself slightly over the suprarenal capsule.

The amount of hæmorrhage thus appeared to be remarkably small for such an extensive injury to the gland, and, moreover, it lay behind and not within the lesser omental sac, into which the gaping wound in the gland directly opened. When we remember how closely the peritoneum covers the anterior surface of the gland, we would naturally expect the hæmorrhage from an anterior rupture to flow into the lesser omental sac. On other grounds, also, I was prepared to find some fluid within this sac, as many of the ducts of the gland must have been torn across, and it is at least probable that some pancreatic juice was secreted, for it will be remembered that the unfortunate little patient lived for about ten hours after the accident. The foramen of Winslow was patent, and some of the fluid in the general peritoneal cavity may have thus come from the lesser sac.

All the other abdominal organs were uninjured. The stomach contained a few ounces of material similar to that seen in the duodenum. Had it been distended, it might not so readily have escaped injury. I was much interested, also, to find that the aorta had not suffered in any way. It was clear that it lay directly in the line of the impact, and presumably had been suddenly and violently pressed against the vertebral column. It would not, I think, have been surprising to find some injury of the external or middle coat.

The liver and kidneys were markedly pale, as were also the lungs in part, suggesting a large rather than a small hæmorrhage. This was certainly not present. The bowel contents only showed some blood-stained mucous for about 18 inches below the site of rupture. The cranial sinuses were congested, but the brain and its membranes were healthy.

The special points of interest in the case are the nature of the injury, the comparative absence of serious signs for some time after its infliction, their subsequently rapid onset and gravity, the absence of any marks of violence upon the abdominal wall and of pain, the large amount of fluid in the peritoneal cavity, the severity of the rupture in the pancreas, and the smallness in amount and anatomical position of the hæmorrhage. If the shock and collapse had been due to the injury acting directly upon the solar plexus, or more indirectly through the nerves of the pancreas and peritoneum, we would have expected their onset to have been practically immediate, and we are therefore led to suggest that they are referable rather to the changes occurring in the peritoneal cavity subsequent to the injury. The dark-coloured fluid, about 1 pint in amount, had probably not come from the ruptured gut, as it was different in character from that found in the neighbourhood of the tear. There remains then only the inflamed peritoneum or the torn pancreas to explain its presence. It is decidedly unusual to find such a large quantity of fluid associated with a simple early peritonitis, and it is thus quite as probable that the pancreas was responsible for some of it at any rate. It is probable that pancreatic secretion has under certain circumstances a peculiarly irritating effect upon the peritoneum, and its gradual and steady escape into the general peritoneal cavity would largely explain the phenomenon observed in the present case. The other points of interest will be considered in conjunction with the other cases.

CASE 2 [Goldmann].—A young man received a violent blow upon the abdomen from the fall of a heavy packing case upon him. It is believed that the corner of the case struck him in the epigastric region. On his admission to the hospital his chief symptoms pointed to abdominal hæmorrhage and intestinal obstruction. A tumour gradually formed in the mesogastrium resembling that formed by a pancreatic cyst. There were no marks of bruising externally upon the skin of the abdominal wall. The general condition of the patient was too grave to admit of laparotomy. He died a few hours after the accident. At the necropsy the pancreas was found to be transversely ruptured. Profuse hæmorrhage had occurred into the cavity of the lesser omentum, and given rise to the pseudo tumour in the mesogastrium. The spleen was also lacerated. The other organs were uninjured.

CASE 3 [Jaun (1 [1])].—A male, a native of India, about 50 years of age, had been subjected to a somewhat curious assault. He was tied up in a sort of lithotomy position; his hands being first tied together, and his knees then forced within the area of the tied arms and secured there by a long lath passing from the one side to the other through the space between the anterior aspect of the elbow and the posterior aspect of the knee. His assailant then

[1] The figures within parentheses refer to bibliography at the end of this paper.

beat him violently with a shoe on the exposed buttocks, genitals, and abdomen, and also kicked him once or twice. On being released he walked home, a distance of about 1 mile, supported between two persons. He was then admitted to the hospital, and died about eighteen hours afterwards. At the necropsy, it was found that the pancreas was ruptured vertically from above downwards, at its right extremity, for about half its breadth. A small clot of blood was found near this, and the rest of the organ looked congested and showed extensive extravasation of blood into its substance. The abdominal cavity contained about six ounces of blood-stained fluid, and the peritoneum in places, especially the transverse mesocolon, showed considerable injection. No other lesion was found, and there was no external sign of injury.

CASE 4 [Wilks and Moxon (2)].—An adult was run over in the street. The pancreas was so crushed in its middle as to be divided into two parts opposite the spinal column. There was but little other sign of injury to the abdominal viscera.

CASE 5 [Cooper (3)].—A 33-year-old man was run over in the street by a light car going very rapidly at the time. He showed no external signs of injury. His symptoms pointed to severe internal hæmorrhage, and he died in less than two hours after the accident. The pancreas was literally smashed and imbedded in coagulated blood. The spleen and kidney were also ruptured, and there was a slight tear on the under surface of the liver. Several ribs were broken.

CASE 6 [Travers (4)].—An intoxicated woman was knocked down by a stage-coach, which, however, did not pass over her, and died a few hours afterwards from internal hæmorrhage. The pancreas was transversely torn across. There were other internal injuries, the liver being lacerated and several ribs were broken.

CASE 7 [Wandesleben (5)].—The pancreas and lung were both injured.

CASE 8 [Störck (6)].—A woman was run over by a coach, and died within a few hours. The pancreas was completely torn in two, and imbedded in a large mass of semi-fluid blood. Several ribs were fractured, and the liver was ruptured.

CASE 9 [M. Le Gros Clark (7)].—A lad showed rupture of the pancreas and other severe injuries which speedily proved fatal.

Edler (8), the latest writer on this subject, could in 1887 find only 3 cases of this lesion, viz., those of Cooper, Travers, and Kuhlenkampff (9). I have not followed him in including the last-named case, as it afforded no evidence that it was a case in point. Kuhlenkampff himself did not claim that the pancreas had been ruptured or lacerated. He believed that the severe blows which the patient had received upon the epigastric region had caused an inflammation of the pancreas, which through resulting obstruction of the main duct had given rise to the mesogastric cyst which he successfully opened and drained. Senn (10), writing a year earlier, mentioned 4 genuine cases, viz., those of Cooper,

Travers, Störck, and Le Gros Clark. I have been able to add 7 cases
to the 2 genuine ones of Edler, and 5 to those of Senn ; but even the
increased knowledge thus afforded us is still sufficiently meagre
to make us exercise much caution in forming any general conclusions. In at least 3 of the cases the injury was caused by their
being run over by a vehicle, and it is interesting to note in almost
the only surgical text-book in which I have found any reference
to rupture of the pancreas, that of Jamain (11), it is said that this
very rare lesion is usually thus caused. A violent and sudden
blow is responsible for 3 more.

Symptoms and Signs.—Shock and collapse would seem to be
the most prominent. They are usually brought about immediately by internal hæmorrhage, as in Cases 2, 5, 6, 8, and 9 ; but
may be due to other and less obvious causes, as in Cases 1 and 3,
where they came on only after a considerable interval. They are
probably due more to the complications than to the pancreas.
In no case have the symptoms pointed to the pancreas as the
main seat of lesion. The absence of any bruising, ecchymosis, or
discoloration of the skin of the abdomen, or any sign of external
violence, is important, and not a little surprising. Its bearing
upon medico-legal cases is obvious. Serious criminal assults may
be made, as in Case 3, without any outward or visible sign of
injury. A similar absence is noted in Cases 1, 2, and 5, and I
have several times observed it in other cases of ruptured viscera.
It may almost be said to be the rule and not the exception. It
may occur also in the thorax, as in the case (12) of a child run
over by a cart, in which the lung was torn without any fracture
of the ribs or injury to the wall of the thorax.

Diagnosis.—This is practically impossible without laparotomy.
The nature of the violence, its exact site of impact and direction,
may make the lesion probable. It can only be verified by laparotomy. I have satisfied myself that upon the cadaver at all events
the anterior surface of the pancreas can be thoroughly explored
by the finger through a vertical incision about 3 inches long, in the
middle line anteriorly, or preferably a little to its left in the epigastric region. If an electric lamp be placed in the interior of a
Ferguson's speculum, both the organ and its covering peritoneum
can be scrutinised.

Prognosis.—The foregoing cases were all rapidly fatal. The
cause of death was internal hæmorrhage in at least 5 of the cases,
viz., 2, 5, 6, 8, and 9 ; but this result was in all probability more
due to the complications than to the lesion in the pancreas. In
Cases 1 and 3 the hæmorrhage was small in amount, and none of
the other parenchymatous organs was ruptured. It is then at
least probable that the hæmorrhage from a rupture of the pancreas
alone will not be severe unless the splenic artery or vein be
ruptured. In themselves they need not be fatal.

Treatment.—It has already been shown that the lesion in the
pancreas is rarely the only one present, and, further, that the

rupture in the gland does not declare itself by any definite signs or symptoms. It follows, then, that ordinary expectant treatment (rest, ice, etc.,) alone can be followed, except in the cases where an exploratory laparotomy is performed. If this be done and a rupture be discovered, it should at once be treated. The hæmorrhage may be arrested by pressure, and the ruptured ends brought close together by comparatively superficial sutures passing through little more than the peritoneal covering of the gland. The covering adheres so closely to the gland without the intervention of any fatty or other tissue that it is easy to bring the separated ends of the gland together by traction exerted alone upon the peritoneum. This procedure is, however, open to the objection that blood or pancreatic juice might collect between the ends and cause their separation again, and lead perhaps to cyst formation or other trouble. Senn (13), from his experiments on animals, recommends that the ends of the ruptured gland be separately ligatured previous to such suturing. This has the advantage of effectually arresting the hæmorrhage and the outpouring of the pancreatic juices, and, further, the close approximation of the ends favours the rapid establishment of the nutrient vascular supply. He would first remove the necrosed portions of the gland. He found that ruptures treated in this way quickly healed, and that there was no danger to be apprehended from the distal part of the gland, as all such physiologically separated portions of gland underwent simple atrophy, and in no case led to cyst formation.

SECOND GROUP.—*Milder Cases.*—We have already seen that such evidence as we are able to bring forward tends to show that ruptures of the pancreas need not in themselves prove fatal, and it is quite conceivable that many such ruptures may occur, and probably have done so, in varying degrees of severity, in cases of abdominal injury which have entirely recovered. Perhaps large ruptures, such as occurred in Case 1, may lead to such an extensive outpouring of pancreatic secretion, mixed with blood-clot and fragments of devitalized pancreatic tissue, that its escape through the foramen of Winslow into the general peritoneal cavity may set up a general chemical, and perhaps also organismal peritonitis. We lack evidence on such a point, however, and it is more probable that the lesion in the gland is followed by inflammation, which results in nothing worse than a certain amount of cicatricial contraction, and the patient recovers entirely without the subsequent occurrence of any other trouble. Cases have been recorded in which even extensive cicatrization of the gland existed without any suspicion of its presence during life. It is obvious, however, that other possibilities exist. There is room for other results between those two extremes. The lesion in the gland may be followed by an inflammation, not restricted to the gland itself, but spreading gradually to other tissues in its neighbourhood, and leading, perhaps

2 k

long afterwards, to subsequent trouble. This supposition is further
strengthened by the fact that many cases of injury received in the
epigastric region have been followed, sometimes long afterwards,
by the appearance of a cyst in this region, and the relation which
the so-called *pancreatic cysts* have to ruptures of the gland itself is
a most interesting one. Increasing attention has been of late
years paid to the subject of these cysts, and a traumatic origin
has been assigned to a large proportion of the reported cases.
These number, so far as I can find, altogether 17, and I have
arranged them in chronological order in the following Table:—

*Table showing the lapse of time between the Injury and the
appearance of the Tumour.*

No.	Year.	Sex	Age.	Nature of Injury.	Time elapsing between the Injury and the appearance of Tumour.	Reference.
1	1882	M.	39	A number of heavy blows upon the abdomen. Patient believed that they were received about the umbilicus in a direction from below upwards.	About 2 months.	Kuhlenkampff, *Ar- l. klin. Wochenschr*, 1882. No. 7, s. 102.
2	1885	M.	19	Patient fell from a waggon, striking the ground on the left side of the abdomen, a heavy keg falling at the same time upon his back.	About 5 weeks.	Senn, *Amer. Journ. Medical Sciences*, New Series. Vol. xc, p. 18.
3	1887	M.	46	Thrown from a waggon.	About 8 years.	Küster, *Deutsche Med Wochenschr.*, Leipzig. Vol. xiii., 1887, p. 189.
4	1888	M.	8	A fall from a horse, bruising the abdomen.	About 3 weeks.	Fenger, *Chicago Med. Journ.*, Feb. 1888.
5	1888	M.	40	A crush between two railway waggons.	About 1 year.	Steele, *Chicago Med. Journ.*, April 1888.
6	1888	M.	Young	Assault by roughs.	...	Freiberg, Karkov, Inaug. Dissert. 1888 (*v. Annals of Surgery*, Nov. 1889).
7	1890	M.	25	A fall upon the left side of abdomen.	About 4 weeks.	Karewsky, *Deutsche Med Wochenschr*, Leipzig, No 46, 1890.
8	1890	M.	56	An injury to the left costal margin.	About 3 months.	Karewsky, *Deutsche Med. Wochenschr.*, Leipzig, No 46, 1890.
9	1890	M.	18	The hind wheel of a lorry carrying coal passed over the upper part of his abdomen.	About 2½ months.	Cathcart, *Edin. Med. Journ.*, July 1890, and *Trans. Med. Chir. Soc.*, Edin., 1889-90, p 73.
10	1890	F.	28	A fall from a great height.	About 3 years.	Riegner, *Berl. klin. Wochenschr.*, No. 42, 1890.
11	1891	M.	21	A kick in the abdomen.	About 8 years.	Pitt and Jacobson, *Trans. Med. Chir. Soc.*, London. 1891, p. 455.
12	1891	M.	50	In lifting a heavy weight he felt something give way in the epigastric region. Shortly afterwards he had a severe fall which knocked his breath out.	About 3 or 4 months after began to feel pain, and later a tumour appeared.	Richardson, *Boston Med. and Surg. Journ.*, 1891, p. 111.
13	1892	M.	38	Horse threw and stamped upon him, striking him over the upper part of the abdomen on the left side.	About 3 weeks.	Littlewood, *The Lancet* 1892, i. 871, and *Trans. Med. Chir. Soc.*, London 1891-92, p. 205.
14	1892	M.	20	Knocked down by a horse at a race meeting.	About 3½ months.	Lloyd, *Brit. Med Jour.*, London. ii. 1892, p. 1051.
15	1892	M.	27	Thrown upon the floor and kept there for a time.	About 10 days. Patient said he noticed it at once.	Lloyd, *Brit Med. Jour.*, London. ii. 1892, p. 1051
16	1894	M.	2	Run over by the wheel of a cab.	About 3 weeks.	J. L. Thomas, *The Lancet*, i. 1894, p. 799.
17	1894	M.	17	Crushed between a locomotive and a truck, the buffers striking his abdomen.	About 3½ months.	Brown, W. H., *The Lancet*, i 1894, p. 21.

The history of the injury is most definite in these cases, and, moreover, the formation of the epigastric tumour followed sufficiently soon after it as in itself to be presumptive of the relationship being cause and effect. The earliest appeared ten days after, and the latest eight years.

In the latter it may reasonably be doubted if there were any connexion between them. It is in a measure, however, supported by two of the cases being delayed for three years, and another for one year. In 6 the interval varied between two and four months, and in other 5 between two and five weeks. It will be noticed that 9 of them were more or less directly related to falls, 6 to blows upon the abdomen, and only 2 to being run over by a vehicle. It is a somewhat curious fact that all but one occurred in males, and this is probably to be accounted for by the greater liability of the male sex to injury. It might justly be brought forward, however, as an additional argument in favour of the causal nature of the injury. Granting, however, that the injury was the primary cause of formation of the cyst, we have still to show that that injury involved the pancreas. The evidence on this point is fairly satisfactory in several of the cases, for the fluid obtained on aspiration or evacuation of the cysts, on being submitted to analysis, gave the reactions characteristic of the pancreatic juice. In other cases the contents failed to give these reactions, and this may point to an origin altogether independent of the pancreas. We know, however, that great changes may occur in the composition of the contents of such cysts, especially if they be of long standing, and it may be that, the connexion with the pancreas having been cut off, the pancreatic characters of the fluid will be gradually lost. We are thus led to look for evidence along other lines. The most conclusive of all, viz., that derived from post-mortem examination, avails us very little here, as of the 17 cases just quoted only 1 ended fatally. The others all recovered after the cyst had been incised and drained. The fatal one, viz., No. 14 of the Table, was reported by Lloyd. An enormous encysted hæmatoma was found situated behind the stomach. It contained 3 or 4 pints of dark blood containing old coagula. The folds of the lesser omentum were so altered that it was hardly possible to say how they entered into the formation of the wall of the sac. No special examination of the pancreas for injury was made.

This case affords us but little if any help, and we are therefore compelled to fall back upon the domain of hypothesis and conjecture in seeking for an explanation. Kuhlenkampff (14) suggested that the injury might cause an inflammation of the gland substance which might lead to closure of the main duct and a consequent extensive cyst. Senn (15) held the same view until he found, from his experiments on animals, that very little distension followed obliteration of the main duct, and that, in short, any part of the gland physiologically separated from the main exit duct underwent simple atrophy. He then suggested that these cysts might have more than one mode of origin, and that the hæmorrhage into them might be variously explained. He gave three main hypotheses,—1st, Hæmorrhage into a pre-existing pancreatic cyst; 2nd, Parenchymatous hæmorrhage producing a cyst, followed by hæmorrhage into the cyst wall; 3rd, That the hæmorrhagic cyst may originate in a dilatation of one of the vessels of the pancreas. Now, the first of these does not get over the difficulty of the first formation of the cyst, and the third, while it may be said to be possible, must be regarded as rare. The second view is at once the most obvious and probable. It was further elaborated by Cathcart (16), who puts it as follows :—" The injury causes a laceration of the gland. This is followed by extravasation of blood, and with this is mixed the pancreatic secretion from the torn ducts. Not only is a constantly increasing fluid thus added to the original hæmatoma, but the collection of fluid probably becomes irritating in character. It will thus tend to excite the formation of a capsule around it, and by chemical irritation and tension would gradually increase in size." This view of the causation and mode of origin of these so-called pancreatic cysts is not only the most natural, but also the most probable which has yet been propounded. It is so obvious that it has doubtless occurred independently to other observers. Indeed, it did so to myself, and I find that Jordan Lloyd (17) has had a similar experience. He says (apparently unaware of Senn and Cathcart having previously suggested it):—" The secretions of the torn gland may be poured into the lesser omental sac with the blood, and that, even if pure pancreatic juice be not irritating to the peritoneum, a mixture of pancreatic juice and devitalized bloodclot may have a very different effect, and that chemical changes of a digestive kind may then be started, which may irritate the serous lining of the sac and cause it to pour out its secretions, and thus gradually distend its cavity."

Now, obvious and simple as this explanation is, we have to remember that it is hypothetical, and must be carefully tested before we can accept it as being satisfactory. Before we can accept it as being the mode of origin of these pancreatic cysts we must exclude the possibility of other and neighbouring structures acting as primary factors in their formation. We cannot do this, for we find that many cases of similar cysts in this region arise apparently spontaneously. No connexion with the pancreas may be suspected until an analysis of the cyst contents suggests it. Such cases are much more numerous than those apparently of traumatic origin. Some of them may originate in retention cysts, as seemed to be the case in a woman, æt. 35, referred to by Sharkey (18). A tumour, said to have been in existence for twelve to fifteen years, was found in the left hypochondrium. It was remarkably mobile. On opening the abdomen it shot out of the wound, dragging with it the tail of the pancreas. On enucleating the cyst, the pancreas bled very freely.

It is at least improbable, however, that even the majority have a similar origin, and we must inquire if no other way is open which would still allow them to retain a connexion with the pancreas. Such a way is perhaps to be found in the spontaneous hæmorrhages which occasionally arise from the pancreas or suprarenal bodies. It is quite well known that hæmorrhage may take place spontaneously into and around the pancreas. It has been met with not infrequently in varying degrees of severity and standing. If recent, the infiltrated parts have the dark colour of ordinary venous blood-clot; if old, they have a brown or slaty colour. Such hæmorrhages may even speedily prove fatal. Zenker (19) describes 3 such cases occurring in strong, healthy men; and Draper (20) 5 somewhat similar cases. Challand (21), Prince (22), Gussenbauer (23), etc., have also discussed the subject. Minor cases are, doubtless, still more common, and may result in the formation of a blood cyst. If the hæmorrhage ruptures any of the pancreatic ducts, we may get a mixture of pancreatic juice as well, and hence the mode of origin of such cysts may come to closely simulate traumatic ones. Störck (24) and Parsons (25) each record a case which somewhat supports this contention. In both a sanguineous cyst connected with the pancreas was present, and the tissue of the gland was infiltrated with hæmorrhage that had taken place into its substance. The parenchymatous hæmorrhage may have been the first thing here, and may have led to the formation of the cyst, which increased by further hæmorrhage taking place from its wall. It is, of course, possible, though not so probable, that the cyst preceded the hæmorrhage.

In some cases the hæmorrhage is more manifest in the neighbourhood of the pancreas than within the organ itself. Harris (26) mentions a case of sudden death in an alcoholic patient where the hæmorrhage was into the adjoining subjacent peritoneal tissue as well as into the pancreas; and Biggs (27) another case of a man who fell dead on coming out of a beer saloon in which he had taken a few glasses of beer. There was hæmorrhage around the pancreas, and a number of minute hæmorrhages within it. We will not stay to discuss the causes of such spontaneous hæmorrhages. The question is an obscure one. Signs of acute inflammation of the gland substance were found in some, while in others the gland was apparently quite healthy. It is not necessary, however, for the blood to come from the pancreas; it may come from the suprarenals. Virchow (28) describes a form of acute hæmorrhagic inflammation of the supra-renal capsules, and several cases of large spontaneous hæmorrhages into and around these organs have been put on record. Further, we have evidence that hæmorrhage may be found in the neighbourhood of the pancreas without having any apparent connexion with either of these glands. Rolleston (29) mentions the case of a man, aged 30, in which hæmorrhage was found around the pancreas, the source of which could not be determined.

We see, then, that we may have the first step in the formation of a cyst arising in a variety of ways, and it is conceivable that such a cyst, in the course of its gradual increase and extension, may come to acquire a connexion with the pancreas, though it originally possessed none. Fischer (30) suggests " that a pancreatic cyst may originate as a blood effusion in the neighbourhood of the gland, it being supposed that the tension of the sanguineous effusion may cause atrophy of part of the gland substance and escape of fluid from opened ducts." He cites as a probable instance a case recorded by Merigot de Treigny (31), where a sanguineous cyst was found adherent to the pancreas, which was atrophied at the position of contact. This anatomical connexion is certainly suggestive, but it is far from conclusive, as it is capable of explanation by other and perhaps more probable modes of origin.

So far we have restricted our observations to hæmorrhages from the region of the pancreas, but in considering the possibilities of cyst formation in this region we have to remember other conditions of etiological importance. Blood has not been present in all these cysts, even in all the traumatic ones, and as some cysts arise in connexion with the spleen, liver, supra-renals, and even lesser omentum, it is obvious that this latter class must be taken into account when dealing with the origin of epigastric cysts. We have to include also hydronephrosis, echinococcus, retroperitoneal dermoid cysts, or even ovarian cysts. The mere mentioning of most of these possible origins is all that is required for our present purpose. Their occurrence is well enough established, and the only one requiring further consideration is the lesser omentum. Its surface extent is the greatest of all the structures in the epigastric region, and if cysts can arise in it independently of any other structure, we see at once what a frequent source of origin it may become. It will facilitate our investigation if we first consider whether either traumatic or spontaneous cysts may arise from the peritoneum at a distance from the pancreas. We find that there is fair evidence on the subject. Godlee (32) has recorded 3 cases of cysts following upon injury whose origin was very possibly peritoneal. In the first, a girl of 4, the cyst had formed on the right side of the abdomen about three weeks after she was run over by a cab. He believed that this cyst was primarily renal, due possibly to a ruptured ureter. In the second, a man of 23, the cyst formed on the left side, and was aspirated about four weeks after the injury. In the third, a boy of 7, the cyst formed first on the left side, and later, about eleven months after the accident, spread to the epigastric region. It was incised. All the 3 cases recovered, and there was no special evidence, in the latter 2 at any rate, to connect them with any particular organ.

Again, in the case recorded by Brown (vide No. 17 of the Table), there was reason to believe that a similar peritoneal cyst, separate from and independent of the pancreatic one, was present as the result of an earlier injury. The evidence in support of similar peritoneal cysts arising spontaneously is still more conclusive. Terrier (33) gives the case of a man, aged 34, who had suffered from attacks of colic and diarrhœa for about five months previous to the detection of a swelling in the hypogastric region. This was tapped, and 450 grammes of blood-stained fluid withdrawn. The cyst refilled, and formed a rounded swelling, reaching from the pubis to the umbilicus, and to within two fingerbreadths of the iliac spines on either side. Laparotomy was performed, and the cyst removed. It was about the size of a fœtal head, and was apparently connected with the mesentery. It contained what looked like pure blood, and its walls were of some thickness, coated internally with fibrin. The patient recovered. Freutzel (34) records another in a woman, aged 20, where the cyst, about the size of a child's head, was situated about the middle of the right side, and was very movable. It was found to be between the layers of the mesentery, and to contain sero-sanguineous fluid. The patient recovered. Simon (35) found a cyst of the great omentum in a man who died of Asiatic cholera. It was adherent above to the greater curvature of the stomach. It had thin walls, and contained granular rust-coloured blood coagula. The arteries and veins of the omentum were normal. With the exception of a few small ulcers in the colon, the organs of the body appeared to be healthy.

It thus, I think, becomes clear that cysts, both traumatic and spontaneous, may arise from the peritoneum, and hence many of those recorded as present in the mesogastric region may be fairly enough referred to the lesser omentum as their source of origin. Thus Sutherland (36) mentions the case of a girl of 8 who was run over by a cab. Three weeks later a swelling appeared in the epigastrium, which disappeared after aspiration about five weeks after the injury. Richet (37) relates a case in a man, aged 42, who had been knocked down by an omnibus, and about six months later developed a cyst in the epigastric and left hypochondriac regions. He died of peritonitis caused by injecting the cyst, after aspiration, with a weak cauterising fluid. The lesser omentum was occupied by a cyst limited above by the liver, below by the pancreas, and in front chiefly by the small omentum, but partly by the stomach. All the surrounding organs were healthy. Rendu (38), Gullois (39), and Méry (40) have recorded somewhat similar traumatic cases, in none of which could any connexion with any of the surrounding organs be detected at the necropsy, nor any satisfactory explanation of the origin of the cyst be given. We might in a like manner cite instances of similar cysts of a spontaneous origin. Pomier (41) opened and drained one in the left hypochondrium. It contained 1500 grammes of purely serous fluid.

It is unnecessary to multiply instances, nor is it incumbent upon us at present to explain the origin of such cysts. Rouiller (42) suggests that a sclerosis of the peritoneum, of alcoholic origin, first causes hæmorrhage and then a cyst; and **Fischer** that the lesion is nervous, probably having its origin in the solar plexus. The latter holds that the hæmorrhage is not really situated within the pleural cavity, but between the omental or mesenteric layers. Be this as it may, however, it is obvious that they come to simulate pancreatic cysts more closely than any others; and if the record of pancreatic cysts be scrutinised, it will be seen that many of them, both traumatic and spontaneous, have no real right to their name, as they had probably no connexion with the pancreas. It is not generally appreciated how many the fallacies are. Not only have we to exclude the cysts of the various surrounding organs —*e.g.* spleen, kidney, supra-renal, and liver—but we have the great body of peritoneal or retroperitoneal cysts also to take into account before we can assert that any cyst is of pancreatic origin. Chemical analysis and microscopic examination will indeed help us in many cases, and they are of the greatest value when they give us positive evidence; but when they fail us, as they often do, we are not entitled thereby to exclude a pancreatic origin, as the contents of the cysts may become much altered in the course of time. Indeed, in the absence of some such direct physiological or anatomical evidence, we have no right to either assert or deny a connexion with the pancreas. In any such case the possibilities are many, and we are not entitled to do more than suggest the likelihood of its being of pancreatic origin. Its greater frequency makes this source the most probable, but it would perhaps be better not to use the term *pancreatic* as descriptive of any such doubtful cyst. The term *epigastric* is fairly distinctive, and has the advantage of in no way begging the question. On prognostic and therapeutical grounds, a perfectly accurate diagnosis is not after all so much of a desideratum, as all cases, whether pancreatic or not, seem to be equally amenable to treatment.

Treatment.—Wherever we have a collection of fluid about whose boundaries and connexions we are somewhat in doubt, the natural tendency is to evacuate the fluid with the least possible disturbance of parts. Hence we find that the first procedure adopted was an emptying of the cyst by means of aspiration. Experience has shown, however, that this is both ineffectual and dangerous. The cyst gradually refills, and attempts to secure its obliteration by means of the injection of iodine, etc., have been somewhat disastrous. A fatal peritonitis has resulted more than once,—indeed, the simple aspiration itself has been followed by somewhat similar serious consequences, brought about doubtless by the rupture of the cyst walls when thin, and the sudden escape of the contents into the peritoneal cavity.

Aspiration has thus been abandoned in favour of laparotomy, which is the favourite method of treatment at the present day. The cyst is brought forward to the anterior abdominal wall, incised, and emptied. Drainage is secured by means of a pancreatic fistula, which discharges for a variable time and then heals.   This was the method followed in all the 17 cases recorded in the foregoing table of traumatic pancreatic cysts, in all of which except one it was successful.   It has been followed with like success in many other cases.   Krecke (43) says that out of 27 cases treated by section and drainage, all recovered; and out of 6 cases treated by dissecting out the cyst, 3 died.   The advisability of trying to dissect out the cyst is very doubtful.

Excision may be easy in some cases, but will be difficult in most, and experience does not favour its recommendation.   The method of anterior incision and drainage, notwithstanding its success, is not altogether perfect.   It has actually failed to cure in a few cases, and other objections may be urged against it.   It is much more suitable for the somewhat movable cysts which come forward to the anterior abdominal wall.   These are generally broader anteriorly than posteriorly, and are thus readily opened from the front.   It is not nearly so suitable for that other division which are somewhat sessile, broader posteriorly than anteriorly, and much less movable.   They are not easily reached by an anterior incision, and, moreover, it is by no means easy to bring the wall of such a cyst forward to the anterior incision, and thus to secure its safe evacuation.   In addition we have to urge the obvious disadvantage of the anterior incision, alike for men and women, in so far as it interferes with the natural usefulness of the abdominal walls, and provides for a drainage of the most imperfect character, allowing of a cure only after a more or less protracted period of time.   Further, the possibility of the pancreatic fistula becoming permanent must not be entirely denied.   Senn in his experiments found that it never occurred, but actual experience in the human subject does not quite bear this out.   Gould (44), indeed, mentions a case in which not only did the pancreatic fistula remain permanent, but malignant disease appeared around it.   It appears to me, therefore, not only reasonable, but most advisable, that we seek for some other method of reaching these cysts free from these objections.   Cathcart and Littlewood have spoken of the ease with which a counter-opening could be made posteriorly in these cases, and it occurred to me that they might be primarily reached and drained by posterior operation.   I thereupon verified this suggestion many times upon the cadaver.   I found it much easier than I expected to cut down upon the tail of the pancreas and lesser omental sac.   A vertical incision, about 3 inches long, is made at the outer border of the left rectus, beginning above at the twelfth rib.   After cutting through the skin and fascia, the thin fibres of the latissimus dorsi are first recognised, and then the strong fascia at the outer border of the rectus.   This is incised, and the upper border of the quadratus lumborum is next seen running downwards and outwards.   The finger is inserted above it, and feels for the posterior surface of the kidney through the fat and cellular tissue. It then defines the position of the renal vessels. The tail of the pancreas and the postero-lateral wall of the lesser omental sac lie just above and inside them, and by inserting a probe I was able to enter the cavity of this sac, either through the mesocolon below the lower border of the pancreas, or through the posterior peritoneum above this gland, at will, according to the obliquity upwards given to the probe. In no case was the supra-renal capsule or any other structure in the neighbourhood injured. When the lesser omental sac was distended with fluid, fluctuation could be distinctly felt by the exploring finger working upwards above the renal vessels, and the fluid could be evacuated with ease by means of a drainage-tube, made to enter the sac with the help of a director and pair of dressing forceps. This procedure will be found to be quite as easy in cases of pancreatic cysts, and probably of others in this neighbourhood. The cyst wall may be in some cases thick, and thus a little difficult to penetrate ; but that need not cause much trouble, while the long-existent distension will have brought the cyst within more easy reach. It may even extend downwards below the line of the renal vessels, and thus be reached by the surgeon whether he goes above or below these structures.

This method of reaching these cysts from behind was adopted by Mr Cotterill with complete success in a case now under his care in the wards of the Royal Infirmary of Edinburgh. He entered the sac below the renal vessels. The patient is doing well. Others have adopted a posterior incision after an anterior one has failed. Thus Gould mentioned that in a case where the cyst was fixed and could not be brought to the surface, with a finger in the cyst he cut down behind below the twelfth rib and drained it posteriorly. The fistula rapidly closed up. A better proof could hardly be given of the advantages of the posterior incision. He would doubt-less have easily reached the cyst had he tried the posterior incision at first. I would strongly advocate this method of procedure, not only because of its ease, but because of the advantages of a posterior over an anterior incision, and of the more perfect drainage and much more rapid convalescence and cure which it promises. Even if it were to fail to reach the cyst, it would in no way prejudice the success of an anterior exploration, and would, more-over, even in such a case allow of the rapid establishment of posterior drainage.

––––––

BIBLIOGRAPHY.

1. JAUN.— *Indian Annals of Medical Science*, vol. iii., 1855, p. 721.
2. WILKS and MOXON.—*Pathological Anatomy*, 3rd edit., p. 491.
3. COOPER.—*The Lancet*, London, 31st December 1839, vol. i. p. 486.

4. TRAVERS.—*The Lancet*, London, June 23, 1827, vol. xiii. p. 384.

5. WANDESLEBEN.—*Gen. Ber. d. k. rhein. Med. Coll.* 1842, Koblenz, 1845, s. 120-123; and *Wochenschr. f. d. ges Heilk. Berl.*, 1845, s. 729-732.

6. STÖRCK.—*Annus Medicus*, 1836, p. 244.

7. LE GROS CLARK.—*Lect. Prin. Surg. Diag.*, 1870, p. 298.

8. EDLER.—"Die traumatischen Verletzungen der parenchymatösen Unterleibsorgane (Leber, Milz, Pancreas, Nieren)," *Archiv für klin. Chir.*, 1887.

9. KUHLENKAMPFF.—"Ein Fall von Pancreasfistel," *Berl. klin. Wochenschr.*, February 13, No. 7, 1882, s. 102.

10. SENN.—*International Journal of Medical Science*, vol. xcii., 1886, p. 423.

11. JAMAIN.—*Man. de path. et de Chir. klin.*, 1870, 2nd ed., tome ii. p. 493.

12. WILKS and MOXON.—*Loc. cit.*, p. 324.

13. SENN.—*International Journal of Medical Science*, vol. xcii., 1886.

14. KUHLENKAMPFF.—*Loc. cit.*

15. SENN.—*Loc. cit.*, vol. xc., 1885, p. 34.

16. CATHCART.—*Trans. Med. Chir. Soc. Edin.*, 1889-90, p. 80.

17. JORDAN LLOYD.—*Brit. Med. Journ.*, London, vol. ii. 1892, p. 1053.

18. SHARKEY.—*The Lancet*, London, vol. ii., Dec. 3, 1892, p. 1273.

19. ZENKER.—*Häemorrhagie: Tagebl. d. 47 Naturforscherversamml in Breslau*, 1874.

20. DRAPER.—*Trans. Assoc. Amer. Physic.*, 1886, pp. 243-251.

21. CHALLAND.—*Bull. de la Soc. méd. de la Suisse romande*, 1877.

22. PRINCE.—*Bost. Med. and Surg. Journ.*, vol. cvii., 1882, p. 55.

23. GUSSENBAUER.—*Wien. Med. Wochenschr.*, No. 13, 1883; *Med. Times*, vol. i., 1883.

24. STÖRCK.—*Archiv gén. de Paris*, Mai et Juillet, 1836.

25. PARSONS.—*Brit. Med. Journ.*, London, 1857.

26. HARRIS. — *Boston Med. and Surg. Journ.*, 1889, vol. cxxi., p. 606.

27. BIGGS.—*New York Med. Rec.*, 1890, vol. xxxvii., p. 362.

28. VIRCHOW.—*Die Krankheiten Geschwülste*, ii.

29. ROLLESTON.—*Trans. Pathol. Soc. London*, 1893, p. 74.

30. FISCHER.—*Guy's Hospital Rep.*, 1892, p. 328.

31. MERIGOT DE TREIGNY.—*Bull. de la Soc. Anat.*, Paris, 1885.

32. GODLEE.—*Trans. Med. Soc. London*, 1887, p. 219.

33. TERRIER.—*Soc. de Chir.*, 1890, p. 383.

34. FRENTZEL.—*Deutsche Zeitschr. für Chir.*, 1892, and *La Semaine médicale*, May 25, 1892.

35. SIMON.—*Bull. de la Soc. Anat.*, 1858, p. 30.

36. SUTHERLAND.—*The Lancet*, London, vol. ii. 1892, p. 1327.

37. RICHET.—*L'Union médicale*, 1877, tom. xliv. p. 82.

38. RENDU.—*Bull. de la Soc. Anat.*, 1880, p. 120.

39. GULLOIS.—*Bull. de la Soc. Anat.*, 1889, p. 556.
40. MÉRY.—*Bull. de la Soc. Anat.*, 1885, p. 39.
41. POMIER.—*Nouv. Archiv d. Obstét. et de Gynéc.*, October 1892.
42. ROUILLER.—*Les kystes hématiques du Péritoine*, Thèse de Paris, 1885.
43. KRECKE.—*Münch. Med. Wochenschr.*, Nos. 25 and 26, 1892, and *Epit. Brit. Med. Journ.*, July 23, 1892.
44. GOULD.—Discussion upon a paper read by the late Mr Hulke at the Clinical Society, November 25, 1892,—*vide The Lancet*, London, vol. ii. 1892, p. 1273.

Mr Joseph Bell said he could not let this pass without thanking Dr Leith for the very clear and admirable way in which he stated all his points. He had only operated on one case, about two years ago, that of a lady who got a bad injury from the shaft of a dog-cart. He was sent for about a fortnight after it happened. The only thing one could do was to lay open the abdomen carefully. He opened the omentum, and found nothing ; then scraped cautiously through the gastro-hepatic omentum, and found a cyst with a thickish wall ; scraped cautiously through that with his nail, and got rid of about a pint of the most abominably smelling pus that ever any one smelt. The patient had been perfectly well since. There had been no fatty stools. Mr Cathcart said that, if necessary, one could drain easily from behind. She was a large, well-formed woman, and he could have made his own place for a drain, being able to get his hand quite freely under her liver. These cases were pretty rare. He might have neglected his opportunities in failing to examine while washing out the cyst whether there was a rupture of the pancreas or not ; but with the lady *in articulo mortis*, and two wise provincial practitioners standing by who were doubtful about operating at all, his neglect was excusable.

Dr Leith, in reply, said that Mr Bell's case was extremely interesting. Might he ask what time intervened between the injury and the operation? (Mr Bell replied, about three weeks.) He thought the case was worthy of a more permanent record.

3. STATISTICS CONCERNING THE PATIENTS ADMITTED WITH ALCOHOLIC SYMPTOMS TO THE ROYAL INFIRMARY, EDINBURGH, FOR THE FIVE YEARS FROM OCTOBER 1, 1889, TO SEPTEMBER 20, 1894.

By A. LOCKHART GILLESPIE, M.D., F.R.C.P. Ed., Medical Registrar to the Royal Infirmary, Edinburgh ; Lecturer on Materia Medica.

THE following statistics deal with the total admissions, both into the medical side and into the surgical side, of patients suffering from the recent effects of alcoholic excess. It is self-

CHART IV.

Monthly admissions of Alcoholic Neuritis, Pneumonia, Delirium Tremens and Surgical Cases.

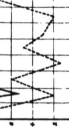
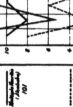
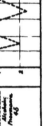
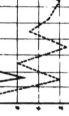
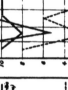

CHART III.

Monthly deaths from Alcoholism and Delirium Tremens in the eight large Towns of Scotland from Oct. 1889 to Sep. 1894.

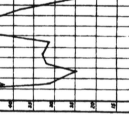
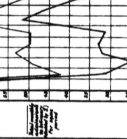
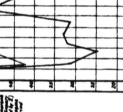
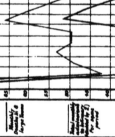
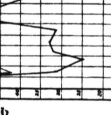
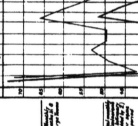
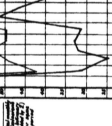
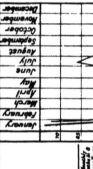

John Bartholomew & Co. Edin?

CHART I.

Monthly admissions of Alcoholic Patients into the Royal Infirmary during the five years from October 1st 1889 to September 30th 1894.

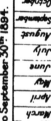
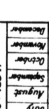
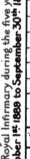
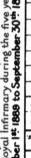
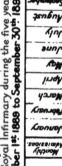
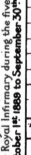
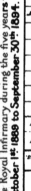
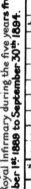
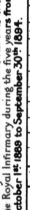
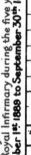
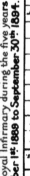
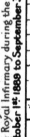
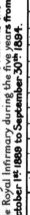
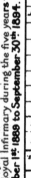
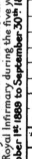
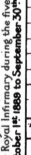
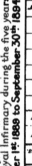
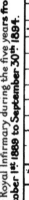

evident that an attempt to include the remote effects, as, for instance, cirrhosis of the liver or of the kidneys, would vitiate the results, not to speak of the difficulty of obtaining trustworthy data of these cases on which to form a reliable opinion.

The total number of such cases was 1264, with 44 deaths, or a mortality of 3·4 per cent.

Of the 1264, 935 were males, with 38 deaths, or 4 per cent., and 329 females, of whom only 6 died, or 1·8 per cent.

The totals in the different years were as follows :—

1889–90...............268, or 3·3 per cent. of total admissions.
1890–91...............198, „ 2·4   „   „   „
1891–92...............208, „ 2·5   „
1892–93...............301, „ 3·4   „
1893–94...............289, „ 3·1   „   „   „

The years 1889–90 and 1892–93 (a very warm season) were the most drunken.

I have worked out the figures for each month for the five years, a graphic Chart (No. I.) of which I now hand round. You will see that the largest number of admissions occurred in January (143), the next largest in July, while August is only a little way behind. I would ask you also to note the small subsidiary rise in the month of April. The large number of cases in January is explained, of course, by the New Year's drinking, and many of them were patients suffering from cut heads and other minor injuries while under the influence of drink. The rise in the admissions in July and August is probably due more to the Trades' Holidays and trips than to the warm weather, for it is notorious that June, especially of late years, has been a finer and warmer month than either of these, but still the admissions in June are not so numerous. In November the number of admissions is least (81), though February has not many more (87).

On separating the males from the females admitted during these five years and constructing a graphic chart for the months, it will be seen that the line representing the males closely corresponds to that of the total, but the difference between the January and the July admissions is more accentuated, while February, June, October, and November show the lowest figures. The majority of the females, on the other hand, were admitted from June to October, the earlier part of the year showing a decided minority.

I also show you Charts indicating the monthly admissions in each of the five years (Chart II. not reproduced here), in which you will notice a certain similarity of outline.

For purposes of comparison I have also written out in another Chart (Chart III.) the total deaths per month which occurred during the same period in eight of the principal towns of Scotland as recorded in the Registrar-General's Returns. You will notice a most remarkable similarity between the two, only one month (November) being dissimilar. A maximum in January, a fall in February and March, a small spring rise followed by a greater summer one, an autumn fall, and an increase up to the maximum in January again.

TYPES.

The total of 1264 may be divided into—

Simple alcoholism, . . 649, or 51·3 per cent. ⎱ 871, or 68·9
Alcoholism with surgical ⎰ per cent.
  injury, ... 222, „ 17·5 „
Delirium tremens, . . 179, „ 14·1 „
Alcoholic neuritis, . . 101, „ 7·9 „
Mental symptoms other than ⎱ 49, „ 3·8 „
  D.T., ... ⎰
Alcoholic pneumonia, . . 45, „ 3·5 „
Acute alcoholic dyspepsia, . 19, „ 1·5 „

Simple Alcoholism.—649 cases: 481 males, 168 females.
Monthly admissions.—Jan., 83; Feb., 48; Mar., 46; Ap., 55; May, 47; June, 46; July, 66; Aug., 59; Sept., 38; Oct., 55; Nov., 41; Dec., 65.

Delirium Tremens.—179 cases: 154 males, 25 females. (See Chart (Chart IV.) for the monthly admissions). 107, or 59 per cent., were admitted from April to September.

Surgical Cases.—222 cases: 130 males (13 per cent. of total males), 92 females (28 per cent. of total females). The admissions are more equally distributed in the twelve months. There is, however, an excess in July.

Neuritis.—101 cases: 70 males (7·4 per cent. of total males), 31 females (9·3 per cent. of total females). Of the males, 43, or 61·4 per cent., were admitted in the summer six months from April to September; while of the females, 25, or 80·5 per cent., entered the hospital in the same period of the year. No case of alcoholic neuritis was admitted during the five years in the month of November.

Mental Cases—49: males 37, females 12. There is nothing remarkable about the figures with regard to these, save the usual preponderance in summer.

Pneumonia.—45 cases; only 1 in a female.
Monthly admissions.—Jan., 8; Feb., 2; March, 6; April, 1; May, 5; June, 3; July, 2; Aug., 8; Sept., 3; Oct., 1; Nov., 2; Dec., 4.

Digestive Cases.—19 in number, chiefly occurred in summer.

OCCUPATIONS.

Of the 329 *women,* 169 were housewives.
          33 „ laundresses.
          21 „ charwomen.

Of the 329 *women,* 20 were shopgirls and seamstresses.

          19 „ beggars, tramps, etc.

          18 „ servants.

          18 „ factory hands.

          10 „ girls at home.

Among the others, 5 were barmaids and 2 teachers.

60·9 per cent. of the housewives were admitted during the summer six months.

Of the 935 *males—*

461 were of the labouring class—labourers, 99; skilled labourers, 172; trade labourers, 161; factory workers, 16; railway employés, 13.

119 were of the shopkeeping class—shopkeepers, 85; travellers, 34.

108 were of the professional class—clerks, 49; others, 59.

84 belonged to the liquor trade.

68 were drivers, coachmen, etc.

26 beggars, tramps, etc.

69 had various occupations.

The Labouring Class, 461.

Males.—The labouring class generally were admitted especially in the months of January, April, and July, in that order; those engaged in indoor trade drinking most in the early months of the year, those with more out-of-door employment exceeding in summer. 14·7 per cent. of the whole number developed delirium tremens, this being especially the case with the indoor workers with 17·8 per cent., who again were more prone to this in winter, the others in summer. Seventy-six cases had surgical injuries as well, or 16·4 per cent.; these were more common in those returned as purely labourers (28·1 per cent.), and were more numerous in summer.

The Shopkeeping Class, 119.

Monthly admissions.—Jan., 18; Feb., 9; March, 6; April, 11; May, 7; June, 11; July, 14; Aug., 9; Sept., 5; Oct., 7; Nov., 5; Dec., 5. They show the same maxima, January, July, and April.

Delirium Tremens cases numbered 21, or 12·6 per cent., chiefly in summer (26 per cent).

The Professional Class, 108, was comparatively large, and contained 49 clerks.

Monthly admissions.—Jan., 14; Feb., 5; March, 7; April, 8; May, 8; June, 5; July, 8; Aug., 14; Sept., 10; Oct., 9; Nov., 6; Dec., 13. Show two maxima, December and January, and July to September.

Delirium Tremens cases, 16, or 14·9 per cent.; 69 per cent. of them in the summer months. The mental cases were larger in proportion than in the other classes, 9, or 8·4 per cent.; 3·9 per cent. being the mean. The surgical cases, 7, or 6 per cent., were low.

Liquor Trade, 84.

Monthly admissions.—Jan., 10; Feb., 3; March, 5; April, 11; May, 11; June, 2; July, 12; Aug., 11; Sept., 2; Oct., 6; Nov., 7; Dec., 6. There was a slight preponderance in summer.

Delirium Tremens, 28, or 32·7 per cent. (16 per cent. is the mean for men), distributed equally over the year. There were only 2 cases of neuritis, and 10 surgical.

Drivers, Cabmen, etc., 68.

Monthly admissions.—Jan., 7; Feb., 5; March, 2; April, 1; May, 5; June, 3; July, 10; Aug., 5; Sept., 9; Oct., 8; Nov., 9; Dec., 4. Maxima, July and September to November. These are the wettest months.

Delirium Tremens, 8 cases, or 11·7 per cent. Surgical cases, 15, or 22 per cent.; higher than average, chiefly (73·3 per cent.) in summer.

Beggars and Tramps, 26, chiefly in summer.

Surgical cases, 26·9 per cent., a very high proportion.

Of Various Occupations, 69.

Comprising soldiers, sailors, postmen, etc. Six boys were quite young. Surgical cases, 19·6 per cent.

Delirium Tremens, 18 per cent.

Of the females, in whom the excess is still more marked in summer, the following notes may be made :—

Delirium Tremens, 25, or 7·6 per cent. Surgical cases, 92, or 28 per cent.; in men only 13 per·cent.

The Housewives, 169, or 13·3 per cent. of whole admissions.

    71 were alcoholic.

    16 had D.T., or 9·5 per cent.

    14 „ mental symptoms.

    48 were surgical, or 28 per cent.

    19 had neuritis, or 11·2 per cent., being above the average; all, save 1, occurred in summer.

    1 „ pneumonia.

Charwomen and Laundresses, 54.

Maximum, March, and in summer.

    26 were alcoholic.

    24 „ surgical, 44·4 per cent. The most pugnacious of any.

    2 „ neuritis.

Shopgirls, Milliners, Servants, etc., 56.

Maximum in January and February.

    8 were neuritis, or 14·2 per cent., which is high.

    5   „   delirium tremens.

Other Females.—Girls at home, 10; teachers, etc., 49.

Largely alcoholic simply, and were admitted for the most part in summer.

General Mortality.—Total mortality, 3·4 per cent.

    5 of the 101 neuritic cases died, or 5 per cent.

    28 of the 45 pneumonia cases died, or 55·5 per cent.

These, then, gentlemen, are the statistical notes derived from the Infirmary Registers during the last five years. The striking points about them, in my opinion, are the great excess of pure drunkenness in summer, due in all probability both to the heat and the holidays, the differences seen in the period at which labourers working outside and indoors get drunk, the large number, proportionately, of the professional class admitted, and the very quarrelsome nature of most of the women who were admitted the worse for alcoholic indulgence.

I hope you will derive some little interest from the details. I know that compiling them was to me a very considerable pleasure

———

Dr Laing said that the ability to obtain work and wages might have considerable influence on the relative amount of drunkenness among indoor and outdoor workers.

After slight informal discussion, *The President* complimented Dr Gillespie on his interesting collection of statistics, and *Dr Gillespie* briefly replied.

APPENDIX.

ON RESECTION AND SUTURE OF THE INTESTINE, WITH CASES.[1]

By F. M. CAIRD, F.R.C.S. Ed., Assistant Surgeon, Royal Infirmary ; Lecturer on Surgery, Edinburgh School of Medicine.

FOR several generations the bold, vigorous, common-sense of that most able teacher, John Bell, has moulded and influenced the practice of the Edinburgh Medical School. He inspired the early attempts at ovariotomy; he also by his satire and invective delayed advance in the department of intestinal surgery. He held up to derision the writings of his colleague Benjamin Bell, and states "that if in all surgery there is a work of supererogation, it is this operation of sewing up a wounded gut."

The revolution effected by Lister uprooting the ancient landmarks and limitations, put power in the surgeon's hands far beyond the wildest dreams of the past. It is astonishing to note the wondrous difference between the present day "now" and the past "then" of 1800 when John Bell flourished.

The conditions under which the surgeon is called to operate upon the intestinal canal may be shortly classified under the heads of *Traumatism* and *Obstruction.* The latter may be divided into, first, the forms of obstruction associated with interruption to the vascular supply of the part. Such are strangulated hernia, volvulus, intussusception. The progress of these cases is acute, the result gangrene. Second, obstruction due to diminution of the lumen. Such forms are due to foreign bodies, or to new growths springing from or external to the bowel. In this series the cases are rather subacute than markedly acute. The fatal issue is caused by ulceration at the seat of the obstruction, or it arises during the storm of intestinal peristalsis and its concomitants. As an example of the changes which ensue when a band arrests the circulation in a loop of bowel, we may take the type presented by a case of strangulated hernia (Fig. 1). On opening the sac, dividing the constriction and pulling out the gut, we may recognise the distended, congested entrant gut (A), the proximal anæmic zone of constriction (B), the distended trapped bowel (C), the distal anæmic zone of constriction (D), and the collapsed pale exit gut

---

[1] Read at Meeting IV., 16th January 1895.

(κ). Further, we recognise the two areas of selection where perforation or gangrene take place, namely, the devitalized area at and just above the peripheral constriction, and also that at the extreme convexity, opposite the mesenteric attachment of the trapped loop (F).

Treatment, under the circumstances when gangrene is discovered or perforation is already present, consists primarily in a careful purification of the sac and its contents *prior* to the division of the stricture, and the pulling into view of the gut beyond. According to the condition of the gut, the patient, and the environment, so will the subsequent procedures vary. If we meet with the typical elliptical necrosis of the bowel which runs longitudinally opposite the mesenteric attachment as at F, Plate I., we may, with Lembert sutures, stitch the sound tissue over the unhealthy, thus inverting the gangrenous area into the lumen. The following cases warrant this practice, which obviates the necessity of cutting any part of the bowel away, and requires no special dexterity. In all probability it is not applicable with safety where more than one-third of the circumference is destroyed. In such cases the fear of stricture ensuing rather determines us to resect.

A. *Partial Gangrene of Intestine treated by Inversion of the gangrenous or ruptured portion.*

I. Mrs M. Strangulated femoral hernia. Rupture of gut. Healing, normal course. Patient has enjoyed good health since the operation, now seven years ago.

II. Mrs C. Strangulated femoral hernia. Gangrene; no perforation. Healing, normal course. When about to leave hospital three weeks after operation, she rapidly sank with symptoms of cardiac failure. There was no obstruction, no abdominal tenderness, no distension. The autopsy showed that a moored tag of omentum had served to accentuate, by its external pressure, a narrowing at the site of operation, and at this spot there was some ulceration of the mucosa. Septic absorption from this cause may have determined the fatal termination.

III. Miss L. Strangulated femoral hernia. Rupture of gut. Healing, normal course. Operation five years ago.

IV. Mrs M. Strangulated femoral hernia. Perforation. Healing, normal course. Operation four years ago.

V. Infant, R. S. B., æt. 18 months. Strangulated congenital hernia. Gangrene; no perforation. Child did well at first; bowels acted normally; but he died suddenly forty-eight hours after operation. Autopsy: no peritonitis; gut united firmly. The intestine was found beset with typhoid ulcers of ten to fourteen days' duration.

We have thus, amongst the five cases, narrated one only in which the fatal issue bears any direct relation to the operation, and even in this (the second case), had I not been discouraged from an abdominal exploration it would have been possible to resect the gut under very favourable auspices.[1]

This method of inversion, although easy, cannot be modified to meet the exigencies of every case. It does not lend itself to those instances in which the gut is almost completely divided by the tight grasp of a narrow femoral ring. The vitality of the proximal end has then been too severely tried to admit of such an experiment. We should require to invaginate a few inches of the damaged gut before we come upon healthy tissue to suture; and since it is impracticable to reproduce the successful natural cure occasionally seen in cases of intussusception, we are driven to resect.

It was my privilege to assist the late Angus Macdonald at an operation in 1883, in which he inadvertently cut away 7 inches of small intestine. Nothing daunted, he at once proceeded to unite the severed ends with a continuous catgut suture. This was the first successful case of removal and primary suture of gut in Edinburgh—to my knowledge. The case impressed one greatly, and all the more so because of the uniform fatality of such rare attempts made in the surgical department. These were, however, emergency operations for gangrenous hernia, the patients very ill and far through, the intestines distended with flatus and fæces, congested and worn out with the attempt to overcome an unyielding obstruction. Moreover, the forlorn hope of a resection was made, and the somewhat tedious interrupted sutures were passed, through unhealthy tissue.

Macdonald's operation, on the other hand, was performed on a patient prepared for operation, with empty viscera; healthy bowel was divided and united by means of the rapid continuous suture. The cause of Macdonald's success was thus largely explained. It remained unappreciated. One was slow to learn the lesson that after all resection and suture of intestine should really be a most successful procedure. The following cases serve to illustrate this:—

B. *Resection of Intestine for Gangrene.*

VI. Mrs M'G., aged 43. Right femoral hernia. Strangulated three days. A feeble woman, collapsed and cold. Resection of 4 inches small intestine along with its triangle of mesentery (Nov. 1893). Patient sank twenty-four hours after operation. Autopsy: no peritonitis; the line of suture water-tight.

VII. Mr W., aged 49. Left femoral hernia. Strangulated for four days. A small loop of bowel slipped back into the abdomen on dividing the constriction. The condition of the fluid in the sac showed that gangrene had occurred, and by introducing a pair of padded forceps through the canal the gangrenous portion was withdrawn, and, along with 7 inches of gut, resected. Patient

---

[1] See Paper, *Edinburgh Medical Journal*, 1890.

greatly collapsed; temperature 97° before operation. Thereafter it rose to 102°, and that night he passed flatus. Operation 24th May 1894. Subsequent course normal. Solid stool streaked with blood 28th May.

VIII. Mr S., æt. 24, of unsound mind. Symptoms of obstruction for three days. Laparotomy: volvulus of sigmoid and descending colon found. The bowel black and gangrenous. Resection 2½ feet of bowel. There was no hæmorrhage. The mesenteric vessels were thrombosed. Two Paul's tubes introduced, so that a possible secondary suture might be performed. Operation September 7, 1893. Patient rallied wonderfully, but died September 9.

IX. J. D., æt. 45. Right inguinal acquired hernia of ten years duration; strangulated two days. Right side of scrotum distended to size of swan's egg with the hernial sac, which in its turn was filled with fluid. Into the upper part of this projected a knuckle of bowel with a large elliptical gangrenous patch. Inversion was out of the question; 7 to 8 inches of small intestine resected. Flatus passed next day. Operation 8th November 1894. Healing, normal course.

The great bugbear of the operation is peritoneal contamination, and it is specially in cases complicated with gangrene that this difficulty arises. We therefore dwell upon further details observed during primary resection and suture in cases of gangrene. After the constriction is divided and the gut pulled well out to expose healthy intestine, the ring from which it emerges should be lightly plugged with sterilized gauze to guard the peritoneum. Just beyond the *distal* end of the gangrenous mass a couple of long-bladed pressure forceps should be applied side by side, and the gut completely divided between them. The mesentery should now be severed along its attachment to the portion of gut we wish to remove, and this enables us to hold the free extremity over a vessel, when on removing the forceps its contents escape and the congestion abates. Having thus relieved the distension and emptied the gut, we may now re-apply the forceps on the central healthy gut, and cut away the intervening damaged portion. The mesentery has now to be dealt with. In cases where the gut has not given way, it is not necessary to remove any of the mesentery. As Kocher has indicated, it suffices to suture the free margins to each other. This checks the small amount of hæmorrhage usually present, and serves to approximate the severed ends of intestine. If, however, the mesentery within the sac has been in contact with fæcal matter, it is better to remove entirely the contaminated triangular portion, as we would also deal with omentum under similar circumstances.

We now proceed to suture. This is simplified by the introduction of three or more provisional loops, which serve to steady and approximate the edges which have to be united. The loops pas through the whole thickness of the gut. The first should be inserted at the mesenteric margin, the other two equidistant from it. Any surplus protruding mucous membrane is now snipped away with curved scissors, the ends of the first and second loops are held tense, and a continuous suture is carried through the whole thickness of the gut from the first to the second loop. The second and third loops are now held tense, and the suture continues to close the second segment of the circle, after which there only remains to make the third segment of the gut tense, and the suture now travels on from the third to the first loop, and completes the union of the divided intestine. Now follows over this the most important stitching in the form of a continuous Lembert suture. The provisional loops are then withdrawn, and additional Lembert sutures are inserted over the site they occupied, as well as at any weak spot which seems to require it,—for example, at the mesenteric insertion. It will be observed that even if the pressure forceps have inflicted any permanent damage on the cut margin of the gut, that edge becomes inverted, thanks to the series of Lembert sutures. It is on the Lembert sutures we rely for secure union and safety from leakage. A careful scrutiny is now made of the junction, the gut is carefully cleansed anew with a stream of sterile salt solution and moist gauze. The gauze which plugged the hernial aperture is withdrawn, the gut returned, and a radical cure performed.

The cases most amenable to resection are probably those of the second series, the neoplasms. If there be no *active* obstruction, we can select our own time for operation, prepare the patient, and so deal with empty bowel. Danger of septic infection is thus reduced to a minimum, and the prognosis is decidedly good. If there be acute obstruction, we must content ourselves by resecting or forming a preliminary artificial anus, and a few days thereafter carry out *secondary* suture, resecting if we have not already done so. The prognosis as regards return of the disease is excellent, since malignant stricture of the intestine is usually of slow growth, is markedly circumscribed, and does not give rise at an early date to secondary foci. Such tumours may be thoroughly removed with ease. It would, therefore, appear that an early diagnostic incision should be practised when one has good reason to suspect disease of the ileo-cæcal and sigmoid regions.

C. *Operations for Stricture and Tumour of the Intestine.*

X. Miss K., æt. 47, spare and active. Complains of a lump in the right iliac region, irregular action of the bowels, and that her health is below par. She strained her side in June 1891. From that time onwards she has experienced intermittent pain at the site now occupied by the tumour. After a severe exertion in August 1892 she had renewed pain, more persistent and disabling.

In January 1893 she discovered the tumour. The pain still continued to increase, often crossed to the left side, and tended to pass upwards. There was no starting pain. Latterly there has been sickness and nausea irrespective of food, but no vomiting. Appetite fairly good. She suffers from irregular diarrhœa, which is never exhausting. Formerly during her illness she was rather constipated. She has not lost much flesh. Urine normal. Midway between the umbilicus and right anterior superior spine there is found a hard rounded tumour about the size of the fist, which can be freely moved to a slight extent laterally.

March 25, 1893.—Abdomen opened over the tumour. The colon, adherent at this point, was mistaken for thickened peritoneum, and incised. Digital examination revealed a tumour of the ileo-cæcal valve lying within the gut, which, however, had contracted adhesions to the surrounding textures. The aperture in the colon was clamped. The cæcum, appendix, six inches of colon, and three of ileum were removed. The transversely divided colon was stitched partially up, until its reduced lumen agreed with that of the small intestine, when end-to-end suturing was employed. For the first three days the pulse varied between 150 and 125; respirations, 30 to 17; temperature, 97° to 98°. She had a little nocturnal vomiting, and required strophanthus and a little morphia. Flatus passed on the third day. Healing, normal course. Solid healthy motions on tenth day. A small fæcal fistula formed after this, but speedily closed. She has enjoyed perfect health since.

XI. J. S., æt. 43. Complains of a swelling on right side of abdomen, with intermittent pain, which began fourteen weeks ago, associated with an attack of vomiting and retching. He has been liable to similar attacks ever since, and is gradually getting thinner. He had an attack of pleurisy about twelve weeks ago. At the beginning and end of December 1893 he had rigors and high temperature. This was ascribed to influenza, then very prevalent.

A mass about the size of two fists is found to the right of the umbilicus. It is tender, has an irregular outline, and is fixed; with mainly a resonant note. Urine normal.

The mass was at first supposed to be inflammatory. Under treatment it subsided slightly, became more circumscribed, and then remained stationary. The abdomen was opened in the right linea semilunaris January 12, 1894. A large malignant tumour, involving the ileo-cæcal region and the colon, was exposed, and with difficulty detached from the vascular adhesions which united it to the parietes and adjacent coils of small intestine. It was finally separated by clamping and dividing the free coils of bowel by which it was still continuous, and we were now able to appreciate the somewhat complicated relation (Fig. 2). It appeared that we had divided the bowel transversely at the points A, B, C, D. We now sutured the ileum to the hepatic flexure of the colon (A to D). The remaining portions of bowel lay so imbedded in vascular adhesions that one feared the patient, already exhausted, could not bear a more prolonged operation, and accordingly the ends of the loop were brought out at the incision, a Paul's tube was inserted at each extremity, and the abdomen was closed (see Fig. 3). The patient rallied well after the operation.

January 13.—He passed a good night; is taking small quantities of soda and milk. Requires no morphia.

January 14.—Doing well until 1 A.M., when he began to be troubled with a copious bronchial secretion. Œdema of the lungs rapidly developed, and he died at five o'clock on the morning of 15th January.

There was no sectio.

XII. Mr D., æt. 60, strong and well nourished. Operation for obstruction 19th March 1895.

About three weeks ago he had a similar attack of milder type. He has always been rather costive; latterly he has been losing flesh slightly. There was general distension, marked fulness and tenderness over the cæcum. The rectum had been washed out with enemata, and contained little more than a pint of fluid.

Operation.—Incision as for lumbar colotomy. A coil of distended sigmoid flexure was withdrawn from the wound, and on making traction on its distal end a mass of carcinoma, followed by a loop of collapsed gut, appeared. All this was left protruding from the wound, and an artificial anus formed by tying a Paul's tube above the carcinomatous stricture, with a view to subsequent resection of the affected part.

Patient did well until 25th March, when he was seized with maniacal delirium, due to iodoform poisoning. On removal of the drug, and careful dressing, he rapidly improved. Resection of the growth and end-to-end suture of the gut took place on 9th April. Normal healing; but at a later date a stitch abscess gave rise to a fæcal fistula, which at present is valvular, admits barely a cedar pencil, and although some flatus escapes, he yet pursues his usual avocations without much inconvenience. A plastic operation may be necessary to close the fistula.

XIII. Mrs O. Complains of pain and swelling in her right side. She is a healthy-looking woman, and suffered first two months ago from an attack of supposed appendicitis. At that time she had a rigor, vomiting, diarrhœa, and pain in the right iliac region. She has never been well since; and a swelling which appeared at that time, a little above the mid point between the anterior superior spine and the umbilicus, has been observed to fluctuate in size. She has also continually required purgatives. Ten days ago she had a recurrence of the symptoms. There is an ill-defined irregular mass about the size of a fist, tender on pressure, in the region mentioned. It can be slightly moved from side to side; is somewhat resonant on percussion. Exploratory incision 26th May; distended ileum, traced down to ileo-cæcal valve, where the cæcum, colon, and a mass of mesenteric glands were found so matted together that, after freeing numerous adhesions, the operation was abandoned and the wound closed. The patient progressed favourably; the bowels acted with greater ease.

She died about six weeks after from gradual weakness, and without any recurrence of her former attacks.

XIV. N. S., aged 7, a miserably thin, stunted girl, suffering from swelling of the abdomen and paroxysmal pain in the right iliac region for three and a half years. She has constantly passed light clay-coloured stools. Medical treatment effected no improvement. Dr Stockman advocated an exploratory incision to ascertain the cause of what he diagnosed as chronic obstruction.

June 1, 1895.—Incision through right linea semilunaris. There was found small intestine, distended and remarkably hypertrophied, much resembling the colon; a short, firm stricture at the ileo-cæcal valve, and a thin atrophied colon which simulated the small intestine. Several inches of gut, embracing the ileo-cæcal valve and appendix, were removed. The patient being very weak, a couple of Paul's tubes were introduced, and the patient sent back to bed, in the hope that secondary suture might be practised at a later date. Free stimulation was required after the operation.

June 5.—The tubes were removed, a fresh resection was carried out, and end-to-end suture practised. The patient passed flatus on the following day, and on the 16th June was taken home by the parents. The wound healed, but the child is still in a weakly condition.

D. *Incision for Foreign Body and Suture of Intestine.*

XV. Mrs W., æt. 64, very stout, flabby, with fatty heart, suffers from obstruction, three days' duration.

Operation, September 25, 1893.—Abdomen opened in middle line. Collapsed small intestine found, due to an impacted gall-stone about the size of a walnut. The calculus could not be crushed by external pressure, and so the gut was incised along its extremity, the gall-stone expressed, and the gut closed with Lembert sutures. At night the patient had peculiar choreic jerkings of the right side of the head.

September 26.—Patient doing well, but much annoyed by the jerking movements of the head and shoulder. She passed flatus, and her breath acquired a peculiar ethereal odour. Some urine was collected, and found to contain 1 grain of sugar to the ounce. She remained in much the same condition, the bowels moving freely, until the 28th, when diabetic coma supervened, and she died on the following day.

The autopsy showed marked fatty degeneration of all the organs; the heart, more especially, was so changed that one marvelled how it could perform its functions. She took chloroform admirably, but we must blame the anæsthetic for determining the diabetic coma.

It is a difficult question to estimate the comparative advantage of primary and secondary suture. When the condition of the patient gives rise to anxiety during the resection one naturally desires to hasten the operation, and postpones suturing till a later date; and there can be no question that this is the proper course to pursue, more especially when we dread shock from a prolonged operation. It does not appear, however, that the element of shock is so extremely pronounced or need be so greatly dreaded as is often supposed. In several of the above cases, even when the patient had been a couple of hours on the table, shock was not at all marked. It is preferable to complete the operation by primary suture at one sitting when possible.

The fewer and simpler the drugs of the physician, the more art he displays in their use, and this holds good of the surgeon and his instruments. It may be that the best results in the surgery of the intestine will be gained with needle and thread. Many of the present ingenious inventions employed in uniting the bowel will then share the fate of the too greatly neglected device of Quatre Maître, who in the thirteenth century employed a calf's trachea for a purpose similar to that which led Ramhdor to use a tallow candle and Senn to employ bone plates.

EXPLANATION OF ILLUSTRATIVE PLATE.

FIG. 1.—Bowel resected in Case IX.
  A, Congested entrant gut; B, Proximal anæmic zone of constriction; C, Distended strangulated gut, which is at F gangrenous, devoid of tension and lustre, and about to give way, the mucosa ulcerated and sloughing; D, Distal anæmic zone of constriction.

FIG. 2.—Relation of parts prior to operation in Case XI.
  A, B, C, Colon and cæcum; D, Small intestine. The tumour is indicated by the cross hatching. The bowel was divided at the points indicated by the letters.

FIG. 3.—Relation of parts at conclusion of operation in Case XI.
  The colon A united to the small intestine B after removal of the tumour. The intervening loop of bowel with Paul's tubes inserted, B and C protruding through the abdominal wound.

Mr Cathcart said that Mr Caird was to be congratulated on the brilliant success of his abdominal cases. There were few cases of success in resection of gangrenous hernia. It was, however, in suitable cases the best operation,—far more satisfactory than an artificial anus. In the latter case the patient very often sank, shortly after the operation, from defective nutrition and sepsis. The use of the silk suture without bone plates was coming more

into vogue both in America and on the Continent. Abbé now advocated nothing but the silk suture. Senn's plates would not pass through a hernial opening, unless it were unjustifiably enlarged. Maunder and other surgeons advocated more complicated methods, such as opening the intestine some little distance from line of suture, pulling the intestine through, and working through the second opening. Mr Caird's method, however, was quite as efficient, and simpler. He was to be complimented on having described so clearly his very successful methods. If the india-rubber tube were used from the beginning, it ought to obviate the necessity for the clamping forceps, which might prove injurious to the bowel.

Mr Stiles said that two summers ago he saw Professor Kocher resect the pylorus. Clamps, resembling somewhat a large pair of his artery forceps, but without the teeth at the extremities of the blades, were used to prevent extravasation; they also facilitated the section, and were valuable in temporarily arresting the hæmorrhage. The divided end of the stomach was completely closed by means of a continuous suture which penetrated all the coats,—a Lembert's suture, also continuous, being afterwards applied to secure inversion. The divided duodenum was then sutured to the edges of a special opening made in the posterior wall of the stomach. He pointed out that although the clamp forceps were sufficiently closed to arrest hæmorrhage, yet there was no danger of them interfering with the subsequent healing. The patient made a good recovery. Out of nine cases in which Kocher has operated in this way, seven recovered. In resecting the intestine, he points out the importance of cutting across the intestine obliquely, more of the gut being removed from the side opposite the mesentery, where the blood supply is more liable to be defective.

Mr Wallace asked, with regard to the infolding of the gangrenous area opposite the mesentery, whether Mr Caird, before he put in the stitches, punctured and emptied the gut, as distended gut was often very difficult to suture. He had a case, just the other day, where a small opening took place in the distended gut, and a quantity of the contents became extravasated. He thoroughly washed away the extravasated material and introduced sutures, bringing peritoneum to peritoneum, but without requiring to invaginate. The hernial sac contained a very large quantity of bowel, and he had great difficulty in returning the contents, but the patient made an uninterrupted recovery. Mr Caird had not dwelt on the great difficulty that might arise from the existence of adhesions in cases of large tumour, when it was very difficult to recognise the gut in its continuity.

Mr Caird, in reply, said that the use of an elastic band or forceps was a matter of convenience. It depended on the assistance. The use of forceps enabled one to manipulate the parts more easily. With regard to longitudinal gangrene opposite the mesenteric attachment, it should be invaginated and stitched, the advantage of that being that we did away with clipping and cutting. Sutures were introduced through healthy gut. The contents could be eased along in one direction or the other. The loop of healthy gut, when once pulled out, was again slightly constricted, and consequently grew thick from venous turgescence, the dead part remaining thin. If the gut were thin all round then resection was necessary.

INDEX.

PRINTED BY OLIVER AND BOYD, EDINBURGH.